INTERVENTIONAL CARDIOLOGY CLINICS

www.interventional.theclinics.com

Editor-in-Chief

MATTHEW J. PRICE

Updates in Peripheral Vascular Intervention

April 2020 • Volume 9 • Number 2

Editor

HERBERT D. ARONOW

ELSEVIER

1600 John F. Kennedy Boulevard • Suite 1800 • Philadelphia, Pennsylvania, 19103-2899

http://www.theclinics.com

INTERVENTIONAL CARDIOLOGY CLINICS Volume 9, Number 2
April 2020 ISSN 2211-7458, ISBN-13: 978-0-323-75506-1

Editor: Stacy Eastman
Developmental Editor: Donald Mumford

Interventional Cardiology Clinics (ISSN 2211-7458) is published quarterly by Elsevier Inc., 360 Park Avenue South, New York, NY 10010-1710. Months of issue are January, April, July, and October. Subscription prices are USD 209 per year for US individuals, USD 495 for US institutions, USD 100 per year for US students, USD 209 per year for Canadian individuals, USD 590 for Canadian institutions, USD 100 per year for Canadian students, USD 296 per year for international individuals, USD 590 for international institutions, and USD 150 per year for international students. To receive student/resident rate, orders must be accompanied by name of affiliated institution, date of term, and the *signature* of program/residency coordinator on institution letterhead. Orders will be billed at individual rate until proof of status is received. Foreign air speed delivery is included in all *Clinics* subscription prices. All prices are subject to change without notice. **POSTMASTER:** Send address changes to *Interventional Cardiology Clinics*, Elsevier Health Sciences Division, Subscription Customer Service, 3251 Riverport Lane, Maryland Heights, MO 63043. **Customer Service: Telephone: 1-800-654-2452** (U.S. and Canada); **1-314-447-8871** (outside U.S. and Canada). **Fax: 1-314-447-8029. E-mail: journalscustomerservice-usa@elsevier.com (for print support); journalsonlinesupport-usa@elsevier.com (for online support).**

Reprints. For copies of 100 or more of articles in this publication, please contact the Commercial Reprints Department, Elsevier Inc., 360 Park Avenue South, New York, NY 10010-1710. Tel.: 212-633-3874; Fax: 212-633-3820; E-mail: reprints@elsevier.com.

CONTRIBUTORS

EDITOR-IN-CHIEF

MATTHEW J. PRICE, MD
Director, Cardiac Catheterization Laboratory,
Division of Cardiovascular Diseases, Scripps
Clinic, La Jolla, California

EDITOR

**HERBERT D. ARONOW, MD, MPH, FACC,
FSCAI, FSVM**
Director, Interventional Cardiology,
Lifespan Cardiovascular Institute, Director,
Cardiac Catheterization Laboratories,
Rhode Island and The Miriam
Hospitals, Associate Professor of
Medicine, Warren Alpert Medical
School of Brown University,
Providence, Rhode Island

AUTHORS

SAHIL AGRAWAL, MD
Attending Cardiologist, Warren Clinic
Cardiology of Tulsa, Saint Francis Hospital,
Tulsa, Oklahoma

MAHESH ANANTHA-NARAYANAN, MD
Section of Cardiovascular Medicine, Yale New
Haven Hospital, New Haven, Connecticut

EHRIN J. ARMSTRONG, MD, MSc, MAS
Cardiology Section, Rocky Mountain Regional
VA Medical Center, Director, Interventional
Cardiology, Director, Vascular Laboratory,
Rocky Mountain Regional VA, Professor of
Medicine, Division of Cardiology, University of
Colorado, University of Colorado School of
Medicine, Aurora, Colorado

TAMUNOINEMI BOB-MANUEL, MD
Department of Cardiovascular Diseases, John
Ochsner Heart and Vascular Center, Ochsner
Medical Center, The Ochsner Clinical School,
The University of Queensland, New Orleans,
Louisiana

LARRY J. DíAZ-SANDOVAL, MD
Professor, Department of Medicine, Michigan
State University, East Lansing, Michigan;
Metro Health-University of Michigan Health,
Grand Rapids, Michigan

DMITRIY N. FELDMAN, MD
Greenberg Division of Cardiology, Weill
Cornell Medical College, NewYork-
Presbyterian Hospital, New York, New York

MATTHEW T. FINN, MD, MSc
Instructor, Department of Cardiology,
Columbia University Irving Medical Center,
New York, New York

JAY GIRI, MD, MPH
Division of Cardiovascular Medicine,
University of Pennsylvania, Penn
Cardiovascular Outcomes, Quality,
and Evaluative Research Center,
University of Pennsylvania Perelman
School of Medicine, Philadelphia,
Pennsylvania

ANDREW M. GOLDSWEIG, MD
Assistant Professor, Division of
Cardiovascular Medicine, University
of Nebraska Medical Center, Omaha,
Nebraska

KAMAL GUPTA, MD
Professor, Department of Cardiovascular
Medicine, University of Kansas School of
Medicine, Kansas City, Kansas

BEAU M. HAWKINS, MD
Department of Medicine, Cardiovascular
Section, University of Oklahoma Health
Sciences Center, Oklahoma City,
Oklahoma

JOSEPH J. INGRASSIA, MD
Instructor, Department of Cardiology,
Columbia University Irving Medical Center,
New York, New York

SAUD KHAN, MD
Department of Medicine, Cardiovascular
Section, University of Oklahoma Health
Sciences Center, Oklahoma City, Oklahoma

SAMEER KHANDHAR, MD
Division of Cardiovascular Medicine,
University of Pennsylvania, Philadelphia,
Pennsylvania

LUKE K. KIM, MD
Greenberg Division of Cardiology, Weill
Cornell Medical College, NewYork-
Presbyterian Hospital, New York, New York

SAMUEL M. KIM, MD, MS
Greenberg Division of Cardiology,
Weill Cornell Medical College,
NewYork-Presbyterian Hospital, New
York, New York

ANDREW J. KLEIN, MD, FACC, FSCAI
Adjunct Professor of Medicine, Saint Louis
University, Saint Louis University School of
Medicine, St Louis, Missouri; Piedmont Heart
Institute, Atlanta, Georgia

TAISEI KOBAYASHI, MD
Division of Cardiovascular Medicine,
University of Pennsylvania, Penn
Cardiovascular Outcomes, Quality, and
Evaluative Research Center, University of
Pennsylvania Perelman School of Medicine,
Philadelphia, Pennsylvania

CARLOS MENA-HURTADO, MD
Section of Cardiovascular Medicine, Yale New
Haven Hospital, New Haven, Connecticut

SAMEER NAGPAL, MD
Section of Cardiovascular Medicine, Yale New
Haven Hospital, New Haven, Connecticut

AMMAR NASIR, MD, FSCAI
John Cochran VA Medical Center, Section 2B
Cardiology, St Louis, Missouri

SAHIL A. PARIKH, MD
Associate Professor of Medicine, Director of
Endovascular Services, Columbia University
Irving Medical Center, New York, New York

STEVEN PUGLIESE, MD
Division of Pulmonology and Critical Care,
University of Pennsylvania, Philadelphia,
Pennsylvania

WALID SABER, MD, FACC, FSCAI, RPVI
Chief of Cardiology, Director of Vascular
Medicine, Interventional Vascular Services,
Non-invasive Vascular Lab, Medical Director of
the Wound Center and Hyperbaric Chamber,
Landmark Medical Center, Woonsocket,
Rhode Island; Clinical Assistant Professor,
Brown University, Providence, Rhode Island;
Partner, Oceanstate Cardiovascular & Vein
Center, Woonsocket, Rhode Island

TAUFIQ SALAHUDDIN, MD
Post-doctoral Research Fellow, Cardiology
Section, Rocky Mountain Regional VA Medical
Center, Aurora, Colorado

ERIC A. SECEMSKY, MD, MSc
Assistant Professor, Division of Cardiovascular
Medicine, Harvard Medical School, Boston,
Massachusetts

PRINCE SETHI, MD
Department of Cardiovascular Medicine,
University of Kansas School of Medicine,
Kansas City, Kansas

AKSHIT SHARMA, MD
Department of Cardiovascular Medicine,
University of Kansas School of Medicine,
Kansas City, Kansas

CHRISTOPHER J. WHITE, MD, MACC,
MSCAI, FAHA, FESC, FACP
Department of Cardiovascular Diseases, John
Ochsner Heart and Vascular Center, The
Ochsner Clinical School, The University of
Queensland, Professor and Chairman of
Medicine and Cardiology, Medical Director
Value Based Care, System Chair for
Cardiovascular Diseases, Department of
Cardiology, Ochsner Medical Center, New
Orleans, Louisiana

ROBERT ZHANG, MD
Department of Medicine, University of
Pennsylvania, Philadelphia, Pennsylvania

CONTENTS

Peripheral arterial interventions require safe and effective vascular access and closure. The sites, techniques, and equipment used may vary depending on patient and procedural factors. To minimize the risk of procedural complications, arterial access should use micropuncture technique, ultrasound and fluoroscopic guidance, a compressible arterial access site, and the smallest diameter sheath necessary. Hemostasis at an arteriotomy site may be achieved by manual compression, device-mediated compression, an intravascular closure device, or an extravascular closure device. Although closure devices improve patient comfort and expedite hemostasis, they have not been shown to reduce complications in comparison with compression.

Plaque modification (PM) for atherosclerotic peripheral vascular lesions includes a variety of device types to alter the vessel structure with the aim of enhancing procedural success. PM device utilization has expanded significantly in the United States in recent years despite limited high-quality clinical trials. This article reviews societal guidelines for PM, evaluates currently available trial evidence, examines various pathologic subsets in which PM may be used, and discusses future areas for research.

Carotid atherosclerosis most frequently manifests in the proximal internal carotid artery and the common carotid artery bifurcations. Subclavian artery atherosclerosis affects the proximal segments with a relatively higher incidence on the left and becomes clinically important in the presence of vertebrobasilar insufficiency or coronary steal. Atherosclerosis of the vertebral artery can lead to posterior circulation stroke. The authors review the major trials on carotid carotid, brachiocephalic and vertebral artery stenosis along with the various available diagnostic and interventional techniques.

Most abdominal aortic aneurysms are treated with endovascular repair (EVAR) in current practice. EVAR has lower periprocedural mortality and morbidity than open surgical repair. Aneurysm neck morphology, iliac anatomy, and access vessel anatomy need careful assessment for the successful performance of EVAR. Regular and long-term follow-up with imaging is mandatory after EVAR, and patients who are less likely to comply are less favorable EVAR candidates. Endoleaks are the most frequent complication of EVAR. Most can be managed with transcatheter or endovascular means. Evolving technology and techniques are allowing more patients to be treated with EVAR with better long-term outcomes.

Atherosclerotic renal artery stenosis is the most common cause of secondary hypertension and may cause progressive renal disease and cardiac destabilization syndromes. Guideline-directed medical therapy is advised in all patients. Patients with refractory symptoms and hemodynamically significant stenoses are more likely to benefit from renal artery stent placement. Chronic mesenteric ischemia (CMI) is an infrequent and difficult to diagnose illness. Due to robust collateralization, clinical symptoms from mesenteric artery stenosis or occlusion is uncommon. Atherosclerosis is the most common etiology of CMI. Current evidence suggests that, compared with open surgical repair, endovascular therapy is the most cost-effective choice for CMI.

Endovascular revascularization for aortoiliac occlusive disease (AIOD) is now considered first-line therapy for patients with claudication and critical limb ischemia and in asymptomatic patients in whom large-bore access is required (eg, mechanical circulatory support or transcatheter aortic valve replacement). The authors review the data supporting endovascular therapy for AIOD, indications and contraindications for AIOD revascularization, as well as the procedural techniques required to safely perform endovascular therapy in this vascular bed. They review prevention and management of the major complications that can occur during these procedures. Finally, they discuss postprocedural management to maintain patency and optimize patient outcomes.

Endovascular intervention devices for femoral-popliteal arterial disease have evolved in the last decade to more effectively treat patients with symptoms of claudication, improve tissue healing, and prevent amputation in patients with critical limb ischemia. Drug-eluting stents and drug-coated balloon therapies have demonstrated significant improvements in short- and mid-term patency and decreases in future target vessel interventions over uncoated balloon angioplasty. Adjunctive lesion preparation options including atherectomy devices are available to treat more complex and calcified lesions, but comparative data are still required.

Chronic limb-threatening ischemia represents end-stage peripheral artery disease. It is underdiagnosed; it relies on clinical symptoms and traditional noninvasive tests, which significantly underestimate the severity of disease. Innovative techniques, approaches, technologies, and risk-assessment tools have significantly improved our ability to treat these patients and to better understand their complex disease process. For patients with chronic limb-threatening ischemia considered without options, the reengineering of deep venous arterialization procedures has shown promising results. Finally, the creation of interactive and multidisciplinary teams in centers of excellence is of paramount importance to significantly improve the care and outcomes of these patients.

Acute limb ischemia (ALI) is a sudden decrease in limb perfusion that threatens limb viability. Using the Rutherford classification, limbs can be categorized as threatened but viable, or irreversibly damaged, which aids clinicians in selecting appropriate therapy. Treatment options for threatened limbs include catheter-directed thrombolysis, percutaneous mechanical thrombectomy, and surgical revascularization. Potential complications from ALI and treatment include ischemia-reperfusion injury, compartment syndrome, systemic inflammatory response syndrome, multiple organ dysfunction syndrome, hyperkalemia, and bleeding.

Treatment of acute pulmonary embolism (PE) historically included anticoagulation and systemic thrombolytic therapy. More recently, catheter guided interventions provided promise of mitigating bleeding risks usually associated with systemic thrombolysis in intermediate to high risk PE patients. Catheter based interventions can broadly be divided into catheter directed thrombolysis and catheter based embolectomy. Both modalities are currently undergoing active research and each has their respective risks and benefits. The decision to administer these advanced therapies for acute PE can be challenging but can be accomplished via a multi-disciplinary PE response team.

May-Thurner syndrome, also known as iliac vein compression syndrome, may cause symptoms of venous hypertension and is a predisposing factor for the development of iliofemoral deep vein thrombosis (DVT). Iliofemoral DVT is associated with high rates of development of postthrombotic syndrome, a potentially debilitating condition associated with development of symptoms related to venous outflow obstruction and resulting in reduced quality of life. In this Clinics article, we review procedural intervention with catheter-directed thrombolysis and stenting for iliofemoral DVT and iliac vein compression.

Chronic venous insufficiency is a common and a highly prevalent vascular disorder, that occurs as a result of venous reflux owing to defective venous valves, which in turn causes venous hypertension with significant symptom burden that can interfere with quality of life. Therapeutic strategy involves lowering the venous pressure by lifestyle changes, compression therapy, and conventional catheter-based thermal ablation and novel nonthermal, nontumescent techniques of ablating the affected veins.

UPDATES IN PERIPHERAL VASCULAR INTERVENTION

RELATED SERIES

Cardiology Clinics
Cardiac Electrophysiology Clinics
Heart Failure Clinics

THE CLINICS ARE NOW AVAILABLE ONLINE!

Access your subscription at:
www.theclinics.com

PREFACE

Peripheral Vascular Intervention from Head to Toe: Navigating the Turns

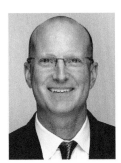

Herbert D. Aronow, MD, MPH, FACC, FSCAI, FSVM
Editor

Tremendous inroads have been made in the treatment of peripheral artery and venous disease over the past 2 decades. As our understanding of these disease states has evolved and as newer tools have become available, there has been a paradigm shift away from open surgical toward "endovascular-first" revascularization strategies. In the vascular world, much effort has been put forth toward reaching cross-specialty consensus in this crowded arena, through development of disease management guidelines, expert consensus statements on device selection, and appropriate-use criteria, and locally in the emergence of multidisciplinary vascular teams. The vascular universe looks much different in 2020 than it did in 2000.

We begin our endovascular tour with an article on vascular access and closure by Goldsweig and Secemsky, who review newer, safer techniques for gaining access to the vasculature through both traditional and novel ports of entry as well as an array of currently available vascular closure devices. Next, Finn, Ingrassia, and Parikh teach us about atherosclerotic plaque modification tools to facilitate arterial revascularization before we embark upon a revascularization journey from head to toe, and from arterial to venous. Anantha-Narayanan, Nagpal, and Mena-Hurtado review carotid, brachiocephalic, and vertebral artery intervention, including the latest techniques for primary and secondary stroke prevention and

symptom mitigation, and newer hybrid open-endo approaches to managing extracranial carotid artery disease. Sharma, Sethi, and Gupta provide an overview of endovascular aortic repair for abdominal aortic aneurysm, an approach offering less morbidity and mortality than that associated with open surgical repair and one that now dominates the landscape. Bob-Manuel and White discuss the remaining indications for the ever-controversial renal artery revascularization, providing us with helpful procedural tips and tricks, including the use of radial artery access, before embarking upon mesenteric artery intervention for symptom relief in chronic mesenteric ischemia. Klein and Nasir cover aortoiliac intervention for claudication, for critical/chronic limb ischemia (CLI), and to facilitate large-bore access for coronary and structural heart procedures. Kim, Kim, and Feldman place structured exercise therapy in context as an upfront strategy for the claudicant and summarize the evidence supporting drug-containing balloons and stents for symptomatic femoropopliteal disease. Diaz reviews below-the-knee (also known as "infrapopliteal") intervention for limb salvage in CLI, including advanced antegrade, retrograde, and inframalleolar techniques. Khan and Hawkins summarize pharmacomechanical approaches and outcomes in the ever-feared patient with acute limb ischemia. Finally, we travel to the "other side" to review

Intervent Cardiol Clin 9 (2020) ix–x
https://doi.org/10.1016/j.iccl.2020.01.001
2211-7458/20/© 2020 Published by Elsevier Inc.

the latest developments in venous disease treatment, where Zhang, Kobayashi, Pugliese, Khandahar, and Giri discuss catheter-directed therapies for submassive and massive acute pulmonary embolism; Salahuddin and Armstrong outline current treatment approaches to iliofemoral deep vein thrombosis and May-Thurner syndrome; and Agrawal and Saber speak of noninvasive and minimally invasive catheter-based therapies for disabling chronic venous insufficiency. We hope the reader will enjoy this comprehensive review of the indications, techniques, and outcomes associated with contemporary catheter-based arterial and venous revascularization.

Herbert D. Aronow, MD, MPH, FACC, FSCAI, FSVM
Warren Alpert Medical School of Brown University
593 Eddy Street, RIH APC 730
Providence, RI 02903, USA

E-mail address:
herbert.aronow@lifespan.org

Twitter: @herbaronowMD (H.D. Aronow)

Vascular Access and Closure for Peripheral Arterial Intervention

Andrew M. Goldsweig, MD[a,*],
Eric A. Secemsky, MD, MSc[b,1]

KEYWORDS

- Peripheral artery disease • Peripheral vascular intervention • Endovascular • Vascular access
- Closure device

KEY POINTS

- Peripheral arterial interventions require safe and effective vascular access and closure. The sites, techniques, and equipment used may vary depending on patient and procedural factors.
- To minimize the risk of procedural complications, arterial access should use micropuncture technique, ultrasound and fluoroscopic guidance, a compressible arterial access site, and the smallest diameter sheath necessary.
- Hemostasis at an arteriotomy site may be achieved by manual compression, device-mediated compression, an intravascular closure device, or an extravascular closure device.
- Although closure devices improve patient comfort and expedite hemostasis, they have not been shown to reduce complications in comparison with compression.

INTRODUCTION

All peripheral arterial interventions require safe and effective vascular access and closure. The sites, techniques, and equipment used may vary depending on patient and procedural factors. Much of the collective experience with vascular access and closure is derived from coronary artery intervention, and many techniques are merely "best practices," with limited supporting data.[1] This review details arterial access and closure with a particular focus on peripheral arterial intervention.

ARTERIAL ACCESS

Sterile Preparation and Local Anesthesia

The patient should be prepared and draped using standard sterile technique. We recommend cleaning an area of at least 5 cm in every direction from the intended access site with an iodine or chlorhexidine solution.

For patients not receiving general anesthesia, subcutaneous local anesthesia should be administered with 1% to 2% lidocaine without epinephrine. For procedures with long expected duration or access greater than 8 French, we favor an equal mixture of lidocaine with bupivacaine, colloquially called "now-and-later," because lidocaine has a rapid onset and bupivacaine has a long duration of action, thus providing anesthesia both during and after the procedure. In cases of small target arteries, a mixture containing equal parts of subcutaneous local anesthetic and nitroglycerine may dilate the target artery to facilitate successful access.

Fluoroscopy-Guided and Ultrasound-Guided Access

The access site should be identified using both fluoroscopy of a radiopaque object placed over bony landmarks and direct ultrasonographic

---

[a] Division of Cardiovascular Medicine, University of Nebraska Medical Center, 982265 Nebraska Medical Center, Omaha, NE 68198, USA; [b] Division of Cardiovascular Medicine, Harvard Medical School, Boston, MA, USA
[1] Present address: 375 Brookline Avenue, Suite 400, Boston, MA 02215.
* Corresponding author.
E-mail address: andrew.goldsweig@unmc.edu

Intervent Cardiol Clin 9 (2020) 117–124
https://doi.org/10.1016/j.iccl.2019.11.001

visualization of the target vessel. Typically, for common femoral artery access, a Kelly clamp is used to identify fluoroscopically the inferior border of the femoral head, and the overlying skin is marked with a surgical pen. This mark corresponds to the inferior border of the "compressible zone" where manual hemostasis can be achieved with compression. Ultrasonography can confirm that access is adequately distant from an arterial bifurcation, an area of diseased vessel, and other nearby neurovascular structures; ultrasonography also facilitates direct visualization of a single anterior wall puncture. The Femoral Arterial Access with Ultrasound trial, compared ultrasound-guided with fluoroscopy-guided common femoral artery access for coronary intervention.[2] Although it was negative with respect to its primary endpoint, successful common femoral artery cannulation, a number of its secondary endpoints were suggestive of benefit. Ultrasound guidance was associated with fewer attempts necessary to obtain access (1.3 vs 3 times, $P<.001$) and a lower incidence of vascular complications (1.4% vs 3.4%, $P = .04$). Many operators have also extrapolated these observations to peripheral arterial intervention.

Seldinger and Modified Seldinger Techniques

Almost every percutaneous vascular access procedure begins with the Seldinger or modified Seldinger technique, which have replaced surgical cutdown. As initially described by Swedish radiologist Dr Sven Ivar Seldinger in 1953, the Seldinger technique involves inserting a catheter with a central needle completely through an artery to determine its depth, removing the needle, withdrawing the catheter to the lumen of the artery, confirming blood flow through the catheter, passing a guidewire through the catheter into the arterial lumen, removing the catheter, and finally placing an access sheath over the guidewire.[3] The modified Seldinger technique involves inserting a needle directly into the arterial lumen without puncturing the posterior wall, passing a guidewire through the needle into the arterial lumen, and placing an access sheath over the guidewire. Because of its simplicity and avoidance of posterior wall puncture, which could result in bleeding, the modified Seldinger technique has generally eclipsed the classic Seldinger technique for most arterial access procedures.

Micropuncture

As opposed to the 18-gauge needle traditionally used for the modified Seldinger technique to permit the passage of a 0.035-inch guidewire, the micropuncture technique uses a 21-gauge needle and 0.021-inch guidewire to obtain vascular access. A 4- or 5-French microcatheter is advanced over the wire into the vessel, and an angiogram may be performed through the microcatheter to confirm placement before exchanging the microcatheter for a larger interventional sheath over a 0.035-inch guidewire. If the access location is angiographically suboptimal, the micropuncture sheath may be removed and manual compression applied to achieve hemostasis, allowing reaccess in a more favorable location. Although limited available data have not confirmed a reduction in vascular complications associated with the micropuncture technique,[4,5] it is intuitively appealing and has been widely adopted as a best practice.

Common Femoral Artery Access

The arterial access site depends on the intervention being performed. Historically, the common femoral artery has been the preferred access site for interventions to most peripheral arteries, including carotid, upper extremity, renal, mesenteric, aortoiliac, femoropopliteal, tibial, and pedal. The common femoral artery should be accessed overlying the femoral head to allow for compression against the femoral head to achieve hemostasis. Access at a level above the femoral head, where the vessel dives deep into the pelvis, is associated with a greater risk of retroperitoneal bleeding, whereas access below the femoral head may result in arteriovenous fistula formation where the femoral vein is located anterior to the common femoral artery. The location of the femoral head may be confirmed by fluoroscopy. Ultrasound guidance can confirm that the access site is remote from the bifurcation of the superficial femoral and profunda femoris arteries, the femoral vein, and the femoral nerve, and may help identify a nondiseased area of the vessel.

Ipsilateral retrograde access is most common for aortoiliac interventions. Contralateral retrograde common femoral arterial access is the most commonly used strategy for femoropopliteal interventions. In this strategy, a long sheath is placed "up-and-over" the aortic bifurcation to approach the target lesion in the antegrade direction.

Alternatively, ipsilateral antegrade common femoral arterial access with sheath insertion directed toward the foot may be used in cases of inhospitable contralateral or ipsilateral iliac vessels, a narrow aortic bifurcation angle, previous "kissing" aortoiliac stent placement, or greater need for catheter support. This strategy provides greater stability and pushability than the up-and-over strategy. However, antegrade common femoral access site may be more difficult both to obtain and to compress because the sheath track runs a long distance through the soft tissue of the pelvis. Additional local anesthesia is useful for patient comfort. As with antegrade puncture, a micropuncture approach may also be used to facilitate safer access for retrograde puncture. A stiff 0.035-inch wire is sometimes required to advance the sheath when subcutaneous tissue cannot be moved out of the way.

Alternative Lower Extremity Arterial Access

Ultrasound-guided antegrade micropuncture access may also be obtained directly into the superficial femoral or popliteal arteries. Additional care must be taken when obtaining hemostasis as these sites are relatively less compressible.

When a lower extremity arterial lesion cannot be crossed in an antegrade fashion, retrograde access may be obtained via the dorsalis pedis or posterior tibial arteries.[6,7] Dedicated kits similar to the micropuncture kit have been developed specifically for pedal access. For example, the Cook (Bloomington, IN) pedal access kit includes a 21-gauge 4-cm needle, a 0.018-inch guidewire, and a 2.9-French inner diameter 7-cm introducer microsheath for low-profile access to a small, diseased pedal vessel.[8] Ultrasound guidance is almost universally necessary to identify the pedal vessels for access. Ultrasound-guided retrograde micropuncture access may also be obtained directly into the tibial, popliteal, and superficial femoral arteries with or without use of a sheath.

Alternative Upper Extremity Arterial Access: Radial and Ulnar

Interest has grown in using the transradial approach for peripheral arterial intervention[9] given the lower risk of access site complications when compared with the transfemoral approach, as demonstrated in randomized coronary interventional trials.[10] The radial artery may be accessed 1 to 2 cm proximal to the flexor crease, guided by palpation of the radial pulse or by ultrasonographic visualization as necessary. Device manufacturers have begun to produce extra-long equipment to permit peripheral intervention from radial artery access. Specifically, Terumo (Tokyo, Japan) has released a product line called "R2P" for radial to peripheral procedures, including 119- and 149-cm sheaths as well

as balloons and a self-expanding stent mounted on 200-mm delivery systems, allowing access to the superficial femoral artery. Cardiovascular Systems, Inc (St. Paul, MN), also make an extended shaft orbital atherectomy device for femoropopliteal intervention via radial access. The feasibility of transradial intervention has been demonstrated in the iliac and superficial femoral,[11] subclavian,[12] carotid,[13] renal,[14] and mesenteric[15] arteries. At present, the R2P approach is limited by a lack of balloons and stents on delivery systems of adequate length to reach below the knee from the radial access site.

Distal radial artery access in the anatomic snuffbox has become increasingly common for coronary intervention because the site is compressible against the scaphoid bone and the patient may be comfortably positioned for left distal radial artery access by a right-handed operator standing in the usual position on the right side of the procedure table.[16] Recently, the distal radial artery has been adopted by peripheral arterial interventionalists also.[17]

Transulnar access may be used when radial access cannot be achieved, although the greater depth of the ulnar artery and the adjacent ulnar nerve make it a less-favorable access site than the radial artery.[18] If the patient's entire wrist is prepped before a procedure, an operator unable to obtain radial artery access may quickly switch to obtain ulnar artery access. Because the hand is well collateralized, ipsilateral radial artery occlusion does not seem to increase the risk of ischemic vascular complications associated with ulnar artery access.[19]

Access to the central circulation from the radial or ulnar artery may be limited by anatomic variants, such as accessory arteries and arterial loops, as well as by subclavian and brachiocephalic artery tortuosity and stenosis. Arterial loops may be crossed and straightened using floppy-tipped 0.035-inch wires with stiff shafts (eg, Versacore [Abbott, St. Paul, MN] or Wholey [Medtronic, Dublin, Ireland]) or by using hydrophilic, stiff 0.018-inch (eg, V-18 [Boston Scientific, Marlborough, MA]) or 0.014-inch (eg, Pilot 50 [Abbott]) wires. Steerable 0.035-inch wires (eg, Angled GlideWire [Terumo]) may facilitate navigation of challenging subclavian and brachiocephalic anatomy.

Alternative Upper Extremity Arterial Access: Brachial, Axillary, and Subclavian

The brachial, axillary, and subclavian arteries may be accessed when other access sites are not possible. Although their larger size in comparison with the radial and ulnar arteries offers the ability to place a larger sheath and deliver larger equipment, it is generally more difficult to compress these arteries, so the increased risk of bleeding complications makes them less favored. These arteries are most frequently used as alternative access sites for transcatheter aortic valve replacement (TAVR) or mechanical circulatory support when transfemoral access is not possible. When performing mesenteric, renal, and lower extremity interventions from a brachial or subclavian artery access site, the left-sided arteries may be preferred because they are located 10 to 15 cm closer to the lower extremities, permitting endovascular tools to reach further down the target vessel.

Alternative Arterial Access: Transcarotid

Recent single-arm trial evidence has emerged to support transcarotid artery revascularization, in which carotid artery stenting is performed via antegrade access to the common carotid artery.[20] Retrograde carotid artery access may be used as alternative access site for TAVR and, rarely, for other endovascular interventions. Although surgical cutdown is the most common method of carotid artery access, ultrasound-guided micropuncture has also been described.[21]

Sheath Selection

Interventional sheath selection depends on the path from the access site to the target lesion, the access site artery size, and the equipment to be delivered. To provide adequate support, the sheath must often extend from the vascular access site to within a few centimeters of the target vessel to provide adequate support to deliver interventional tools to the target lesion. A long portion of the sheath should not be left outside the body as this will limit device reach. Precurved sheaths may facilitate access to particular arteries. A sheath with a hydrophilic coating, such as the Destination (Terumo), Flexor (Cook), or Shuttle (Cook), may be preferred to traverse long subcutaneous tracts and narrow, tortuous arteries. When the sheath must bend considerably, such as in highly angulated vasculature, a braided metal sheath, such as the Arrow (Teleflex, Wayne, PA), may be preferred to prevent kinking, which might occur with a traditional plastic sheath. Stiff 0.035-inch wires, such as the Amplatz SuperStiff (Boston Scientific) or Lunderquist (Cook) wires, may be used facilitate sheath advancement. A short sheath or sheathless approach may be used when secondary retrograde pedal access is

employed for lower extremity lesion crossing, with larger equipment being delivered in the antegrade direction through a primary access site in a larger artery.

The sheath diameter must be appropriate for the access site artery. In general, to reduce the risk of complications, the smallest possible sheath diameter should be selected. A useful parameter is the sheath-to-artery ratio, which refers to the ratio between the sheath outer diameter and the minimal arterial lumen diameter in millimeters. In transcatheter aortic valve implantation (TAVI), a sheath-to-femoral-artery ratio of greater than 1.05 has been shown to predict a higher rate of vascular access complications.[22] This concept has also been extended to radial artery access for coronary artery interventions, with a cutoff sheath-to-artery ratio of 1.5 predicting a higher risk of radial artery occlusion.[23] If a sheath with a diameter approaching or greater than the access site artery's diameter is needed for a prolonged period, such as for an infusion catheter, placement of an ipsilateral antegrade perfusion catheter should be considered to prevent ischemia from arterial flow obstruction by the sheath. Such an antegrade perfusion catheter is typically necessary for extracorporeal membrane oxygenation.[24]

The sheath circumference must also be appropriate to accommodate the equipment to be used. Although catheters and balloons may only require 5-French sheaths, certain crossing devices, atherectomy devices, and stents may require sheath circumferences of 7 French or larger. In addition, potential bailout equipment should be considered when selecting a sheath size: although balloon angioplasty may be the planned intervention, a stent may become necessary should a dissection occur, or a covered stent may be required to treat a perforation. Table 1 describes characteristics of several common sheaths used for peripheral arterial intervention.

VASCULAR ACCESS CLOSURE

Manual Compression

After the completion of an arterial intervention, equipment must be removed and hemostasis achieved at the vascular access site. The most basic and time-tested hemostatic method is prolonged compression of the arterial access site, which results in thrombotically mediated occlusion of the arterial puncture site. Hemostatic pads made of gauze infused with thrombogenic agents may facilitate this process and may reduce bleeding from capillaries near the skin surface of the subcutaneous track.

Table 1
Selected endovascular sheaths commonly used for peripheral arterial interventions

Product	Manufacturer	Available Lengths (cm)	Available French Sizes	Noteworthy Features
Destination	Terumo	45, 65, 90, 119, 149	5, 6, 7, 8	Hydrophilic; preshaped curves available
Flexor	Cook	45, 55, 70, 90, 110	4, 5, 6, 7, 8, 10, 12	Hydrophilic; preshaped curves available
Shuttle	Cook	80, 90, 110	4, 5, 6, 7, 8	Hydrophilic
Pinnacle	Terumo	10, 25	4, 5, 6, 7, 8, 9, 10, 11	Hydrophilic; preshaped curves available; 119 and 149 cm lengths available
Prelude	Merit	11, 23	4, 5, 6, 7, 8	With/without hydrophilic coating
Arrow	Teleflex	11, 23	4, 5, 6, 7, 8, 9	Braided metal
Input	Medtronic	7, 11, 23	5, 6, 7, 8, 9, 10, 11	Silicone coating
DrySeal	Gore	33, 34, 65	12, 14, 15, 16, 18, 20, 22, 24, 26	Inflatable gasket, radiopaque tip

Before performing manual compression, procedural anticoagulation should be allowed to dissipate: an activated clotting (ACT) time less than 160 seconds or a partial thrombolastin time (PTT) less than 45 seconds (when heparin is used) is desirable,[25] although ACT and PTT assays vary by device, so local thresholds should be determined. Manual compression is performed by an operator pushing at the arterial access site against a bony structure. A simple rule is to compress the arterial access site at suprasystolic pressure for several minutes corresponding to 3 times the French size (millimeters circumference) of the sheath being removed (ie, 18 minutes for a 6-French sheath). The common femoral artery may be compressed against the femoral head, the radial and ulnar arteries may be compressed against the carpal bones, the dorsalis pedis and posterior tibial arteries may be compressed against the tarsal bones, and, with some difficulty, the brachial artery may be compressed against the humerus. However, the subclavian and axillary arteries may be difficult to compress, and if the preclose technique (described below) or a closure device is not used, many operators prefer either surgical cutdown or balloon tamponade from a second access site to achieve hemostasis.

Compression Devices

Prolonged manual compression may be uncomfortable for both patients and operators. Accordingly, specialized mechanical compression devices have been developed for this purpose. The FemoStop (Abbott) is a belt-like device that wraps around a patient's hips to facilitate pressure on the common femoral artery by an air bladder with a pressure manometer. The air bladder is inflated to supersystolic pressure for several minutes and then maintained at subsystolic pressure for several hours to facilitate hemostasis, with inflation times dependent on the size of the arteriotomy and the degree of anticoagulation. Similarly, the ClampEase (Pressure Products, Ranco Palos Verdes, CA) device functions like a C-clamp, pushing on the arteriotomy site with a pressure pad connected by a curved arm to a flat metal panel placed under the patient. Bracelet-like devices may be applied to compress the radial (including distal transradial) and ulnar arteries. Such devices include the TR Band (Terumo), PreludeSYNC (Merit, Jordan, UT), and TRAcelet (Medtronic). These devices may also be used off-label for compression at pedal access sites. The SafeGuard family of devices (Merit) are comprised of adhesive bandages with built-in air bladders and are manufactured in various shapes and sizes to accommodate different access sites. Mechanical compression devices also permit "patent hemostasis," in which the pressure applied is adequate to prevent extravasation of blood from the access site while also permitting distal perfusion. Patent hemostasis may be confirmed by pulse palpation, Doppler ultrasonography, or plethysmography distal to the compression device while collateral circulation is manually occluded (ie, ulnar artery manually occluded while radial artery patency is tested). Leaving compression devices in place for too long at high pressure can result in distal ischemia and local skin necrosis.

Closure Devices

To facilitate more rapid closure of arterial access sites, a variety of vascular closure devices have been developed. Compared with compression, the use of a closure device has been associated with reduced time to hemostasis, reduced time to ambulation, and improved patient comfort. However, it is important to note that use of a closure device has never been demonstrated to reduce bleeding complications. This finding was confirmed by the 4524-patient ISAR-CLOSURE trial, which demonstrated noninferior complication rates with closure devices compared with manual compression following coronary artery intervention,[26] and has also been confirmed by retrospective analysis of real-world procedure data.[27] Closure devices may generally be considered in 2 categories: extravascular closure devices that mechanically seal the puncture site and intravascular closure devices that plug the arterial access track. Table 2 presents vascular closure devices commonly used in the United States.

Intravascular Closure Devices

The Angio-Seal (Terumo), which consists of a bioabsorbable anchor placed on the intimal surface of the vascular wall and a collagen plug placed on the external adventitial surface. The device, available in 6- and 8-French sizes, is favored for its ease of use and relatively short learning curve. The Perclose ProGlide (Abbott) deploys a suture across the arterial access site to bring together the edges of the punctured arterial wall. Perclose is the only device approved in the United States to close venous access, and it is the only device that allows the operator to maintain wire access to the vessel during deployment, which may facilitate bailout options in the case of device failure. StarClose (Abbott) implants a permanent nitinol clip, which grasps tissue immediately superficial to the arterial puncture site and draws it together in a purse-string fashion.

Head-to-head studies of intravascular closure devices are extremely limited. The small, but adequately powered, compression, Angio-Seal, or ProGlide trial randomized 200 patients undergoing transfemoral coronary intervention to manual compression, Angio-Seal, or Perclose[28]: there were 10 failures to deploy Perclose and none for Angio-Seal (P<.01); time to hemostasis

was shorter with Angio-Seal (5.3 vs 46.8 minutes, P<.01). However, there was no significant difference in major vascular complications between the 3 groups.

Extravascular Closure Devices

A frequent concern in peripheral arterial intervention is substantial atherosclerotic burden near the vascular access site, which may increase the risk of intravascular closure device failure or vessel closure with device deployment. In such case, an extravascular closure device (or manual compression) may be preferred over an intravascular closure device.

The most frequently used extravascular closure device is Mynx (Cardinal Health, Dublin, OH), which delivers a polyethylene glycol (PEG) sealant to the subcutaneous track near the arterial puncture site. Osmotically active PEG rapidly absorbs water from blood and interstitial fluid, causing the sealant to swell in size and occlude the hole. A large, propensity-matched analysis of 73,124 patients undergoing vascular closure found that the Mynx device showed a significantly greater risk of any vascular complication than alternative endovascular or extravascular closure devices (absolute risk, 1.2% vs 0.8%; relative risk, 1.59; 95% CI, 1.42–1.78; P<.001).[29]

Exoseal (Cardinal Health) is an alternative extravascular closure device and consists of a plug made of polyglycolic acid, which increases platelet aggregation and traps erythrocytes to form a thrombus-like network inside the matrix of the plug. In a 168-patient trial of Exoseal following antegrade common femoral artery access for peripheral arterial disease intervention, there was a 1.8% rate of pseudoaneurysm and a 5.4% rate of hematoma formation.[30] Another device, named Vascade (Cardiva, Santa Clara, CA), places a collagen plug in the subcutaneous track near the arterial puncture site. Similar to PEG, the collagen becomes hydrated and expands to fill the tissue defect. In addition, the collagen is thrombogenic, potentiating clot formation around the plug to seal the subcutaneous track.

Large-Bore Vascular Closure

For procedures requiring sheath sizes greater than 8 French, 1 or more Perclose devices may be used with the "preclose" technique.[31] In this technique, a 6-French arteriotomy is made, the device sutures are deployed but not tightened, a larger sheath is deployed, the procedure is performed, and finally the device sutures are tightened on sheath removal.

Table 2
Selected vascular closure devices commonly used following peripheral arterial interventions

	Product	Manufacturer	Access Sizes Closed (French)	Mechanism
Intravascular	Angio-Seal	Terumo	6, 8	Intravascular anchor, extravascular collagen plug
	Perclose ProGlide	Abbott	6–8, larger with preclose technique	Suture through the arterial wall
	StarClose	Abbott	5, 6	Nitinol clip
	Manta	Teleflex	12–25	Intravascular anchor, extravascular collagen plug
Extravascular	Mynx	AccessClosure	5, 6, 7	Polyethylene glycol plug
	ExoSeal	Cardinal	5, 6, 7	Polyglycolic acid plug
	Vascade	Cardiva	5, 6, 7	Collagen plug

The Manta device (Teleflex) is approved for closure of access sites with sheaths of 12 to 25 French outer diameter. Similar to Angio-Seal, Manta is composed of a bioabsorbable endovascular anchor and an extravascular collagen plug that sandwich the access site. A pivotal clinical study demonstrated the safety and efficacy of this device,[32] and a head-to-head trial called MASH-TAVI comparing Manta and Perclose following TAVI is underway, although a small, nonrandomized, single-center study reported lower complication rates using the preclose technique.[33]

SUMMARY

Successful arterial access and closure are critical components of any peripheral arterial intervention. The risk of procedural complications may be minimized with arterial access using micropuncture technique, both ultrasound and fluoroscopic guidance, a compressible arterial access site, and the smallest diameter sheath necessary. Closure of an arteriotomy site may be achieved by manual compression, device-mediated compression, an intravascular closure device, or an extravascular closure device. Although closure devices improve patient comfort and expedite hemostasis, they have not been shown to reduce complications in comparison with manual compression. Careful attention to the intricacies of access and closure facilitates safe and effective endovascular interventions.

DISCLOSURE

A.M. Goldsweig reports that he has no conflicts of interest to disclose. E.A. Secemsky has served as a consultant for Medtronic, Cook Medical, Philips, CSI and has received grants to institution from Medtronic, Cook Medical, CSI, AstraZeneca, BD Bard.

REFERENCES

1. Shroff A, Pinto D. Vascular access, management, and closure: best practices. Washington, DC: Society for Cardiovascular Angiography and Interventions; 2019.
2. Seto AH, Abu-Fadel MS, Sparling JM, et al. Real-time ultrasound guidance facilitates femoral arterial access and reduces vascular complications: FAUST (Femoral Arterial Access With Ultrasound Trial). JACC Cardiovasc Interv 2010;3(7):751–8.
3. Seldinger SI. Catheter replacement of the needle in percutaneous arteriography; a new technique. Acta Radiol 1953;39(5):368–76.
4. Ambrose JA, Lardizabal J, Mouanoutoua M, et al. Femoral micropuncture or routine introducer study (FEMORIS). Cardiology 2014;129(1):39–43.
5. Ben-Dor I, Maluenda G, Mahmoudi M, et al. A novel, minimally invasive access technique versus standard 18-gauge needle set for femoral access. Catheter Cardiovasc Interv 2012;79(7):1180–5.
6. Sanghvi KA, Kusick J, Krathen C. Retrograde tibiopedal access for revascularization of lower-extremity eripheral artery disease using a 6 Fr slender sheath: the "Pedal-First" Pilot project. J Invasive Cardiol 2018;30(9):334–40.
7. Bazan HA, Le L, Donovan M, et al. Retrograde pedal access for patients with critical limb ischemia. J Vasc Surg 2014;60(2):375–81.
8. El-Sayed HF. Retrograde pedal/tibial artery access for treatment of infragenicular arterial occlusive disease. Methodist DeBakey Cardiovasc J 2013;9(2):73–8.
9. Yamashita T, Imai S, Tamada T, et al. Transradial approach for noncoronary angiography and interventions. Catheter Cardiovasc Interv 2007;70(2): 303–8.

10. Ferrante G, Rao SV, Juni P, et al. Radial versus femoral access for coronary interventions across the entire spectrum of patients with coronary artery disease: a meta-analysis of randomized trials. JACC Cardiovasc Interv 2016;9(14):1419–34.

11. Sanghvi K, Kurian D, Coppola J. Transradial intervention of iliac and superficial femoral artery disease is feasible. J Interv Cardiol 2008;21(5):385–7.

12. Yu J, Korabathina R, Coppola J, et al. Transradial approach to subclavian artery stenting. J Invasive Cardiol 2010;22(5):204–6.

13. Folmar J, Sachar R, Mann T. Transradial approach for carotid artery stenting: a feasibility study. Catheter Cardiovasc Interv 2007;69(3):355–61.

14. Trani C, Tommasino A, Burzotta F. Transradial renal stenting: why and how. Catheter Cardiovasc Interv 2009;74(6):951–6.

15. Patel T, Kuladhipati I, Shah S. Successful percutaneous endovascular management of acute post-traumatic superior mesenteric artery dissection using a transradial approach. J Invasive Cardiol 2010;22(4):E61–4.

16. Kiemeneij F. Left distal transradial access in the anatomical snuffbox for coronary angiography (ldTRA) and interventions (ldTRI). EuroIntervention 2017;13(7):851–7.

17. van Dam L, Geeraedts T, Bijdevaate D, et al. Distal radial artery access for noncoronary endovascular treatment is a safe and feasible technique. J Vasc Interv Radiol 2019;30(8):1281–5.

18. Hahalis G, Tsigkas G, Xanthopoulou I, et al. Transulnar compared with transradial artery approach as a default strategy for coronary procedures: a randomized trial. The Transulnar or Transradial Instead of Coronary Transfemoral Angiographies Study (the AURA of ARTEMIS Study). Circ Cardiovasc Interv 2013;6(3):252–61.

19. Kedev S, Zafirovska B, Dharma S, et al. Safety and feasibility of transulnar catheterization when ipsilateral radial access is not available. Catheter Cardiovasc Interv 2014;83(1):E51–60.

20. Kwolek CJ, Jaff MR, Leal JI, et al. Results of the ROADSTER multicenter trial of transcarotid stenting with dynamic flow reversal. J Vasc Surg 2015;62(5):1227–34.

21. Bergeron P. Direct percutaneous carotid access for carotid angioplasty and stenting. J Endovasc Ther 2015;22(1):135–8.

22. Hayashida K, Lefèvre T, Chevalier B, et al. Transfemoral aortic valve implantation new criteria to predict vascular complications. JACC Cardiovasc Interv 2011;4(8):851–8.

23. Isawa T, Horie K, Inoue N. Cutoff value of the sheath-to-artery ratio for radial artery occlusion in patients undergoing transradial percutaneous coronary interventions using sheathless guiding catheters for acute coronary syndrome. New Orleans (LA): American College of Cardiology; 2018.

24. Vallabhajosyula P, Kramer M, Lazar S, et al. Lower-extremity complications with femoral extracorporeal life support. J Thorac Cardiovasc Surg 2016;151(6):1738–44.

25. Bangalore S, Bhatt DL. Femoral arterial access and closure. Circulation 2011;124(5):e147–56.

26. Schulz-Schupke S, Helde S, Gewalt S, et al. Comparison of vascular closure devices vs manual compression after femoral artery puncture: the ISAR-CLOSURE randomized clinical trial. JAMA 2014;312(19):1981–7.

27. Wimmer NJ, Secemsky EA, Mauri L, et al. Effectiveness of arterial closure devices for preventing complications with percutaneous coronary intervention: an instrumental variable analysis. Circ Cardiovasc Interv 2016;9(4):e003464.

28. Martin JL, Pratsos A, Magargee E, et al. A randomized trial comparing compression, Perclose Proglide and Angio-Seal VIP for arterial closure following percutaneous coronary intervention: the CAP trial. Catheter Cardiovasc Interv 2008;71(1):1–5.

29. Resnic FS, Majithia A, Marinac-Dabic D, et al. Registry-based prospective, active surveillance of medical-device safety. N Engl J Med 2017;376(6):526–35.

30. Hackl G, Gary T, Belaj K, et al. Exoseal for puncture site closure after antegrade procedures in peripheral arterial disease patients. Diagn Interv Radiol 2014;20(5):426–31.

31. Michaels AD, Ports TA. Use of a percutaneous arterial suture device (Perclose) in patients undergoing percutaneous balloon aortic valvuloplasty. Catheter Cardiovasc Interv 2001;53(4):445–7.

32. Wood DA, Krajcer Z, Sathananthan J, et al. Pivotal clinical study to evaluate the safety and effectiveness of the MANTA percutaneous vascular closure device. Circ Cardiovasc Interv 2019;12(7):e007258.

33. Hoffmann P, Al-Ani A, von Lueder T, et al. Access site complications after transfemoral aortic valve implantation—a comparison of Manta and Pro-Glide. CVIR Endovasc 2018;1(1):20.

Plaque Modification in Endovascular Procedures in Patients with Infrainguinal Disease

Matthew T. Finn, MD, MSc, Joseph J. Ingrassia, MD,
Sahil A. Parikh, MD*

KEYWORDS

- Atherectomy • Plaque modification • Laser • Rotational atherectomy • Directional atherectomy
- Orbital atherectomy • Vascular lithotripsy • Peripheral artery disease

KEY POINTS

- Plaque modification uses a variety of devices/mechanisms to debulk, soften, crack, or "otherwise modify" the vessel structure seeking to improve results with angioplasty balloons or stents.
- Plaque modification therapies have proliferated in recent years despite limited high-quality data.
- Further studies, particularly head-to-head trials, will aid in developing consensus guidelines and specific scenarios for utilization of plaque modification.

INTRODUCTION

Endovascular plaque modification (PM) uses a variety of mechanisms to debulk, soften, crack, or "otherwise modify" the vessel structure to improve device passage and increase luminal gain with angioplasty balloons or stents. These benefits come at a cost of higher risk of distal embolization and vessel perforation. Herein, we (1) examine the evidence base for PM technologies, including that supporting their use in various pathologic vessel subsets (ie, calcified plaque, noncalcified plaque, and in-stent restenosis), to provide a better understanding of the associated risks and benefits; (2) review consensus guidelines for PM devices; and (3) highlight future research needs that should drive device evolution.

PLAQUE MODIFICATION DEVICE UTILIZATION

PM device utilization has expanded in recent years, growing from approximately 10% of cases

in 2010 to 18% in 2016.[1] This increase has occurred despite limited randomized trial data. Many of the existing studies are small registries assessing PM in diverse patient populations and vascular lesion types (eg, short vs long lesions, calcific vs noncalcific disease, claudicants vs critical limb ischemia). This has led to significant treatment variation in PM use across endovascular operators in the United States, as exemplified by a study that found that use ranged from 0% to 32% of cases by geographic region.[1]

SCIENTIFIC STATEMENTS ON PLAQUE MODIFICATION

Given the lack of head-to-head trials evaluating PM devices, there is currently little consensus guiding PM device use. The 2018 the American College of Cardiology (ACC)/American Heart Association/Society for Cardiac Angiography and Interventions (SCAI)/Society of Interventional Radiology/Society for Vascular Medicine

Department of Cardiology, Columbia University Irving Medical Center, 161 Fort Washington Avenue, 6th Floor, New York, NY 10032, USA
* Corresponding author.
E-mail address: sap2196@cumc.columbia.edu

Intervent Cardiol Clin 9 (2020) 125–137
https://doi.org/10.1016/j.iccl.2019.12.004

2018 Appropriate Use Criteria for Peripheral Artery Intervention[2] afford atherectomy an "M" classification for "may be appropriate" in femoropopliteal and below the knee (BTK) lesions. However, in patients with iliac arterial disease, atherectomy carries an "R" for rarely appropriate given a lack of sufficient data to recommend its clinical use.

The SCAI consensus statement on device selection for femoropopliteal disease emphasizes that PM therapies are not definitive, but rather adjunctive (ie, for lesion preparation before definitive balloon or stent treatment) (Table 1).[2,3] The writing group suggested PM for severely calcified vessels (Fig. 1), but did not specifically define how to classify calcium severity. There are several calcium classification schemes, including that from the Peripheral Academic Research Consortium,[4] which have been developed from inclusion criteria for various PM trials in the peripheral and coronary space (Table 2).

The Society of Vascular Surgery Guidelines, ACC guidelines on peripheral arterial disease, and the Trans-Atlantic Inter-Society Consensus Document on Management of Peripheral Arterial Disease II guidelines also mention PM as an important adjuvant for successful endovascular treatment but do not offer additional specific guidance for use.[5–7]

EVIDENCE BASE SUPPORTING PLAQUE MODIFICATION

A variety of available PM device options exist, including those using laser, directional, rotational, orbital, and lithotripsy treatments. In this article, we review the mechanisms, technical specifications and standard use, safety, and efficacy of various PM technologies for treatment of peripheral arterial disease (PAD) in general and among various pathologic subsets in particular (Tables 3 and 4).

LASER

Laser-guided PM (Excimer; Spectranetics, Colorado Springs, CO, Fig. 2A) uses pulses of monochromatic light to soften or "vaporize" a tissue layer of approximately 10 µm. Laser was the first extensively studied PM device and has been deployed in the coronary arteries as well as in the periphery.

The single-arm CELLO study[8] examined outcomes in 65 patients with moderate to severely calcified femoropopliteal disease, almost a quarter of whom requiring stenting. The study demonstrated a primary patency rate of 76.9% at 1 year. The 2014 EXCITE study[9] randomized 250 patients with femoropopliteal in-stent restenosis (ISR) to excimer laser plus percutaneous transluminal angioplasty (PTA) versus PTA alone. Freedom from target lesion (TLR) revascularization at 6 months was 73.5% versus 51.8% in favor of laser + PTA ($P = .05$). This pivotal trial demonstrated superiority of laser atherectomy for treatment of ISR and supported this additional Food and Drug Administration indication.

ROTATIONAL

There are several available rotational PM devices on the market in the United States. The

Table 1
Society for Cardiac Angiography and Interventions consensus guidelines for plaque modification device treatment in various lesion subsets

Lesion Type	Laser	Directional	Orbital/ Rotational
Moderate to severe calcified, undilatable, focal lesion	IIB	III	IIA
Moderate to severe calcified, undilatable, intermediate lesion	IIB	III	IIA
Moderate to severe calcified, undilatable, diffuse lesion	IIB	IIA	IIB
Moderate to severe calcified, dilatable, focal lesion	III	III	IIB
ISR, focal lesion	IIA	III	III
ISR, intermediate lesion	IIA	III	III
ISR, diffuse lesion	IIA	III	III

Abbreviations: Class I, device is recommended; IIA, device use is reasonable; IIB, device use may be reasonable however benefits are in question; III, device use not recommended; ISR, in-stent restenosis.
From Bailey, Steven R., Joshua A. Beckman, Timothy D. Dao, Sanjay Misra, Piotr S. Sobieszczyk, Christopher J. White, L. Samuel Wann, et al. 2019. "ACC/AHA/SCAI/SIR/SVM 2018 Appropriate Use Criteria for Peripheral Artery Intervention." Journal of the American College of Cardiology; with permission.

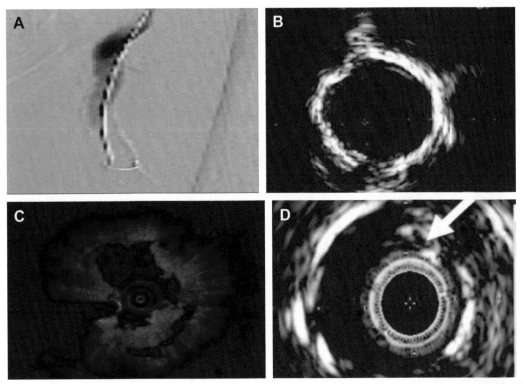

Fig. 1. Examples of significant calcification on (A) angiography and (B) intravascular ultrasound imaging. Depicted intravascular ultrasound imaging demonstrates greater than 270° of calcification. (C, D) Demonstrate calcified lesions on OCT and intravascular ultrasound respectively after PM with ShockWave lithotripsy. The arrow in (D) represents fractured calcium nodule.

Table 2
Peripheral Academic Research Consortium classification of severity of vascular calcification

Degree of Lesion Calcification	Calcium Quantification
Focal	<180 (1 side of vessel) and less than one-half of the total lesion length
Mild	<180 and greater than one-half of the total lesion length
Moderate	≥180 (both sides of vessel at the same location) and less than one-half of the total lesion length
Severe	≥180 (both sides of the vessel at the same location) and greater than one-half of the total lesion length

From Patel, Manesh R., Michael S. Conte, Donald E. Cutlip, Nabil Dib, Patrick Geraghty, William Gray, William R. Hiatt, et al. 2015. "Evaluation and Treatment of Patients with Lower Extremity Peripheral Artery Disease: Consensus Definitions from Peripheral Academic Research Consortium (PARC)." *Journal of the American College of Cardiology* 65 (9): 931–41.; with permission.

rotablator system (**Fig. 2**B), which initially was used in the coronary arteries, is now also available for use in infrainguinal (particularly BTK) disease.

There are limited contemporary data evaluating rotablator in the peripheral vasculature. A 1995 single-center French study of 150 patients reported a high complication rate (25%), but complications were broadly defined as significant spasm, thrombosis, dissection, perforation, distal emboli, or no reflow.[10] Primary patency after rotablator plus PTA at 14 months was 76%.

JetStream atherectomy (Boston Scientific, Marlborough, MA, **Fig. 2**C), which uses rotational atherectomy combined with active aspiration of released debris, has been studied in 2 registries: JET and JET-SCE.[11,12] In JET, 241 patients with de novo or restenotic (non-ISR) femoropopliteal lesions ≥4 cm in length received PM with the Jetstream device. At 12-month follow-up, primary vessel patency was 77.2% based on duplex ultrasound. JET-SCE was a single-center study examining Jetstream atherectomy plus drug-coated balloons (DCB) versus Jetstream atherectomy plus PTA. The 12-month incidence of TLR-free survival was

Table 3
Summary major of studies examining plaque modification technologies by year

Study	Year	Trial Design/Device/N	Pathologic Subset	Primary Patency at 1 y (Unless Noted Otherwise)	Other Major Outcomes	Conclusion/Major Limitations
Disrupt PAD II[22]	2019	Nonrandomized, multicenter, single arm ShockWave Lithotripsy N = 60	Femoropopliteal Mod-Sev calcification 93.3% CTO 16.7%	12-mo patency was 54.5%,	30-d MAE rate was 1.7% with one grade D dissection. Clinically driven TLR at 12 mo was 20.7%	Low rates of TLR and excellent safety data with 0% distal embolization despite only 3% embolic protection use
Liberty 360[21]	2019	Prospective, multicenter registry divided by rutherford class Diamondback 360 N = 1204	Femoropopliteal and BTK lesions 58.5% with calcification CTO in approximately one-third of patients	1-y freedom from MAE: 82.6% in RC2,3, 73.2% in RC4,5, and 59.3% in RC6 patients	Quality-of-life scores improved significantly across all groups	Endovascular treatment had high success and low MAE across all Rutherford groups Rutherford class 6: unplanned amputation is frequently not necessary with 91% amputation-free at 1 y
JET-SCE[12]	2018	Single center Jetstream N = 75	Femoropopliteal de novo or ISR (18%) 80% significant calcium CTO 30%	12-mo TLR-free survival: Jetstream + DCB vs Jetstream with PTA (94.7% vs 68.0%, P = .002)	Distal embolization requiring treatment occurred in 1.2% of patients	Jetstream + DCB had superior 1-y TLR rates compared with Jetstream + PTA alone
JET[11]	2018	Prospective, multicenter registry Jetstream atherectomy N = 241	Femoropopliteal de novo and ISR lesions	12-mo patency was 77.2% based on duplex ultrasound		In patients with complex, long lesions, Jetstream-based intervention had a high primary patency at 1 y and low complication rate
EASE[13]	2017	Single arm, Registry Multicenter The Phoenix system N = 128	Infrainguinal de novo and ISR lesions	6-mo TLR freedom: 88%	Device success was 99%	Adequate safety and efficacy per authors

Study	Year	Design	Vessel/Characteristics	Procedural Success	Outcomes	Conclusions
VISION[19]	2017	Single-arm registry Pantheris directional (OCT guided) N = 158	Infrainguinal vessels Mod-Sev Calcium excluded 20% CTOs	Procedural success (stenosis <30% after Pantheris + adjunctive treatment): 97%	MAEs after 6 mo: 16.6% TLR: 4% device-related events Quality-of-life metrics improved at 6 mo compared with baseline	High rate of procedural success with low rate of TLR
DEFINITIVE-AR[18]	2017	Multicenter RCT Pilot SilverHawk or TurboHawk + DCB vs DCB alone N = 102	Femoropopliteal 84% severe calcification CTOs ≥5 mm excluded	DA + DCB: 84.6% DCB: 81.3% $P = .88$	Flow-limiting dissection 2% vs 19% in favor of DA + DCB	DA + DCB safe and effective but there was no significant difference in 1-y outcomes (underpowered)
DEFINITIVE-LE[17]	2014	Single-arm registry SilverHawk Directional N = 797 (596 claudicants, 201 CLI)	Infrainguinal vessels 37% calcified 17% CTO	78% in the claudicant group, 71% in patients with CLI	Perforation: 5.3% Stent rate: 3.2% Target vessel femoropopliteal: 81.6% Infrapopliteal: 18.5% Limb salvage 95% in CLI population	Acute safety and 12-mo durability in claudicants and CLI
CONFIRM Series (I, II, & III)[23]	2014	Prospective registry single arm Diamondback360, Predator360, and Stealth360 N = 3135	"All comers" 81.1% Mod-Sev Calcium CTO percentage not defined			Variety of subanalyses regarding orbital atherectomy on outcomes
COMPLIANCE 360[20]	2014	Multicenter RCT Pilot Diamondback 360 + Balloon angioplasty vs BA alone N = 50	Femoropopliteal Sig Calcium	Freedom from TLR in 77.1% of lesions in the PM group vs 11.5% in the PTA group ($P<.001$) at 6 mo, 12 mo no significant difference remained	Lower max ATM for balloon inflations in the PM group (4 atm vs 9.1 atm) $P<.001$ Lower rate of bail-out stenting in the orbital atherectomy arm	At 12 mo, TLR or restenosis was similar in both groups despite the large difference in stent use at the time of initial treatment

(continued on next page)

Study	Year	Trial Design/Device/N	Pathologic Subset	Primary Patency at 1 y (Unless Noted Otherwise)	Other Major Outcomes	Conclusion/Major Limitations
EXCITE[9]	2014	Multicenter RCT Excimer laser PM + PTA vs PTA alone for ISR N = 250	Femoropopliteal bare metal stent ISR CTO 30.5% in laser arm and 36.8 in PTA arm (P = .37)	6-mo primary patency 71.1% vs 56.4%, in favor of laser P = .004. Freedom TLR 6 mo: 73.5% vs 51.8% in favor of laser (P<.005)	30-d MAE rates were 5.8% vs 20.5% (P<.001 in favor of Laser + PTA)	Superiority of Laser + PTA over PTA alone in ISR
PATENT[24]	2014	Single arm Laser for ISR N = 90	Femoropopliteal bare metal stent ISR Mod-Sev Calcification 76% CTO 34.1%	37.8% duplex patency at 12 mo	9 (10.0%) patients experienced distal embolization Freedom from TLR at 6 and 12 mo were 87.8% and 64.4%	High procedural success rate but low primary patency rate at 1 y suggests laser alone does not sufficiently treat ISR
CALCIUM 360[25]	2012	Multicenter, multiarm registry Diamondback 360 + Balloon angioplasty vs PTA alone N = 50	CLI patients Infrapopliteal	Freedom from mortality at 1 y 100% in Diamondback + PTA vs 68.4% in PTA alone (P = .01)	No difference in procedural success rate or bail-out stenting	No difference in freedom from target lesion revascularization but lower mortality in orbital atherectomy + PTA vs PTA alone Authors encourage larger confirmatory studies
Pathway VD[26]	2009	Single arm, registry Pathway PV system followed by PTA N = 172	Mostly SFA/Pop. Few BTK (9%) Mod-Sev calcium 51% CTO 31%	61.8% patency at 12 mo by duplex	99% technical success	Adequate safety and efficacy per authors Single-arm study
CELLO[8]	2009	Single arm, registry Turbo-Booster/Turbo-Elite laser catheters N = 65	Femoropopliteal 61.5% Mod-Sev calcium CTO 20%	76.9% at 1 year	23% had stenting although not clearly due to dissection/recoil, etc	Adequate safety and efficacy per authors Single-arm study

| Henry et al,[10] 1995 | 1995 | Single arm, registry Rotablator N = 150 | Femoropopliteal 50% and BTK 50% | After an average of 14-mo follow-up 76% patent | Broadly defined complication rate was high at 25% 97% reported technical success | High rates of success with good patency result; however, with high complication rates although broadly defined |

Abbreviations: BTK, below the knee; CLI, critical limb ischemia; CTO, chronic total occlusion; DA, directional atherectomy; DCB, drug-coated balloon; ISR, in-stent restenosis; MAE, major adverse events per trial design; Mod-Sev, moderate-severe; N, number; OCT, optical coherence tomography; PM, plaque modification; PTA, percutaneous transluminal angioplasty; RC, Rutherford class; RCT, randomized controlled trial; SFA, superficial femoral artery; TLR, target lesion revascularization; pop, popliteal artery.

Table 4
Major plaque modification/atherectomy devices, specifications, and utilization for peripheral arterial disease

Device	Mechanism	Rail Guidewire Size (Inches)	Sheath Size	Eccentric Calcium	CTO Lesion with Subintimal Segment	Thrombotic Lesion Efficacy	ISR Lesions	BTK Lesions
Excimer laser	Monochromatic light to dissolve/soften plaque	0.014	6 Fr	Yes	Yes	Yes	Yes	Yes
Rotablator	Rotational	Specialty wire: tapered wire with 0.014 spring tip	Depends on burr size; 6-Fr sheath generally acceptable					Yes
JetStream	Rotational	0.014	7 Fr	Yes		Yes	Yes	
Phoenix	Rotational	Specialty wire: 0.014	5–7 Fr depending on device size	Yes		Yes		
Ocelot	Rotational - OCT image guided	0.014	6 Fr	Yes	Yes			
Pantheris	Directional- OCT image guided	0.014	7 or 8 Fr	Yes	Yes			
SilverHawk	Directional	0.014	6 or 7 Fr	Yes	Yes			
TurboHawk	Directional	0.014	6–8 Fr	Yes	Yes			
HawkOne	Directional	0.014	7 Fr	Yes	Yes			
Diamondback 360	Orbital	0.14 with 0.18 tip	4 Fr 1.25 mm burrs 5 Fr 1.25 mm, 1.75 mm burrs and all radial compatible burrs 6 Fr 2.0 mm Burr	Yes				Yes

| ShockWave | Lithotripsy | 0.014 | M5 device 3.5–6.0 6 Fr; 6.5–7.0 7 Fr S5 device 3.0–4.0 5 Fr | Yes | Yes | Yes (S4 device) |

Abbreviations: BTK, below the knee; CTO, chronic total occlusions; Fr, French; ISR, in-stent restenosis; OCT, optical coherence tomography.

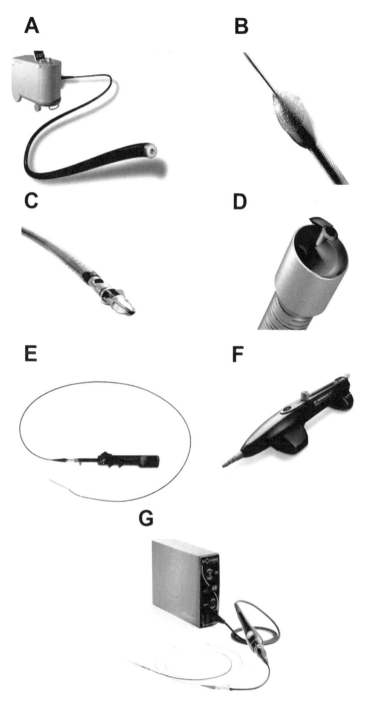

Fig. 2. Commonly used devices for PM. Clockwise from top left: (A) Excimer laser, (B) Rotoblator, (C) Jetstream, (D) Phoenix, (E) Silver-Hawk, (F) Diamondback360, and (G) ShockWave. Images compliments of their respective device companies. ([A, D] *Courtesy of* Royal Philips; and [B, C] © 2019 Boston Scientific Corporation or its affiliates. All rights reserved. and [E] *Courtesy of* Medtronic, Inc., Minneapolis, MN; with permission; and [F] © 2019 Cardiovascular Systems, Inc. CSI®, Diamondback 360®, GlideAssist®, ViperWire Advance® and ViperSlide® are registered trademarks of Cardiovascular Systems, Inc., and used with permission.)

94.7% for Jetstream + DCB versus 68.0% for Jetstream plus PTA (*P* = .002).

An additional rotational PM option is the Phoenix system (Philips, Amsterdam, Netherlands, **Fig. 2**D), which also combines front-end lesion cutting with debris clearance. This device was studied in the 2014 EASE registry,[13–15] which demonstrated an 88% 6-month freedom from TLR and a very low rate of procedural embolization (<1%).

DIRECTIONAL

SilverHawk, TurboHawk, and HawkOne systems (Medtronic, Minneapolis, MN, **Fig. 2**E), and Pantheris (Avinger, Redwood City, CA) are examples of directional atherectomy devices that use rotating cutting disks to resect and then remove the atherosclerotic plaque. The SilverHawk uses a 1-directional cutting blade consisting of a rotating blade inside a housing with a collection area. The TurboHawk functions similar to the SilverHawk, but has 4 atherectomy blades, facilitating increased plaque removal per pass and is recommended for use in highly calcified vessels.[16]

In the single-arm DEFINITIVE-LE,[17] 797 patients with claudication or critical limb ischemia (CLI) underwent SilverHawk Directional Atherectomy. At 1 year, primary patency rate was 78% among claudicants and 71% in patients with CLI. The subsequent DEFINITIVE-AR[18] multicenter randomized controlled pilot trial compared SilverHawk or TurboHawk + DCB versus DCB alone in 102 patients with calcified femoropopliteal lesions. The study showed no difference between treatment arms, but was underpowered. However, DEFINITIVE-AR did find that directional atherectomy plus DCB had a significantly lower incidence of flow-limiting dissection compared with DCB alone ($P = .01$). There were only 2 patients with distal embolization requiring treatment in the atherectomy arm, although distal embolic protection devices were used in more than 80% of cases. The ongoing multicenter, single-arm REALITY study (clinicaltrials.gov NCT02850107) will assess 1-year primary patency and freedom from major adverse events among patients treated with HawkOne or SilverHawk directional atherectomy plus DCB.

The Avinger Pantheris directional atherectomy system combines optical coherence tomography (OCT) with directional atherectomy. The OCT imaging component is designed to allow for targeted atherectomy of diseased vessel segments. The Pantheris device was studied in the 2017 VISION trial. This study showed a 97% procedural success rate with only a 4% rate of target lesion revascularization at 6 months, although lesions with moderate to severe calcification were excluded.[19]

ORBITAL

The Diamondback360 orbital atherectomy (Cardiovascular Systems Inc., St. Paul, MN, Fig. 2F) device has a diamond-coated tungsten crown that orbits inside the vessel in a 360-degree arc allowing for differential PM based on vessel size. Diamondback360 atherectomy is available in multiple crown sizes, shapes, and lengths, and is compatible with sheaths as small as a 4-Fr sheath for smaller 1.25-mm burrs.

Longer shaft length devices have been developed to allow for treatment of femoropopliteal and tibial lesions from the radial artery.

Compliance 360 was a randomized, multicenter pilot study of 50 patients with calcified femoropopliteal disease comparing Diamondback360 orbital atherectomy plus PTA versus PTA alone.[20] At 6 months, the study's primary endpoint, freedom from TLR (including adjunctive stenting) or restenosis was achieved in 77.1% of the orbital atherectomy group and 11.5% of balloon angioplasty group lesions ($P<.001$). However, at 12 months these differences were no longer significant (81.2% vs 78.3%, $P>.99$). Nevertheless, investigators observed that much lower balloon pressure inflations were required at the time of the procedure in the OA plus PTA arm resulting in significantly less need for bail-out stenting (5.3% vs 77.8%, $P<.001$).

The subsequent Liberty 360 study, a large, multicenter, "all comers" and "all device" registry found that 91% of Rutherford class 6 patients remained amputation-free at 1 year.[21] In addition, an unpublished analysis from the registry presented at the 2018 Amputation Prevention Symposium demonstrated that 1-year freedom from major adverse events was 73.2% in Rutherford class 4 or 5 and was in 59.3% in Rutherford class 6 patients.[21]

ENDOVASCULAR LITHOTRIPSY

ShockWave balloon lithotripsy (ShockWave Medical, Santa Clara, CA, Fig. 2G), uses pulsatile ultrasound energy to modify calcific plaque beyond the intimal layer. DISRUPT PAD II,[22] a nonrandomized, multicenter single-arm trial assessed intravascular lithotripsy in 60 patients with moderate to severe femoropopliteal calcific stenosis. The incidence of the study's primary safety endpoint 30-day major adverse events was 1.7% with only 1 grade D dissection and no distal embolization events despite use of embolic protection in only 3%. The study's primary effectiveness endpoint, primary patency at 12 months, was 54.5%, whereas clinically driven TLR at that time point was 20.7%.

KNOWLEDGE GAPS AND FUTURE DIRECTIONS

Randomized controlled device trials, are the current gold standard. However, across atherectomy devices, RCTs are underrepresented, with only 3 such studies as described previously, 2 of which were underpowered. It is clear that future research must include head-to-head randomized studies of PM devices in different patient, anatomic, and lesion subsets (eg, claudicants, CLI, BTK disease, ISR). In addition, most PM studies in PAD have been conducted in patients with at least moderate calcific stenosis. Their use in soft plaque or thrombus and in non-ISR lesions remains controversial. Additional studies to provide evidence for or against PM use in these scenarios are needed. Last, the comparative efficacy of newer PM technologies, when used alone or in combination with DCB, remains to be determined. Studies such as the ongoing DISRUPT PAD III randomized trial and DISRUPT OS registry (clniicaltrials.gov NCT02923193) may help address these issues.

SUMMARY

PM can be an important adjuvant tool to treat complex lesions, particularly in the setting of moderate or greater vascular calcification or ISR. The role of these devices in noncalcific or nonrestenotic lesions is unclear. Emerging data should help operators better understand which lesion subsets may benefit from the use of PM. The rising utilization of these devices has resulted in a proliferation of device iterations using various mechanisms. Without adequately designed and sized head-to-head efficacy and safety trials, choosing between devices remains challenging.

DISCLOSURE

Dr S.A. Parikh reported serving on the advisory boards of Abbott Vascular, Medtronic, Boston Scientific, Philips, and CSI Inc. He has also reported serving as a paid consultant for Terumo, and Merrill LifeSciences and receiving grants and/or institutional research support from Abbott Vascular, Boston Scientific, Silk Road Medical, Shockwave Medical, TriReme Medical, and Surmodics Inc. All other authors have no disclosures.

REFERENCES

1. Mohan S, Flahive JM, Arous EJ, et al. Peripheral atherectomy practice patterns in the United States from the vascular quality initiative. J Vasc Surg 2018;68(6):1806–16.
2. Bailey SR, Beckman JA, Dao TD, et al. ACC/AHA/SCAI/SIR/SVM 2018 appropriate use criteria for peripheral artery intervention. J Am Coll Cardiol 2019;73(2):214–37.
3. Feldman DN, Armstrong EJ, Aronow HD, et al. SCAI consensus guidelines for device selection in femoral-popliteal arterial interventions. Catheter Cardiovasc Interv 2018;92(1):124–40.
4. Patel MR, Conte MS, Cutlip DE, et al. Evaluation and treatment of patients with lower extremity peripheral artery disease: consensus definitions from Peripheral Academic Research Consortium (PARC). J Am Coll Cardiol 2015;65(9):931–41.
5. Norgren L, Hiatt WR, Dormandy JA, et al. Inter-Society Consensus for the Management of Peripheral Arterial Disease (TASC II). J Vasc Surg 2007;45(Suppl S):S5–67.
6. Conte MS, Pomposelli FB, Clair DG, et al. Society for Vascular Surgery practice guidelines for atherosclerotic occlusive disease of the lower extremities: management of asymptomatic disease and claudication. J Vasc Surg 2015;61(3):2S–41S.e1.
7. Hirsch AT, Haskal ZJ, Hertzer NR, et al. ACC/AHA 2005 guidelines for the management of patients with peripheral arterial disease (lower extremity, renal, mesenteric, and abdominal aortic): executive summary a collaborative report from the American Association for Vascular Surgery/Society for Vascular Surgery, Society for Cardiovascular Angiography and Interventions, Society for Vascular Medicine and Biology, Society of Interventional Radiology, and the ACC/AHA Task Force on Practice Guidelines (Writing Committee to Develop Guidelines for the Management of Patients With Peripheral Arterial Disease) endorsed by the American Association of Cardiovascular and Pulmonary Rehabilitation; National Heart, Lung, and Blood Institute; Society for Vascular Nursing; TransAtlantic Inter-Society Consensus; and Vascular Disease Foundation. J Am Coll Cardiol 2006;47(6):1239–312. Available at: http://www.onlinejacc.org/content/47/6/e1.abstract.
8. Dave RM, Patlola R, Kollmeyer K, et al. Excimer laser recanalization of femoropopliteal lesions and 1-year patency: results of the CELLO registry. J Endovasc Ther 2009;16(6):665–75.
9. Dippel EJ, Makam P, Kovach R, et al. Randomized controlled study of excimer laser atherectomy for treatment of femoropopliteal in-stent restenosis: initial results from the EXCITE ISR trial (EXCImer Laser Randomized Controlled Study for Treatment of FemoropopliTEal In-Stent Restenosis). JACC Cardiovasc Interv 2015;8(1 Part A):92–101.
10. Henry M, Amor M, Ethevenot G, et al. Percutaneous peripheral atherectomy using the rotablator: a single-center experience. J Endovasc Surg 1995;2(1):51–66.
11. Gray WA, Garcia LA, Amin A, et al, JET Registry Investigators. Jetstream Atherectomy System treatment of femoropopliteal arteries: results of the post-market JET Registry. Cardiovasc Revasc Med 2018;19(5 Pt A):506–11.
12. Shammas NW, Shammas GA, Jones-Miller S, et al. Long-term outcomes with Jetstream atherectomy with or without drug coated balloons in treating

femoropopliteal arteries: a single center experience (JET-SCE). Cardiovasc Revasc Med 2018;19(7 Pt A):771–7.

13. Davis T, Ramaiah V, Niazi K, et al. Safety and effectiveness of the Phoenix Atherectomy System in lower extremity arteries: early and midterm outcomes from the prospective multicenter EASE study. Vascular 2017;25(6):563–75.

14. Liu J, Li T, Huang W, et al. Percutaneous mechanical thrombectomy using Rotarex catheter in peripheral artery occlusion diseases–experience from a single center. Vascular 2019;27(2):199–203.

15. Freitas B, Steiner S, Bausback Y, et al. Rotarex mechanical debulking in acute and subacute arterial lesions: single-center experience with 525 patients. Angiology 2017;68(3):233–41.

16. Charitakis K, Feldman DN. Atherectomy for lower extremity intervention: why, when, and which device. 2016. Available at: https://www.acc.org/latest-in-cardiology/articles/2015/06/16/07/58/atherectomy-for-lower-extremity-intervention.

17. McKinsey JF, Zeller T, Rocha-Singh KJ, et al. Lower extremity revascularization using directional atherectomy: 12-month prospective results of the DEFINITIVE LE study. JACC Cardiovasc Interv 2014;7(8):923–33.

18. Zeller T, Langhoff R, Rocha-Singh KJ, et al. Directional atherectomy followed by a paclitaxel-coated balloon to inhibit restenosis and maintain vessel patency: twelve-month results of the DEFINITIVE AR study. Circ Cardiovasc Interv 2017;10(9). https://doi.org/10.1161/CIRCINTERVENTIONS.116.004848.

19. Schwindt AG, Bennett JG Jr, Crowder WH, et al. Lower extremity revascularization using optical coherence tomography-guided directional atherectomy: final results of the evaluation of the pantheris optical coherence tomography imaging atherectomy system for use in the peripheral vasculature (VISION) study. J Endovasc Ther 2017;24(3):355–66.

20. Dattilo R, Himmelstein SI, Cuff RF. The COMPLIANCE 360 trial: a randomized, prospective, multicenter, pilot study comparing acute and long-term results of orbital atherectomy to balloon angioplasty for calcified femoropopliteal disease. J Invasive Cardiol 2014;26(8):355–60.

21. LIBERTY 360° two-year data show high freedom from major amputation. Vascular News 2018. Available at: https://vascularnews.com/liberty-360-two-year-data/. Accessed October 19, 2019.

22. Brodmann M, Werner M, Holden A, et al. Primary outcomes and mechanism of action of intravascular lithotripsy in calcified, femoropopliteal lesions: results of Disrupt PAD II. Catheter Cardiovasc Interv 2019;93(2):335–42.

23. Lee MS, Yang T, Adams G. Pooled analysis of the CONFIRM registries: safety outcomes in diabetic patients treated with orbital atherectomy for peripheral artery disease. J Endovasc Ther 2014;21(2):258–65.

24. Schmidt A, Zeller T, Sievert H, et al. Photo ablation using the turbo-booster and Excimer laser for in-stent restenosis treatment: twelve-month results from the PATENT study. J Endovasc Ther 2014;21(1):52–60.

25. Shammas NW, Lam R, Mustapha J, et al. Comparison of orbital atherectomy plus balloon angioplasty vs. balloon angioplasty alone in patients with critical limb ischemia: results of the CALCIUM 360 randomized pilot trial. J Endovasc Ther 2012;19(4):480–8.

26. Zeller T, Krankenberg H, Steinkamp H, et al. One-year outcome of percutaneous rotational atherectomy with aspiration in infrainguinal peripheral arterial occlusive disease: the multicenter pathway PVD trial. J Endovasc Ther 2009;16(6):653–62.

Carotid, Vertebral, and Brachiocephalic Interventions

Mahesh Anantha-Narayanan, MD, Sameer Nagpal, MD,
Carlos Mena-Hurtado, MD*

KEYWORDS

- Carotid endarterectomy • Vertebral artery stenosis • Brachiocephalic interventions

KEY POINTS

- Carotid artery stenting and endarterectomy are equally safe and efficacious methods of revascularization in patients with asymptomatic or symptomatic carotid stenosis.
- Subclavian steal syndrome causing vertebrobasilar insufficiency or coronary subclavian steal syndrome with internal mammary artery bypass are the two major indications for subclavian intervention.
- Restenosis is common with vertebral artery angioplasty, so stenting is preferred, although long-term follow-up data are limited.

INTRODUCTION

Atherosclerotic disease of coronary and carotid arteries leading to ischemic heart disease and stroke accounts for almost one-third of deaths worldwide.[1] Incidence of ischemic stroke ranges between 8% and 15%.[2,3] Carotid atherosclerosis most frequently manifests in the proximal internal carotid artery and the common carotid artery bifurcations. Subclavian artery atherosclerosis affects the proximal segments with a relatively higher incidence on the left and becomes clinically important in the presence of vertebrobasilar insufficiency or coronary steal. Atherosclerosis of the vertebral artery can lead to posterior circulation stroke. Both endovascular and open surgical therapies are options for treating carotid, brachiocephalic, and vertebral lesions. The authors review the major trials on carotid, brachiocephalic, and vertebral artery stenosis along with the various available diagnostic modalities and interventional techniques, with an in-depth review of endovascular interventions.

EPIDEMIOLOGY: CAROTID DISEASE

The prevalence of significant carotid artery stenosis is in the range of 4.5% to 7%.[4] Most carotid disease results from atherosclerosis, although a minority is related to trauma[5] or fibromuscular disease.[6] Traditional risk factors include age, sex, diabetes mellitus, hypertension, and hyperlipidemia.[7,8] Carotid stenosis is more common in patients who have atherosclerosis involving other vascular beds, including peripheral artery disease and coronary artery disease,[9,10] and shares pathophysiology of atherosclerotic progression.

DIAGNOSIS OF CAROTID ARTERY DISEASE
Ultrasound
Duplex ultrasound is the mainstay for noninvasive diagnosis of carotid stenosis.[11] It is a low-cost modality, has high temporal and spatial resolution, and provides both anatomic and flow velocity information about the degree of stenosis and morphologic characteristics of the

Funding: None.
Section of Cardiovascular Medicine, Yale New Haven Hospital, New Haven, CT 06511, USA
* Corresponding author.
E-mail address: carlos.mena-hurtado@yale.edu
Twitter: @Mahesh_maidsh; @Yalecards (M.A.-N.)

Intervent Cardiol Clin 9 (2020) 139–152
https://doi.org/10.1016/j.iccl.2019.12.008

plaque. The major limitations are poorer visualization in the presence of significant calcification, patient body habitus, and a high carotid bifurcation. The ultrasound velocity criteria for diagnosing carotid stenosis are shown in Fig. 1.

Computed Tomographic Angiography

Computed tomographic angiography (CTA) is the primary cross-sectional imaging modality for suspected anatomic carotid stenosis in clinical settings, such as trauma, stable atherosclerosis, or stroke.[12] The major limitations of CTA are exposure to ionizing radiation and use of iodinated contrast, which limits use in patients with renal dysfunction. Conventional CTA includes static images performed in the arterial phase acquiring images of the head and neck with a single contrast bolus. Newer multiphasic CTA with rapid sequential imaging allows for visualization of flow within vessels analogous to the catheter-based digital subtraction angiography (DSA).[13] CT perfusion imaging can be used adjunctively in the assessment of significance of carotid stenosis.[14]

Magnetic Resonance Angiography

Magnetic resonance angiography (MRA) does not use ionizing radiation or intravenous contrast but cannot be obtained in patients with older pacemakers or implantable cardioverter-defibrillators, unless they are compatible.[15] Contrast MRA improves the visualization of small residual vascular lumen and helps differentiate between complete occlusion versus high-grade stenosis. MRA can accurately assess plaque characteristics particularly when thin-section high-resolution imaging algorithms are applied.

Digital Subtraction Angiography

DSA involves acquiring high-resolution images using conventional radiograph with digital acquisition of images in rapid sequence using intraarterial injection of contrast. This helps to evaluate both anatomic and real-time physiologic depiction of flow dynamics. DSA, although invasive, remains the gold-standard imaging technique and is the modality of choice used to define carotid stenosis in most of the published randomized trials. Carotid artery stenosis according to arteriography was defined by in the North American Symptomatic Carotid Endarterectomy Trial (NASCET).[16] According to this technique, the percentage of carotid stenosis was defined by comparing the minimal residual lumen at the level of the stenotic lesion with the diameter of the more distal internal carotid artery at which the walls of the artery first becomes parallel (beyond any poststenotic dilatation). The formula used to calculate degree of stenosis is $(1 - A/B) \times 100\%$, where A is the diameter at the point of maximum stenosis and B is the diameter of the arterial segment distal to the stenosis where the walls first become parallel. This method has been subsequently applied to CTA as well.

APPROACH TO ASYMPTOMATIC CAROTID ARTERY DISEASE

Asymptomatic carotid stenosis refers to the presence of narrowing in the extracranial

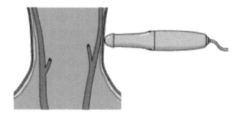

Degree of Stenosis	Unstented carotid artery	Carotid artery after stenting
0-19%	PSV <130 cm/s	PSV <150 cm/s and ICA/CCA ratio<2.15
20%–49%	PSV 130–189 cm/s	PSV 150–219 cm/
50%–79%	PSV 190–249 cm/s and EDV <120 cm/s	PSV 220–339 cm/s and ICA/CCA ratio = 2.7
80%–99%	PSV = 250 cm/s and EDV = 120 cm/s, or ICA/CCA ratio = 3.2	PSV = 340 cm/s and ICA/CCA = 4.5

Fig. 1. Degree of stenosis based on carotid ultrasound. CCA, common carotid artery; EDV, end diastolic velocity; ICA, internal carotid artery; PSV, proximal systolic velocity.

internal carotid artery in individuals without transient ischemic attack (TIA) or ipsilateral ischemic stroke in the prior 6 months.

Most ischemic strokes in patients with asymptomatic carotid stenosis are preceded by TIAs.[17–19] As a result, some experts recommend watchful waiting of patients with asymptomatic carotid stenosis until they experience a TIA.[20,21] However, the risk of stroke without warning was about 1% to 2%, suggesting that watchful waiting may not be an optimal strategy and early intervention may be beneficial instead.[22–24] There is a substantial amount of controversy surrounding the management of patients with asymptomatic carotid stenosis. Therapeutic modalities include the following:

1. Intensive medical therapy
2. Carotid endarterectomy (CEA)
3. Carotid artery stenting (CAS)

WHAT DO THE GUIDELINES SAY?

The American Heart Association/American Stroke Association (AHA/ASA) guidelines for primary prevention of stroke recommend the following for patients with asymptomatic carotid artery disease[25]:

1. Treatment with aspirin and statin daily along with appropriate lifestyle changes (Class I, level of evidence [LOE] C).
2. Consider CEA in asymptomatic patients who have greater than 70% stenosis of the internal carotid artery if the risk of perioperative stroke, myocardial infarction, and death is low (<3%). It should be noted that the efficacy of CEA compared with medical therapy has not been well established in patients with asymptomatic carotid stenosis (Class IIa, LOE A).
3. Patients undergoing CEA should receive both preoperative and postoperative aspirin (Class I, LOE C).
4. Annual duplex ultrasonography is reasonable in patients with greater than 50% carotid stenosis (Class IIa, LOE C).
5. Prophylactic CAS might be considered in highly selected patients with asymptomatic carotid stenosis (≥60% by angiography, ≥70% by Doppler ultrasound) (Class IIb, LOE B).
6. In asymptomatic carotid artery stenosis patients who are at high risk of complications for carotid intervention by either CEA or CAS, the effectiveness of revascularization versus medical therapy alone is not well established (Class IIb, LOE B).

7. It is not recommended to screen low-risk populations for asymptomatic carotid artery stenosis (Class III, LOE C).

The 2011 ASA/ACCF/AHA/AANN/AANS/ACR/ASNR/CNS/SAIP/SCAI/SIR/SNIS/SVM/SVS[26] multisociety guidelines agree with the guidelines from the AHA/ACC but also offer a class I (LOE B) for CAS or CEA in patients with greater than 50% stenosis on catheter angiography. According to a recent report, both CAS and CEA are performed predominantly for patients with asymptomatic carotid stenosis.[27]

MEDICAL THERAPY

Annual rates of ipsilateral ischemic strokes have fallen significantly with medical therapy alone secondary to the increasing use of efficient medical therapy, including aspirin, statin, antiplatelets, and angiotensin-converting enzyme inhibitors/angiotensin receptor blockers, along with lifestyle modifications.[28,29] Effective usage of medical therapy could be seen from the increasing trend of medication usage in the Asymptomatic Carotid Surgery Trial (ACST) in which use of lipid-lowering therapy increased from 17% around 1996 to almost 58% around 2003. Another study reported a decrease in composite endpoint of stroke, death, myocardial infarction, or CEA after onset of symptoms with intensive medical therapy.[30]

CAROTID ENDARTERECTOMY
Major Carotid Endarterectomy Trials
The 3 major trials of CEA plus medical therapy versus medical therapy alone for asymptomatic carotid stenosis include the Veterans Affairs Cooperative Study Group (VA trial),[31] Asymptomatic Carotid Atherosclerosis Study (ACAS),[32] and the ACST.[33] The VA trial[31] assigned 444 male patients with 50% to 99% carotid stenosis by angiography to aspirin alone or aspirin combined with CEA. At 4-year follow-up, CEA significantly decreased the primary end point, ischemic stroke or TIA (relative risk [RR] reduction 0.38, 95% confidence interval [CI] 0.22 to 0.67). The relatively larger ACAS[32] study randomized 1662 patients between the ages of 40 and 79 years with 60% to 99% stenosis to CEA+aspirin or aspirin alone. At 2.7-year follow-up, the incidence of the primary endpoint (ipsilateral stroke and any perioperative stroke or death) was significantly lower with CEA+aspirin compared with aspirin alone (RR 0.53, 95% CI 0.22–0.72). The

largest randomized controlled trial (RCT), ACST,[33] randomized 3120 patients aged 40 to 91 years, who had ≥60% carotid artery stenosis (diagnosed by duplex ultrasound) to immediate CEA or deferred CEA until a definitive indication. Patients in the immediate CEA group received CEA within 1 year of carotid stenosis diagnosis. At 3.4 years, immediate CEA was associated with lower perioperative risk of stroke or death of 3.1%. The 5-year risk for all stroke or perioperative death in the immediate CEA was 6.4% compared with 11.8% in the deferral group, which was a statistically significant difference. Long-term follow-up of the ACST trial showed the net risk for all stroke or perioperative death in the immediate CEA group was much lower when compared with the deferral CEA group, both at 5 years (6.9 vs 10.9%) and at 10 years (13.4 vs 17.9%).[34]

CAROTID ARTERY STENTING
Major Carotid Artery Angioplasty and Stenting Trials

When CAS was introduced, CEA had already become the gold standard for carotid revascularization, and it would have been unethical to randomize patients to CAS versus medical therapy alone. Multiple RCTs have compared CAS to CEA including ACT I,[35] CREST,[36] and SAPPHIRE.[37] ACT I was the only trial on asymptomatic carotid artery disease, whereas the others included both symptomatic and asymptomatic carotid stenosis.

SAPPHIRE[37] randomized 334 high surgical risk patients with symptomatic and ≥50% carotid stenosis or asymptomatic with ≥80% carotid stenosis to CAS or CEA. CAS was noninferior on its primary end point, periprocedural death, stroke, or myocardial infarction within 30 days after the procedure and/or death or ipsilateral stroke within 1 year (12.2% vs 20.1%, 95% CI −0.7%–16.4%).

CREST[36] randomized 2502 standard surgical risk patients with asymptomatic or symptomatic carotid artery stenosis to CAS or CEA. The primary end point, a composite of death, myocardial infarction, or stroke within 30 days plus any ipsilateral stroke during 4-year follow-up, was similar between CAS and CEA (hazard ratio [HR] 1.11, 95% CI 0.83 to 1.44). The overall stroke rates, including periprocedural stroke, were similar between groups. In the immediate postoperative period of 30 days, CAS was associated with higher risk of minor stroke compared with CEA (HR 1.95, 95% CI 1.15–3.30) but a lower risk for periprocedural myocardial infarction (HR 0.5, 95% CI 0.3–0.9).

The ACT I[35] randomized 1453 standard surgical risk patients with asymptomatic 70% to 99% carotid stenosis assigned to either CAS or CEA (3:1). CAS was noninferior to CEA on the primary end point death, myocardial infarction, or stroke within 30 days of the procedure and ipsilateral stroke to 1-year post-procedure (CAS 3.8% vs CEA 3.4%). Five-year cumulative stroke-free survival rates were also not different (CAS 93.1% vs CEA 94.7%).

FEATURES ASYMPTOMATIC CAROTID STENOSIS WITH HIGH RISK OF STROKE

Severity and progression of carotid stenosis on follow-up screening an important factors for both asymptomatic and symptomatic carotid artery stenosis. Patients with asymptomatic embolism and silent infarcts (embolic) have a higher risk of subsequent stroke, and consequently, might benefit from carotid revascularization. In the ACSRS trial, which included 462 patients with asymptomatic carotid stenosis, the presence of silent embolic infarcts on brain computed tomography scan at baseline was associated with higher risk of ipsilateral stroke at follow-up (HR 3.0, 95% CI 1.46–6.29).[38] The presence of high-risk plaque, including carotid ulcers, intraplaque hemorrhage, and echo lucent plaques, has been shown to be associated with higher risk of strokes as well.[39–41] Finally, low cerebral blood flow reserve has been shown to be associated with the development of ischemic strokes in patients with a metaanalysis showing a fourfold increase in risk of ischemic strokes (odds ratio 4.07, 95% CI 2.00–11.07).[42] Whether any of the above features should impact the decision to revascularize or the timing of revascularization remains unknown.

APPROACH TO SYMPTOMATIC CAROTID ARTERY DISEASE

Symptomatic carotid artery stenosis is defined as a sudden onset of focal neurologic symptoms confined to the ipsilateral carotid artery, including one or more TIAs or ischemic strokes in the prior 6 months.

CAROTID ENDARTERECTOMY
Major Trials with Symptomatic Carotid Stenosis

There are extensive randomized data in patients with symptomatic carotid artery stenosis, supporting CEA as a safe and effective treatment for reducing ischemic stroke, when compared with medical therapy alone. CEA is an acceptable therapy for patients with symptomatic carotid stenosis of 50% to 99% stenosis with surgically favorable carotid lesion in the absence of significant cardiopulmonary problems and with no prior ipsilateral CEA with perioperative risk of stroke and death of less than 6%.

There are 2 major randomized trials of CEA in patients with symptomatic carotid stenosis. NASCET randomized 659 patients with TIA or nondisabling stroke with 50% to 99% stenosis in the ipsilateral carotid artery as measured by residual lumen diameter at the most stenotic location of the carotid vessel compared with the lumen in the normal segment of carotid artery distal to the lesion.[16] The study was prematurely terminated because CEA was associated with overwhelming benefit compared with medical therapy over a period of 18 months. At 2-year follow-up, risk of death or stroke was lower (15.8 vs 32.3%) along with the risk of death, ipsilateral stroke, fatal stroke, or major stroke. Follow-up out to 7 years demonstrated a similar reduction in TIA or nondisabling strokes.[43]

The European Carotid Surgery Trial (ECST)[44] randomized 2518 patients with nondisabling ischemic stroke, TIA, or retinal infarct in the ipsilateral carotid artery to either CEA or medical therapy. Degree of stenosis was measured by using the lumen of most of the stenotic segment of the carotid artery compared with the likely original diameter of the carotid bulb. At 3 years, CEA significantly reduced the incidence of ipsilateral stroke when compared with medical therapy alone (2.8% vs 16.8%), which was replicated at 6-[45] and 10-year follow-up.[46] An analysis reporting pooled results of NASCET, ECST, and VAT[47] found that CEA was beneficial in patients with greater than 50% symptomatic carotid stenosis. The analysis also showed that, in patients with near occlusive carotid stenosis, there was no significant benefit of CEA.

TIMING OF SURGERY

Data from the NASCET and ESCT trials suggest patients who received CEA within 2 weeks of nondisabling stroke or TIA had major benefit compared with greater than 2 weeks.[48] However, in patients with disabling moderate or severe stroke, there is a very high risk of stroke with CEA in the immediate postoperative period, as shown by prior published studies,[49,50] especially within 48 hours.[51]

RISK SCORE FOR CAROTID INTERVENTIONS

A few risk factors should be considered before deciding on carotid revascularization in patients with symptomatic carotid stenosis, including age, sex, degree of stenosis, time since stroke or TIA, symptoms, and plaque morphology. An online stroke risk calculator model based on the ECST trial is available online (www.stroke.ox.ac.uk).

CAROTID ARTERY ANGIOPLASTY AND STENTING

Patients with symptomatic carotid stenosis have been included in multiple RCTs comparing CAS and CEA. Patients with moderate or severe stroke/disability were appropriately excluded from these trials. As discussed above, SAP-PHIRE[37] and CREST[36] included patients with both symptomatic and asymptomatic carotid stenosis; in SAPPHIRE, CAS was noninferior to CEA, whereas in CREST, these revascularization modalities were considered equivalent. The 2011 multispecialty guidelines by Brott and colleagues[52] give a class I indication for both CAS and CEA in symptomatic carotid artery stenosis patients with greater than 70% stenosis of the internal carotid artery as documented by noninvasive imaging or greater than 50% as documented by catheter angiography with anticipated periprocedural mortality or stroke rate of less than 6%.

EMBOLIC PROTECTION DEVICES

There are 2 primary types of embolic protection devices (EPD) to prevent cerebral embolization during CAS (Fig. 2). EPD is mandatory for reimbursement by Medicare for carotid interventions.[53]

Distal Embolic Protection
A distal EPD uses a balloon or a filter that is placed in the distal internal carotid artery to provide protection from embolic phenomena, thus isolating the brain from debris during the CAS procedure. Use of a distal balloon requires collateral flow. With the availability of new filters in the market, a distal balloon is rarely used. The distal filters promote blood flow through the filter; thus, ipsilateral cerebral perfusion is maintained throughout the procedure unless the filter becomes overwhelmed with debris. The only disadvantage is that there is no active protection when the lesion is caused before deploying the filter.

Proximal Embolic Protection
With proximal EPD, protection is established first before crossing the target lesion or performing an intervention. The advantage is that a proximal EPD could be used in a tortuous internal carotid artery because the distal landing zone does not

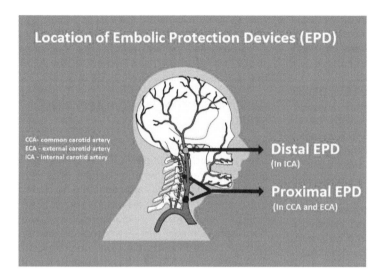

Fig. 2. Location of EPD for CAS.

affect the deployment in the proximal segment. The external and the common carotid arteries are occluded with flow reversal. To use a proximal EPD, the external carotid artery must be patent, and there must be an adequate segment of this vessel to accommodate an occlusion balloon proximal to the takeoff of the superior thyroid artery. The aortic arch and the common carotid configuration must also accommodate a 9F guiding catheter (6F working channel). Like the distal internal carotid balloon, the proximal EPD also requires collateral flow. The common carotid artery balloon is inflated first followed by the external carotid balloon. Debris is then removed with catheter aspiration after the procedure followed by external carotid balloon deflation. Finally, the common carotid artery balloon is deflated, and the EPD is removed. Multiple trials have demonstrated that proximal embolic protection results in less distal embolization than distal embolic protection.[54–57]

TECHNIQUES FOR CAROTID ARTERIAL INTERVENTION WITH CAROTID ARTERIAL ANGIOPLASTY AND STENTING

The preferred access for CAS is femoral access; however, radial, brachial, or direct femoral access may be used in selected patients. A multicenter randomized study by Ruzsa and colleagues[58] has shown that transradial access for CAS appears to be safe with no difference in total procedural and fluoroscopic time. At the authors' institution, if a preprocedural CTA is available, they try to evaluate the aortic arch to evaluate difficult anatomy, including type III

arch or presence of bovine anatomy. The various arch types are shown in **Fig. 3**. All patients receive antiplatelets before the procedure. At the authors' institution, they routinely load their patients with clopidogrel a few days before the procedure and have them on a maintenance regimen of 75 mg per day along with aspirin 81 mg per day. On the day of the procedure, they receive 300 mg of clopidogrel along with aspirin 81 mg. Using femoral access, they insert a pigtail catheter to obtain arch aortography. After visualizing the origin of carotid arteries, they exchange the short sheath for a 6F × 90-cm long destination sheath over an 0.0035" atraumatic j-tip intermediate stiff wire (Rosen wire; Infiniti Medical, LLC, Redwood City, CA, USA).

The authors then perform a selective engagement of the right or the left carotid artery under direct visualization using a 5F Vitek catheter (Cook, Bloomington, IN, USA); many operators will used nonshaped catheters, such as the JR4 instead, given their easier use and lower propensity to embolize. Most operators will then advance a glide wire through the diagnostic catheter into the common carotid artery (for the left) or through the brachiocephalic artery into the common carotid artery (for the right). When greater support is needed and there is not significant distal common carotid artery or ostial external carotid artery stenosis, the guidewire can be advanced into the distal external carotid artery. The diagnostic catheter is then advanced either to the distal internal carotid or to the external carotid artery (depending on the chosen wire position), and the sheath is advanced over the diagnostic catheter or the

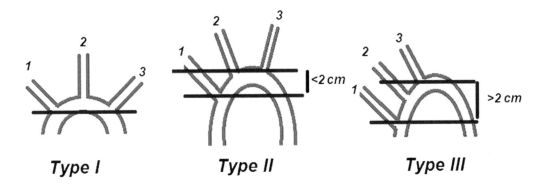

Type I   Type II   Type III

1. Right innominate artery
2. Left common carotid artery
3. Left subclavian artery

Fig. 3. Types of aortic arches.

diagnostic catheter can be removed and the sheath advanced over its dilator instead. The EPD is then deployed with the radiopaque tip in the petrous portion of the internal carotid artery. Once the EPD is deployed, a timer is started in order to keep track of and minimize filter deployment time. Next, stenting of the carotid artery is performed, covering the internal and the common carotid artery, when disease is present in the distal common carotid or ostial internal carotid artery, or deploying the stent in the internal carotid alone when disease is entirely confined to that location. Lesion predilation and lesion postdilation may or may not be performed, balancing the angiographic outcome with the risk of embolization with each balloon inflation. A follow-up angiogram should be obtained before EPD removal to determine whether the filter has been overwhelmed with embolic debris. If flow is less than brisk, aspiration thrombectomy should be performed multiple times to remove as much debris as possible from the stagnant column of blood proximal to the EPD, being mindful for cerebral ischemia resulting from reduced ipsilateral perfusion while doing so. It is important to note that the flow will not improve on angiography once the filter is overwhelmed, so repeat angiography is unnecessary. The EPD is removed, and a completion angiogram is performed, including orthogonal views of the carotid bifurcation and a lateral and anteroposterior intracranial view (modified Townes) to rule out perforation, dissection, and distal embolization. The authors routinely follow up these patients with carotid ultrasound at 1, 6, and 12 months and then yearly after CAS.[59] They continue dual antiplatelet therapy for a month after carotid stenting.

TRANSCAROTID ARTERY REVASCULARIZATION

Transcarotid artery revascularization (TCAR) is a hybrid open and endovascular technique whereby the common carotid is directly visualized by cutdown above the clavicle, and micropuncture access is obtained. Femoral vein access is achieved with a venous return sheath, which serves to create a circuit between the common carotid artery and the femoral vein, in which there is a flow controller and embolic filter. This conduit serves to establish flow reversal during carotid angioplasty, and stenting thus eliminates the need for distal or proximal percutaneous EPD. The single-arm ROADSTER (Reverse Flow Used During Carotid Artery Stenting Procedure) trial determined that the device was safe, with a 99% technical success rate. The Silk Road Enroute Transcarotid Neuroprotection system is commonly used.[60] After flow reversal is established, target lesion angioplasty is performed with a 4-mm balloon (monorail system), as with traditional transfemoral angioplasty and stenting. The stent is then advanced into the ideal position using roadmap or bony landmarks and then deployed. Poststent dilation is performed per operator discretion. Then, antegrade flow is established, and postprocedural angiography is performed to visualize both the carotid and the intracerebral vessels.

Surgical closure of vascular cutdown is performed, and femoral venous access is closed with manual pressure. A study published by Malas and colleagues[61] compared outcomes of TCAR to CAS using the Vascular Quality Initiative database. Rates of in-hospital TIA/stroke were higher with CAS when compared with TCAR. After multivariate adjustment, there was no statistically significant difference between CAS versus TCAR (2.5% vs 1.7%, $P = .25$). A recently published propensity-matched study comparing TCAR to CAS showed TCAR was associated with lower risk of stroke and death when compared with CAS.

CAROTID ENDARTERECTOMY

The CEA surgical procedure is beyond the scope of this article, and the reader is encouraged to review relevant articles.[62–65]

BRACHIOCEPHALIC INTERVENTIONS

Brachiocephalic interventions include those involving the brachiocephalic (innominate) and subclavian arteries, the latter being more common. This review focuses on subclavian interventions. Subclavian stenosis, although uncommon, can be associated with significant morbidity and mortality.[66,67] Left-sided is more common than right-sided subclavian stenosis.[68,69] The most common cause is atherosclerosis, similar to carotid stenosis. Other causes include fibromuscular dysplasia, Takayasu arteritis, thoracic outlet syndrome, radiation, and trauma.

ANATOMY

The left subclavian artery usually originates as the distal-most branch of aortic arch and typically gives rise to vertebral artery, internal mammary artery, and the thyrocervical trunk and then continues as axillary artery. The right subclavian artery is a branch of the brachiocephalic artery.

SUBCLAVIAN ARTERY STENOSIS
Asymptomatic Subclavian Stenosis
Asymptomatic subclavian stenosis is the most common presentation, because most patients have extensive collateral supply that masks significant symptoms.

Symptomatic Subclavian Stenosis
Symptomatic subclavian stenosis is defined as stenosis associated with the following: (1) upper-limb ischemia causing arm claudication and fatigue; (2) subclavian steal syndrome associated with disorientation, loss of balance, dizziness, diplopia, nystagmus, tinnitus, hearing loss secondary to vertebrobasilar insufficiency owing to vertebral-subclavian steal; (3) coronary steal phenomenon in postcoronary artery bypass surgery patients, whereby associated reversal of flow in either the left or the right internal mammary artery causes coronary ischemia.

Evaluation of Subclavian Stenosis
The major clinical clue is the presence of differential in blood pressures in the arms. A greater than 15-mm Hg pressure difference between arms suggests the presence of significant stenosis.[70,71] A second clue is the presence of decreased radial or brachial pulse amplitude, along with nailbed changes. The presence of significant subclavian bruit in the supraclavicular fossa suggests significant stenosis as well.

Imaging for Subclavian Stenosis
Duplex ultrasound with color flow of subclavian artery can provide both anatomic and functional assessment. The presence of waveform dampening, monophasic waveform, flow reversal, color aliasing, or elevated velocities is suggestive of significant obstruction. MRA and CTA are excellent noninvasive modalities with limitations as described above. Both CT and MR provide a better understanding of the type and severity of stenosis and also help to assess surrounding structures. Catheter DSA remains the gold standard for evaluation of patients with subclavian stenosis. A catheter-measured resting pressure gradient of 20 to 30 mm Hg is considered significant.

MEDICAL THERAPY

As with atherosclerosis in any bed, patients with asymptomatic stenosis benefit from medical therapy, including aspirin, angiotensin-converting enzyme inhibitor or angiotensin receptor blocker, and statin.[72]

SUBCLAVIAN ARTERY REVASCULARIZATION

Indications for revascularization include symptoms of arm ischemia, vertebral-subclavian steal syndrome, and coronary-subclavian steal syndrome in patients with coronary artery bypass grafting with internal mammary artery grafting.[73] Revascularization can be performed using either percutaneous or surgical techniques, but the former is preferred given its lower morbidity and mortality. Brachiocephalic angioplasty has a primary and secondary patency of 98% and 93% at 10 years.[74] Restenosis occurs in about 10% of patients after stenting. For more complex tubular lesions, surgical options are preferred, including carotid-subclavian bypass, carotid transposition, and axilloaxillary bypass.

Technique for Subclavian Revascularization

The authors typically load patients with P2Y12 inhibitor at least 24 to 48 hours before the procedure along with full-dose aspirin. The subclavian artery ranges between 7 and 10 mm in diameter, while the brachiocephalic artery ranges between 8 and 11 mm in diameter. A 7 or 8F guide catheter or a 6F 90-cm atraumatic tip sheath is used. After the sheath insertion, a smaller-sized diagnostic catheter (a multipurpose or a Judkins Right or an angled glide catheter) is used to engage ostium of subclavian. A support wire, either a 0.014-in or a 0.018-in wire, is used to cross the lesion. The authors then cross the lesion with the diagnostic catheter. Following this, the wire is exchanged over the catheter for a 0.035-in wire (eg, Wholey or Rosen). Balloon angioplasty is performed with a 5- or 6-mm balloon, avoiding the ostium of the vertebral or internal mammary artery. The authors' practice is to routinely perform sizing of the vessel using intravascular ultrasound (IVUS) before and after stenting (**Fig. 4**). Following balloon angioplasty, balloon-expandable stents are usually used secondary to their radial strength and ability to accurately deliver them, especially for proximal subclavian stenosis (**Fig. 5**). For mid and distal vessels, angioplasty alone is usually preferred because stenting is highly prone to fracture from the clavicle or the first rib. It is important to cover the ostium of subclavian or brachiocephalic artery, and it is ideal to protrude 2 to 3 mm of the stent outside the ostium. It is important to visualize the subclavian artery in orthogonal views during angioplasty. The unsheathing technique is usually used to promote proper positioning of the stent. It is essential to choose stents that are not oversized to avoid risk of dissection or rupture. The authors routinely perform IVUS after deployment to confirm stent expansion and to look for dissection. The authors perform follow-up ultrasounds at 1, 6, and 12 months and then annual follow-up. If restenosis is suspected, they obtain subclavian duplex.

VERTEBRAL ARTERY INTERVENTIONS

Atherosclerotic vertebral artery disease as a cause of posterior circulation ischemia is often underdiagnosed secondary to the vague nature of symptoms. Trauma, fibromuscular dysplasia, dissection, and aneurysm are other causes of

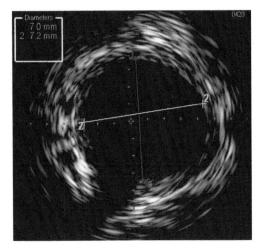

Fig. 4. IVUS of subclavian artery.

vertebral artery disease. Vertebral artery disease can be treated with both surgical and endovascular approaches.

ANATOMY

The vertebral artery is a branch of the subclavian artery, but in a small proportion of patients, it can originate directly from the aortic arch.[75] The vertebral artery is divided into 4 segments V1 to V4: V1 extends from the artery origin to the cervical spinal foramina; V2 is intraforaminal; V3 extends from the cervical foramina to foramen magnum; and V4 is intracranial.

ETIOLOGY

Similar to the carotid arteries, atherosclerosis is the most common cause for vertebral artery stenosis, although fibromuscular dysplasia, Takayasu disease, trauma, osteophyte

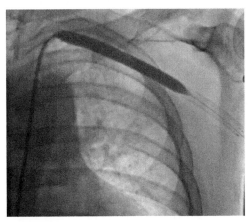

Fig. 5. Balloon-expandable stenting of the left subclavian artery.

compression, or dissections could contribute to vertebral disease. Patients with vertebrobasilar TIAs are at 30% to 35% risk of stroke at follow-up,[76,77] which is in turn associated with 20% to 30% mortality.[78,79] Vertebral artery stenosis causing ischemia can be hemodynamic or embolic. Severe stenosis, including subclavian/vertebral steal, can cause hemodynamic flow reversal in the vertebral artery. Also, conditions such as hyperviscosity or anemia can aggravate posterior circulation ischemia. Embolic phenomenon accounts for one-third of the strokes from vertebral artery.[80]

INDICATIONS FOR VERTEBRAL INTERVENTIONS

The major indications are the following: (1) hemodynamic symptoms with bilateral vertebral artery stenosis if both are patent or unilateral greater than 60% stenosis in the dominant vertebral artery; (2) posterior territory ischemic infarct suspected to be from an embolism from the corresponding vertebral artery; (3) symptomatic vertebral artery aneurysm and asymptomatic aneurysm greater than 1.5 cm.

IMAGING

Selective angiography of the subclavian and the vertebral artery remains the gold standard for evaluation of vertebral artery stenosis. Contrast-enhanced MRI is less invasive but tends to overestimate the lesions. Ability of duplex ultrasound to evaluate vertebral artery is limited secondary to the close proximity to the clavicle and also to the intraosseous course of the artery. It is important to exclude other conditions that could mimic vertebrobasilar insufficiency, including posterior fossa stroke, inner ear pathologic condition, and tumors before planning for vertebral intervention. Finally, a cardiac evaluation is prudent to exclude any hypoperfusion to brain secondary to valve disease, arrhythmia, or low ejection fraction, causing hypoperfusion to the brain with mild or moderate vertebral stenosis.

OPEN SURGICAL VERSUS ENDOVASCULAR INTERVENTION

Surgical intervention is preferred because this is more durable, but the number of surgeons with adequate experience is limited. Various types of surgical interventions include vertebral artery repair, vertebral artery transposition, and vertebral artery bypass. In prior published studies, combined stroke and death rates from open surgical procedures range from 1% to 4%

depending on the location of the vertebral lesion. Long-term outcomes of open surgical interventions are excellent with a patency rate of 90% at 10 years. Data on endovascular interventions are very limited, and endovascular intervention is associated with higher rates of restenosis with angioplasty alone in the range of 15% to 50%, considering the relatively smaller size of the vessel. The carotid and vertebral artery transluminal angioplasty study (CAVATAS 2001) compared endovascular intervention to medical therapy for vertebral stenosis.[81] About 25% of the patients who underwent endovascular intervention had a TIA within 30 days, although there were no major strokes or deaths within 30 days in either group. At 4.5 years, there were no major strokes in either group. Although V1 segment can be approached with either endovascular or open intervention, surgery is not the best option for V2 segment considering the intraosseous course of the vessel. V3 is not an ideal vessel segment for either surgery or endovascular intervention, and endovascular treatment is the preferred option for V4 disease.

SUMMARY

Diseases involving the extracranial cervical common and internal carotid arteries are most commonly related to atherosclerosis but rarely may occur in the setting of trauma, radiation, collagen vascular disease, or compression. Duplex ultrasound remains the most common modality used for diagnosis, whereas DSA remains the gold-standard diagnostic test. There has been a significant improvement in medical therapy for patients with carotid stenosis over time. CEA is associated with a higher incidence of perioperative myocardial infarction, and CAS is associated with an increased risk of perioperative minor stroke. Overall, CAS and CEA are equally safe and efficacious methods of revascularization in patients with asymptomatic or symptomatic carotid stenosis. Percutaneous revascularization of the carotid requires a proximal or distal EPD, and operator experience plays a major role in achieving technical success. Subclavian steal syndrome causing vertebrobasilar insufficiency or coronary subclavian steal syndrome in the presence of an internal mammary artery bypass are 2 major indications for subclavian intervention, and choice of intervention depends on patient's anatomy, the presence of concomitant carotid disease, and comorbidities. Vertebral artery intervention with either open surgery or endovascular intervention carries greater risk than carotid artery intervention and is associated with an overall periprocedural mortality of less than 5%. Restenosis is common with vertebral artery angioplasty, so stenting is preferred, although long-term follow-up data are limited.

CONFLICT OF INTERESTS AND DISCLOSURES

Dr C. Mena-Hurtado is a consultant for Cook Medical, Medtronic, Cardinal Health, and Boston Scientific.

REFERENCES

1. GBD 2013 Mortality and Causes of Death Collaborators. Global, regional, and national age-sex specific all-cause and cause-specific mortality for 240 causes of death, 1990-2013: a systematic analysis for the Global Burden of Disease Study 2013. Lancet 2015;385:117–71.
2. Hajat C, Heuschmann PU, Coshall C, et al. Incidence of aetiological subtypes of stroke in a multi-ethnic population based study: the South London Stroke Register. J Neurol Neurosurg Psychiatry 2011;82:527–33.
3. Kolominsky-Rabas PL, Weber M, Gefeller O, et al. Epidemiology of ischemic stroke subtypes according to TOAST criteria: incidence, recurrence, and long-term survival in ischemic stroke subtypes: a population-based study. Stroke 2001;32:2735–40.
4. Fine-Edelstein JS, Wolf PA, O'Leary DH, et al. Precursors of extracranial carotid atherosclerosis in the Framingham Study. Neurology 1994;44:1046–50.
5. Engelter ST, Traenka C, Lyrer P. Dissection of cervical and cerebral arteries. Curr Neurol Neurosci Rep 2017;17:59.
6. Mettinger KL, Ericson K. Fibromuscular dysplasia and the brain. I. Observations on angiographic, clinical and genetic characteristics. Stroke 1982; 13:46–52.
7. de Weerd M, Greving JP, Hedblad B, et al. Prevalence of asymptomatic carotid artery stenosis in the general population: an individual participant data meta-analysis. Stroke 2010;41:1294–7.
8. De Angelis M, Scrucca L, Leandri M, et al. Prevalence of carotid stenosis in type 2 diabetic patients asymptomatic for cerebrovascular disease. Diabetes Nutr Metab 2003;16:48–55.
9. Simons PC, Algra A, Eikelboom BC, et al. Carotid artery stenosis in patients with peripheral arterial disease: the SMART study. SMART study group. J Vasc Surg 1999;30:519–25.
10. Ahmed B, Al-Khaffaf H. Prevalence of significant asymptomatic carotid artery disease in patients with peripheral vascular disease: a meta-analysis. Eur J Vasc Endovasc Surg 2009;37:262–71.
11. Grant EG, Benson CB, Moneta GL, et al. Carotid artery stenosis: grayscale and Doppler ultrasound diagnosis–Society of Radiologists in Ultrasound consensus conference. Ultrasound Q 2003;19:190–8.
12. Wintermark M, Arora S, Tong E, et al. Carotid plaque computed tomography imaging in stroke and nonstroke patients. Ann Neurol 2008;64:149–57.
13. Menon BK, d'Esterre CD, Qazi EM, et al. Multiphase CT angiography: a new tool for the imaging triage of patients with acute ischemic stroke. Radiology 2015;275:510–20.
14. Roberts HC, Dillon WP, Smith WS. Dynamic CT perfusion to assess the effect of carotid revascularization in chronic cerebral ischemia. AJNR Am J Neuroradiol 2000;21:421–5.
15. Alvarez-Linera J, Benito-León J, Escribano J, et al. Prospective evaluation of carotid artery stenosis: elliptic centric contrast-enhanced MR angiography and spiral CT angiography compared with digital subtraction angiography. AJNR Am J Neuroradiol 2003;24:1012–9.
16. North American Symptomatic Carotid Endarterectomy Trial. Methods, patient characteristics, and progress. Stroke 1991;22:711–20.
17. Pessin MS, Duncan GW, Mohr JP, et al. Clinical and angiographic features of carotid transient ischemic attacks. N Engl J Med 1977;296:358–62.
18. Mohr JP, Caplan LR, Melski JW, et al. The Harvard Cooperative Stroke Registry: a prospective registry. Neurology 1978;28:754–62.
19. Russo LS. Carotid system transient ischemic attacks: clinical, racial, and angiographic correlations. Stroke 1981;12:470–3.
20. Dodick DW, Meissner I, Meyer FB, et al. Evaluation and management of asymptomatic carotid artery stenosis. Mayo Clin Proc 2004;79:937–44.
21. Shanik GD, Moore DJ, Leahy A, et al. Asymptomatic carotid stenosis: a benign lesion? Eur J Vasc Surg 1992;6:10–5.
22. Inzitari D, Eliasziw M, Gates P, et al. The causes and risk of stroke in patients with asymptomatic internal-carotid-artery stenosis. North American Symptomatic Carotid Endarterectomy Trial Collaborators. N Engl J Med 2000;342:1693–700.
23. Goldstein LB, Adams R, Becker K, et al. Primary prevention of ischemic stroke: a statement for healthcare professionals from the Stroke Council of the American Heart Association. Stroke 2001; 32:280–99.
24. Chambers BR, Norris JW. Outcome in patients with asymptomatic neck bruits. N Engl J Med 1986;315: 860–5.
25. Meschia JF, Bushnell C, Boden-Albala B, et al. Guidelines for the primary prevention of stroke: a statement for healthcare professionals from the American Heart Association/American Stroke Association. Stroke 2014;45:3754–832.

26. Brott TG, Halperin JL, Abbara S, et al. 2011 ASA/ ACCF/AHA/AANN/AANS/ACR/ASNR/CNS/SAIP/ SCAI/SIR/SNIS/SVM/SVS guideline on the management of patients with extracranial carotid and vertebral artery disease. Stroke 2011;42: e464–540.

27. Lichtman JH, Jones MR, Leifheit EC, et al. Carotid endarterectomy and carotid artery stenting in the US medicare population, 1999-2014. JAMA 2017; 318:1035–46.

28. Abbott AL. Medical (nonsurgical) intervention alone is now best for prevention of stroke associated with asymptomatic severe carotid stenosis: results of a systematic review and analysis. Stroke 2009;40:e573–83.

29. Spence JD. Management of asymptomatic carotid stenosis. Neurol Clin 2015;33:443–57.

30. Spence JD, Coates V, Li H, et al. Effects of intensive medical therapy on microemboli and cardiovascular risk in asymptomatic carotid stenosis. Arch Neurol 2010;67:180–6.

31. Hobson RW, Weiss DG, Fields WS, et al. Efficacy of carotid endarterectomy for asymptomatic carotid stenosis. The Veterans Affairs Cooperative Study Group. N Engl J Med 1993;328:221–7.

32. Endarterectomy for asymptomatic carotid artery stenosis. Executive Committee for the Asymptomatic Carotid Atherosclerosis Study. JAMA 1995; 273:1421–8.

33. Halliday A, Mansfield A, Marro J, et al. Prevention of disabling and fatal strokes by successful carotid endarterectomy in patients without recent neurological symptoms: randomised controlled trial. Lancet 2004;363:1491–502.

34. Halliday A, Harrison M, Hayter E, et al. 10-year stroke prevention after successful carotid endarterectomy for asymptomatic stenosis (ACST-1): a multicentre randomised trial. Lancet 2010;376:1074–84.

35. Rosenfield K, Matsumura JS, Chaturvedi S, et al. Randomized trial of stent versus surgery for asymptomatic carotid stenosis. N Engl J Med 2016;374: 1011–20.

36. Brott TG, Howard G, Roubin GS, et al. Long-term results of stenting versus endarterectomy for carotid-artery stenosis. N Engl J Med 2016;374: 1021–31.

37. Yadav JS, Wholey MH, Kuntz RE, et al. Protected carotid-artery stenting versus endarterectomy in high-risk patients. N Engl J Med 2004;351:1493– 501.

38. Kakkos SK, Sabetai M, Tegos T, et al. Silent embolic infarcts on computed tomography brain scans and risk of ipsilateral hemispheric events in patients with asymptomatic internal carotid artery stenosis. J Vasc Surg 2009;49:902–9.

39. Madani A, Beletsky V, Tamayo A, et al. High-risk asymptomatic carotid stenosis: ulceration on 3D

ultrasound vs TCD microemboli. Neurology 2011; 77:744–50.

40. Singh N, Moody AR, Gladstone DJ, et al. Moderate carotid artery stenosis: MR imaging-depicted intraplaque hemorrhage predicts risk of cerebrovascular ischemic events in asymptomatic men. Radiology 2009;252:502–8.

41. Topakian R, King A, Kwon SU, et al. Ultrasonic plaque echolucency and emboli signals predict stroke in asymptomatic carotid stenosis. Neurology 2011; 77:751–8.

42. Gupta A, Chazen JL, Hartman M, et al. Cerebrovascular reserve and stroke risk in patients with carotid stenosis or occlusion: a systematic review and meta-analysis. Stroke 2012;43:2884–91.

43. Paciaroni M, Eliasziw M, Sharpe BL, et al. Long-term clinical and angiographic outcomes in symptomatic patients with 70% to 99% carotid artery stenosis. Stroke 2000;31:2037–42.

44. MRC European Carotid Surgery Trial: interim results for symptomatic patients with severe (70-99%) or with mild (0-29%) carotid stenosis. European Carotid Surgery Trialists' Collaborative Group. Lancet 1991;337:1235–43.

45. Randomised trial of endarterectomy for recently symptomatic carotid stenosis: final results of the MRC European Carotid Surgery Trial (ECST). Lancet 1998;351:1379–87.

46. Cunningham EJ, Bond R, Mehta Z, et al. Long-term durability of carotid endarterectomy for symptomatic stenosis and risk factors for late postoperative stroke. Stroke 2002;33:2658–63.

47. Rerkasem K, Rothwell PM. Carotid endarterectomy for symptomatic carotid stenosis. Cochrane Database Syst Rev 2011;(4):CD001081.

48. Rothwell PM, Eliasziw M, Gutnikov SA, et al. Endarterectomy for symptomatic carotid stenosis in relation to clinical subgroups and timing of surgery. Lancet 2004;363:915–24.

49. Blaisdell WF, Clauss RH, Galbraith JG, et al. Joint study of extracranial arterial occlusion. IV. A review of surgical considerations. JAMA 1969;209: 1889–95.

50. Rob CG. Operation for acute completed stroke due to thrombosis of the internal carotid artery. Surgery 1969;65:862–5.

51. De Rango P, Brown MM, Chaturvedi S, et al. Summary of evidence on early carotid intervention for recently symptomatic stenosis based on meta-analysis of current risks. Stroke 2015;46: 3423–36.

52. Brott TG, Halperin JL, Abbara S, et al. 2011 ASA/ACCF/AHA/AANN/AANS/ACR/ASNR/ CNS/SAIP/SCAI/SIR/SNIS/SVM/SVS guideline on the management of patients with extracranial carotid and vertebral artery disease: executive summary: a report of the American College

of Cardiology Foundation/American Heart Association Task Force on Practice Guidelines, and the American Stroke Association, American Association of Neuroscience Nurses, American Association of Neurological Surgeons, American College of Radiology, American Society of Neuroradiology, Congress of Neurological Surgeons, Society of Atherosclerosis Imaging and Prevention, Society for Cardiovascular Angiography and Interventions, Society of Interventional Radiology, Society of NeuroInterventional Surgery, Society for Vascular Medicine, and Society for Vascular Surgery. Developed in collaboration with the American Academy of Neurology and Society of Cardiovascular Computed Tomography. Catheter Cardiovasc Interv 2013;81:E76–123.

53. Giri J, Parikh SA, Kennedy KF, et al. Proximal versus distal embolic protection for carotid artery stenting: a national cardiovascular data registry analysis. JACC Cardiovasc Interv 2015;8: 609–15.

54. Giordan E, Lanzino G. Carotid angioplasty and stenting and embolic protection. Curr Cardiol Rep 2017;19:120.

55. Omran J, Mahmud E, White CJ, et al. Proximal balloon occlusion versus distal filter protection in carotid artery stenting: a meta-analysis and review of the literature. Catheter Cardiovasc Interv 2017; 89:923–31.

56. Cano MN, Kambara AM, de Cano SJ, et al. Randomized comparison of distal and proximal cerebral protection during carotid artery stenting. JACC Cardiovasc Interv 2013;6:1203–9.

57. Montorsi P, Caputi L, Galli S, et al. Microembolization during carotid artery stenting in patients with high-risk, lipid-rich plaque. A randomized trial of proximal versus distal cerebral protection. J Am Coll Cardiol 2011;58:1656–63.

58. Ruzsa Z, Nemes B, Pintér L, et al. A randomised comparison of transradial and transfemoral approach for carotid artery stenting: RADCAR (RADial access for CARotid artery stenting) study. EuroIntervention 2014;10:381–91.

59. Mohler ER, Gornik HL, Gerhard-Herman M, et al. ACCF/ACR/AIUM/ASE/ASN/ICAVL/SCAI/SCCT/ SIR/SVM/SVS/SVU [corrected] 2012 appropriate use criteria for peripheral vascular ultrasound and physiological testing part I: arterial ultrasound and physiological testing: a report of the American College of Cardiology Foundation appropriate use criteria task force, American College of Radiology, American Institute of Ultrasound in Medicine, American Society of Echocardiography, American Society of Nephrology, Intersocietal Commission for the Accreditation of Vascular Laboratories, Society for Cardiovascular Angiography and Interventions, Society of Cardiovascular Computed Tomography, Society for Interventional Radiology, Society for Vascular Medicine, Society for Vascular Surgery, [corrected] and Society for Vascular Ultrasound. [corrected]. J Am Coll Cardiol 2012;60: 242–76.

60. Kwolek CJ, Jaff MR, Leal JI, et al. Results of the ROADSTER multicenter trial of transcarotid stenting with dynamic flow reversal. J Vasc Surg 2015; 62:1227–34.

61. Malas MB, Dakour-Aridi H, Wang GJ, et al. Transcarotid artery revascularization versus transfemoral carotid artery stenting in the Society for Vascular Surgery Vascular Quality Initiative. J Vasc Surg 2019;69:92–103.e2.

62. Little NS, Meyer FB. Carotid endarterectomy—indications, techniques, and Mayo Clinic experience. Neurol Med Chir (Tokyo) 1997;37:227–35.

63. Tokumaru GK. The role of carotid endarterectomy in the management of carotid artery disease and stroke. J Am Optom Assoc 1995;66: 113–22.

64. Levinson MM, Rodriguez DI. Endarterectomy for preventing stroke in symptomatic and asymptomatic carotid stenosis. Review of clinical trials and recommendations for surgical therapy. Heart Surg Forum 1999;2:147–68.

65. Cardona P, Rubio F, Martinez-Yélamos S, et al. Endarterectomy, best medical treatment or both for stroke prevention in patients with asymptomatic carotid artery stenosis. Cerebrovasc Dis 2007; 24(Suppl 1):126–33.

66. Hennerici M, Rautenberg W, Mohr S. Stroke risk from symptomless extracranial arterial disease. Lancet 1982;2:1180–3.

67. Moran KT, Zide RS, Persson AV, et al. Natural history of subclavian steal syndrome. Am Surg 1988; 54:643–4.

68. Rodriguez-Lopez JA, Werner A, Martinez R, et al. Stenting for atherosclerotic occlusive disease of the subclavian artery. Ann Vasc Surg 1999;13: 254–60.

69. Schillinger M, Haumer M, Schillinger S, et al. Outcome of conservative versus interventional treatment of subclavian artery stenosis. J Endovasc Ther 2002;9:139–46.

70. Osborn LA, Vernon SM, Reynolds B, et al. Screening for subclavian artery stenosis in patients who are candidates for coronary bypass surgery. Catheter Cardiovasc Interv 2002;56:162–5.

71. Lobato EB, Kern KB, Bauder-Heit J, et al. Incidence of coronary-subclavian steal syndrome in patients undergoing noncardiac surgery. J Cardiothorac Vasc Anesth 2001;15:689–92.

72. Ochoa VM, Yeghiazarians Y. Subclavian artery stenosis: a review for the vascular medicine practitioner. Vasc Med 2011;16:29–34.

73. Patel SN, White CJ, Collins TJ, et al. Catheter-based treatment of the subclavian and innominate arteries. Catheter Cardiovasc Interv 2008;71:963–8.

74. Hüttl K, Nemes B, Simonffy A, et al. Angioplasty of the innominate artery in 89 patients: experience over 19 years. Cardiovasc Intervent Radiol 2002;25:109–14.

75. Cavdar S, Arisan E. Variations in the extracranial origin of the human vertebral artery. Acta Anat (Basel) 1989;135:236–8.

76. Cartlidge NE, Whisnant JP, Elveback LR. Carotid and vertebral-basilar transient cerebral ischemic attacks. A community study, Rochester, Minnesota. Mayo Clin Proc 1977;52:117–20.

77. Whisnant JP, Cartlidge NE, Elveback LR. Carotid and vertebral-basilar transient ischemic attacks: effect of anticoagulants, hypertension, and cardiac disorders on survival and stroke occurrence–a population study. Ann Neurol 1978;3:107–15.

78. Flossmann E, Rothwell PM. Prognosis of vertebro-basilar transient ischaemic attack and minor stroke. Brain 2003;126:1940–54.

79. McDowell FH, Potes J, Groch S. The natural history of internal carotid and vertebral-basilar artery occlusion. Neurology 1961;11(4 Pt2):153–7.

80. Caplan LR, Wityk RJ, Glass TA, et al. New England Medical Center posterior circulation registry. Ann Neurol 2004;56:389–98.

81. Endovascular versus surgical treatment in patients with carotid stenosis in the carotid and vertebral artery transluminal angioplasty study (CAVATAS): a randomised trial. Lancet 2001;357:1729–37.

Endovascular Abdominal Aortic Aneurysm Repair

Akshit Sharma, MD, Prince Sethi, MD, Kamal Gupta, MD*

KEYWORDS

- Abdominal aortic aneurysm • Endovascular aneurysm repair • Endoleak

KEY POINTS

- Most abdominal aortic aneurysms are treated with endovascular repair (EVAR) in current practice.
- EVAR has lower periprocedural mortality and morbidity compared with open surgical repair.
- Anatomic factors, such as aneurysm neck morphology, iliac anatomy, and access vessel anatomy, need careful assessment for the successful performance of EVAR.
- Regular and long-term follow-up with imaging is mandatory after EVAR, and patients who are less likely to comply are less favorable EVAR candidates.
- Endoleaks are the most frequent complication of EVAR. Most can be managed with transcatheter or endovascular means.

INTRODUCTION

The treatment of abdominal aortic aneurysm (AAA) has evolved significantly over the past several decades. From the 1950s until the 1990s, open surgical repair (OSR) was the only treatment for AAA. Although still considered the gold standard, OSR is associated with relatively high periprocedural morbidity and mortality. Elective OSR has a mean operative mortality of ∼4%.[1,2] In 1986, the first report of endovascular stent graft–based repair was published, paving the way for minimally invasive endovascular aneurysm repair (EVAR).[1,3] Over the last 3 decades, EVAR has become the preferred treatment for AAA repair for most patients. In the United States, about 80% of all AAAs are treated with EVAR.[4]

INDICATIONS

Elective AAA repair is considered in asymptomatic patients with a fusiform aneurysm ≥5.5 cm in diameter and in those with an expanding aneurysm sac (increase in size by ≥5 mm in a 6-month interval or 10 mm in a year). A lower threshold of ≥5 cm may be considered in women because of the higher associated rupture rate at a given size in women compared with men.[5,6] Earlier repair is also reasonable for those with saccular aneurysms. Emergent AAA repair is recommended for symptomatic AAA (embolization, abdominal/back pain, and/or rupture).

CONTRAINDICATIONS

EVAR should not be performed in patients unlikely to adhere with regular noninvasive imaging follow-up to monitor for endoleak. Contraindications for EVAR are primarily based on vessel anatomy.[7] There are very few absolute contraindications because even with adverse anatomic features, EVAR can be performed using newer techniques or investigational devices. However, this may come at a cost of a higher sac growth and rupture risk. Important relative contraindications include the following:

i. Adverse infrarenal aortic neck anatomy (Fig. 1)
ii. Suprarenal aneurysmal disease (unless using fenestrated devices)

Department of Cardiovascular Medicine, University of Kansas School of Medicine, 3901 Rainbow Boulevard, Delp 1001, Kansas City, KS 66160, USA
* Corresponding author.
E-mail address: kgupta@kumc.edu

Intervent Cardiol Clin 9 (2020) 153–168
https://doi.org/10.1016/j.iccl.2019.12.005

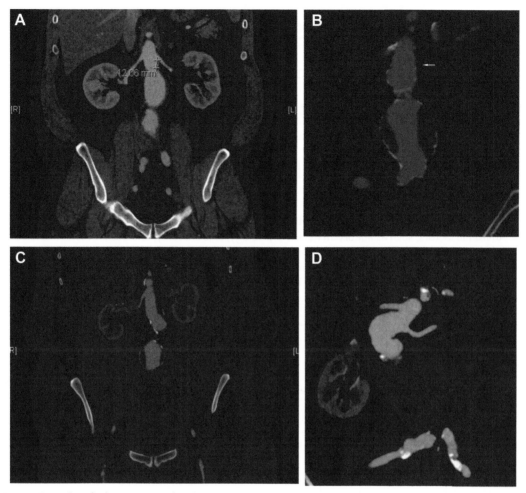

Fig. 1. Examples of adverse proximal neck anatomy. (A) Short (<15 mm) neck, (B) reverse taper neck with shorter proximal diameter (*black arrow*) and larger distal diameter (*white arrow*) of the aneurysm neck, (C) thick thrombus layer and dilated neck, (D) tortuous and angulated neck.

iii. Bilateral internal or external iliac artery aneurysm
iv. Excessive iliac artery tortuosity, especially with associated calcification and stenosis

Late- (but not end-) stage chronic kidney disease is also a relative contraindication given the need for concomitant iodinated contrast. Contrast use can be minimized with the use of intravascular ultrasound imaging.[8,9] OSR also carries a risk of worsening renal function and in some studies is associated with a greater risk of this than EVAR.[10,11] Limited life-expectancy is also a significant contraindication to both EVAR and OSR.

ENDOVASCULAR ANEURYSM REPAIR EVIDENCE BASE

There is a large body of evidence comparing EVAR and OSR for AAA repair. The Dutch Randomized Endovascular Aneurysm Management (DREAM) trial,[12,13] the UK Endovascular Aneurysm Repair versus Open Repair in Patients with Abdominal Aortic Aneurysm (EVAR-1) trial,[14] the US Veterans Open versus Endovascular Repair (OVER) trial,[15] and the Anevrysme de L'aorte abdominale Chirugie vs Endoprosthe (ACE) trial[16] are pivotal trials that have helped establish EVAR as the preferred method for AAA repair for most patients in the current era. The key results of these trials are summarized in Table 1.

Several metaanalyses and systematic reviews have shown improved short-term mortality with EVAR when compared with OSR (1.4% vs 4.2%). These studies have also shown a decreased length of hospital stay and lower incidence of complications, such as bowel ischemia, acute kidney injury, and pneumonia, with the use

Table 1
Summary of randomized controlled trials comparing the endovascular aortic repair and open surgical repair outcomes

Study	Follow-Up (y)	Number of Patients EVAR	OSR	30-d Mortality EVAR (%)	OSR (%)	RR (95% CI; P value)	Outcomes Long-Term Mortality[a] EVAR	OSR	95% CI; P value
DREAM	Range: 5.1–8.2 Mean: 6.4	173	178	1.2	4.6	RR 3.9 (0.9–32.9; 0.10)	31.1%	30.1%	Difference 1% point (−8.8–10.8; 0.97)
EVAR-1	Median: 6.0	626	626	1.8	4.3	OR 0.39 (0.18–0.87; 0.02)	7.5/100-person-years	7.7/100-person-years	HR 1.03 (0.86–1.23; 0.72)
OVER	Mean: 5.2	444	437	0.5	3.0	HR and CI not reported (P = .004)	32.9%	33.4%	HR 0.97 (0.77–1.25; 0.81)
ACE	Median: 3.0	150	149	1.3	0.6	P = NS	11.3%	8%	P = NS

Abbreviations: CI, confidence interval; HR, hazard ratio; NS, not significant; OR, odds ratio; RR, relative risk.
[a] All the data under long term mortality reflect overall deaths through the duration of study follow-up.

of EVAR. However, late mortality is not significantly different between these modalities, raising concerns that late sac growth and rupture because of endoleaks in the EVAR group may explain these observations.[17–22]

ENDOVASCULAR ANEURYSM REPAIR DEVICES

Multiple EVAR devices have been approved for commercial use in the United States.[23,24] Device-specific anatomic selection criteria can be found in the instructions for use for each device.[23] Among other characteristics, these anatomic measurements include neck length, neck diameter, neck angle, and iliac diameter.[24] EVAR devices can be broadly grouped into 2 categories based on the proximal attachment site of the stent graft, namely suprarenal and infrarenal fixation devices.

Infrarenal Fixation
These devices involve placement of the stent graft in the infrarenal aorta without any graft or device material extending superior to the origin of the renal arteries. Most infrarenal fixation devices require a proximal sealing zone of at least 15 mm in length, aortic neck diameter less than 32 mm, and a neck angulation of less than 60°.[25]

Suprarenal Fixation
The suprarenal fixation devices have metallic stents (but not graft material) extending superior to the origin of the renal arteries.[24] The superior stent extension may or may not have hooks/barbs for attachment to the suprarenal aortic wall. Although these devices are meant to be used in all routine cases, some operators prefer their use in patients with more unfavorable neck anatomy, such as a shorter neck or significant neck angulation.[25] Despite concerns for ischemia or infarction resulting from bare-metal struts crossing renal or visceral artery origins and associated embolization, several observational studies have demonstrated that these devices are safe relative to their infrarenal fixation counterparts.[26,27] A recent metaanalysis found no significant differences in renal complication rates with use of suprarenal devices versus infrarenal devices.[28]

Device Innovations
Although EVAR is performed in most patients requiring AAA repair, many do not meet the strict anatomic criteria for Food and Drug Administration (FDA)-approved EVAR devices. In fact, up to 66% of patients with infrarenal AAA may be anatomically ineligible for EVAR using these strict criteria.[24] With improving technology, it is likely that EVAR will become

available for an even greater percentage of patients. One such technology involves endovascular stapling of the graft material to the infrarenal aortic wall to prevent or seal leaks and to prevent graft slippage. The Heli-FX EndoAnchor system (Medtronic Vascular, Santa Clara, CA, USA) is FDA approved for use for this purpose. Real-world registry and retrospective data have confirmed their safety, and they appear effective in preventing and treating proximal type I endoleaks in patients with unfavorable neck anatomy (Fig. 2).[29–31] The Gore Excluder Conformable AAA Endoprosthesis, which would allow for endovascular repair with neck angulations up to 90°, is under investigation in an FDA-approved study (Fig. 3).

PATIENT SELECTION

Suitable aortic and access vessel anatomy are the key determinants of a successful endovascular repair.[32] An AAA is primarily defined by its location related to the renal arteries.[33] Suprarenal AAA involves the renal artery, extends superiorly, and may involve the origins of the superior mesenteric artery and celiac arteries.[33] A juxtarenal aneurysm extends to the renal arteries; however, it does not involve the suprarenal aorta. An infrarenal AAA arises at least 10 mm below the renal arteries.[33] Endovascular repair is best suited for infrarenal AAA whereby renal arteries are not involved. Technologic advances, such as the use of fenestrated grafts, and use of advanced techniques, such as snorkels and chimneys, can allow endovascular repairs of more complex anatomy. However, there is a high incidence of late endoleaks and/or visceral vessel compromise.[34–37] A detailed discussion of this topic is beyond the scope of this article, and the reader is directed to a recent review by Swerdlow and colleagues.[24]

Comorbid Factors

Evaluation of the medical comorbidities is an important component of preprocedure risk assessment and is a key determinant of the patient's eligibility for EVAR. Patients with chronic kidney disease are at increased risk of worsening kidney function from the iodinated contrast used during the procedure. Similar to the OSR, other medical comorbidities, such as coronary artery disease, congestive heart failure, cerebrovascular disease, peripheral vascular disease, uncontrolled diabetes, hypertension, poor baseline functional status, chronic obstructive pulmonary disease, and ongoing tobacco use, predispose the patient to increased periprocedural complications, and as such, might warrant a careful preoperative assessment and potential need for additional testing, such as noninvasive cardiac stress testing and pulmonary function testing before the aneurysm repair. Similarly, patients with low platelet counts ($<150,000/\mu L$) might warrant additional evaluation because of concerns of increased perioperative bleeding. The 2018 Society of Vascular Surgery practice guidelines have a good discussion of this topic.[25]

Anatomic Factors
Aortoiliac vessels

Common femoral and iliac artery anatomy has important implications for vascular access, device introduction, adequate fixation at the distal attachment site, and maintenance of limb patency. Adequate diameter and absence of tortuosity and calcification in the femoral and iliac vessels facilitate introduction of the stent graft. With current generation devices, sheath sizes have been reduced to 14 to 20F for most main bodies and to 12F for iliac limbs facilitating access and reducing the risk of femoral or iliac vessel injury. The diameter of the distal aorta should also be considered during pre-EVAR planning.[38] One recommendation is that the distal aortic diameter should be at least 20 mm for adequate placement of a bifurcated stent graft and allow for expansion of both limbs to prevent stent occlusion.[38] Although possible to

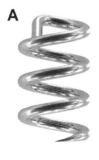
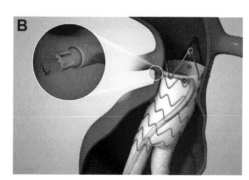

Fig. 2. Heli-FX Endoanchor endostapling system for proximal aortic neck type I endoleak treatment and prophylaxis. (A) Individual endostaple, (B) delivery sheath deploying an endostaple to staple the graft material and aortic wall together. (Reproduced with permission of Medtronic, Inc.)

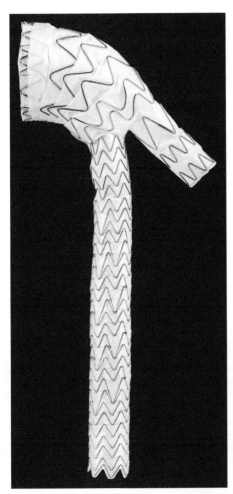

Fig. 3. Main body of the Gore Excluder Conformable bifurcated stent graft. The proximal body can be actively bent or curved during deployment to better conform to an angulated aortic neck. (*Courtesy of W.L. Gore and Associates, Inc., Newark, DE; with permission.*)

safely place stent grafts in smaller aortas, these may need more aggressive after dilatation.

Iliac artery diameter, calcification, tortuosity, iliac angle, and common iliac artery (CIA) length are important anatomic predictors for successful repair.[39] A minimum iliac diameter of 6 to 7 mm is usually needed for main body device delivery.[38] However, some lower-profile devices (14F sheath compatible) can be delivered through even smaller vessels. Stenotic arteries or occlusive iliac disease may necessitate angioplasty and/or stent placement intraprocedurally. A dilated or aneurysmal iliac artery affects the successful distal fixation of the graft limb and may necessitate an extension of the graft limb into the external iliac artery.

Severe tortuosity and iliac artery calcification may make device delivery challenging and predispose to iliac vessel dissection and perforation. A CIA length greater than 3 cm is considered ideal to ensure optimal graft limb positioning and seal. If the CIA is too short, an extension of the aortic stent graft into the external iliac artery may be needed to ensure successful distal fixation.[33]

Aneurysm neck

Suitable aortic neck anatomy is an important predictor for successful EVAR and related outcomes.[40,41] Key anatomic factors include neck length, diameter, angle, shape, and presence of calcification or thrombus.[38,40,41]

Longer infrarenal aortic neck (>1.5 cm), absence of significant calcification (especially protuberant calcific plaque), and thrombus are favorable factors.[33,38,40,41] Short neck length (<10 mm), neck angle greater than 60°, ≥50% circumferential proximal neck thrombus (≥2 mm thick), ≥50% calcified proximal neck, reverse taper neck, and a neck diameter greater than 31 mm are considered unfavorable or hostile neck features for endovascular repair.[40,41] Fig. 1 details examples of some of these neck anatomies.

The presence of a reverse tapered aortic neck is a strong predictor for early type I endoleak.[38] Long-term durability of EVAR depends on the successful seal between the proximal aortic neck and the stent graft. Patients with a larger-diameter aortic neck anatomy have a higher risk of type I endoleaks, higher rate of reinterventions, a higher incidence of aneurysmal sac expansion/rupture, and a lower overall survival compared with patients with a small-diameter aortic neck undergoing EVAR.[32,40–42]

Aneurysm morphology   Aneurysm sac morphology may also influence the success of endovascular repair.[38] The aneurysmal angle, presence of branching vessels, and the presence of intramural thrombus are important anatomic factors. *Aortic aneurysm angle* is defined as the most acute angle in the line to the central lumen between the lowest renal artery and the aortic bifurcation.[33]

Generally, as the aneurysmal tortuosity increases, the aneurysm angle is decreased. Consequently, a small aneurysm angle and increased tortuosity make stent-graft delivery and deployment difficult. The presence of an intraluminal mural thrombus can result in distal embolization during device delivery. Aortic branches arising from the AAA, mainly inferior mesenteric and lumbar arteries, are considered major collateral pathways and predispose to type II endoleak.[38] Furthermore, accessory renal arteries arising from the AAA may be occluded by the placement of the stent graft and may impair renal function. Equally important is evaluation of the superior mesenteric artery. Because the inferior mesenteric artery is routinely covered during EVAR, patients with superior mesenteric artery occlusion or severe stenosis are at risk of gut ischemia after EVAR.[33]

PREPROCEDURAL IMAGING

Computed tomographic angiography (CTA) is the most commonly used imaging modality for preprocedural anatomic assessment and planning of endovascular repair. Advanced software provides a centerline and 3-dimensional image processing, which is essential in patients with complex aortoiliac anatomy. The centerline method allows for very accurate measurements, critical to planning cases with challenging anatomy (Fig. 4). In addition to providing the anatomic extent of the aneurysm and aortoiliac vasculature, unenhanced CT

images are often used to evaluate arterial wall calcification and evaluate for a possible intramural hematoma in the acute setting.[33] MRI provides another option for patients who are unable to receive iodinated contrast.

PROCEDURE
Arterial Access

Historically, EVAR was performed under general anesthesia; however, it is now commonly performed under local anesthesia. Early on, common femoral arterial access was obtained by surgical exposure via "cutdown" skin incision. With the advent of smaller sheaths and suture-mediated arterial closure devices, bilateral percutaneous arterial access is the preferred mode of access. PEVAR was a randomized, multicenter study that compared percutaneous versus open femoral exposure for endovascular aortic aneurysm repair.[43] PEVAR found that percutaneous EVAR was noninferior to the

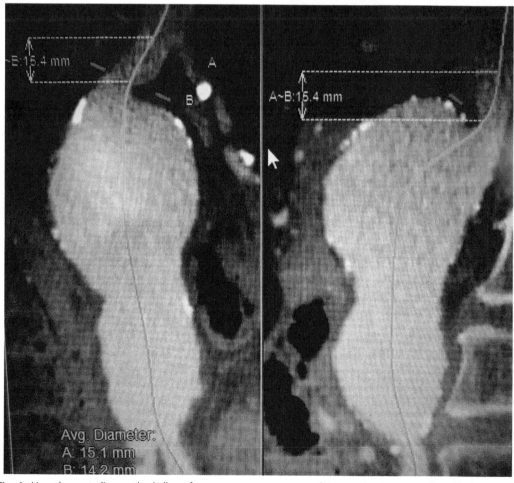

Fig. 4. How the centerline method allows for accurate measurement of the proximal aortic neck and helps in planning the case.

femoral cutdown and was associated with reduced operative time, fewer wound complications, and shorter hospital length of stay.[43]

Stent-Graft Delivery

The decision regarding which common femoral artery to access for main body insertion is influenced by multiple factors. Most often, the iliofemoral arteries of greatest diameter and with the least calcification are preferred for the main body. Other factors include the tortuosity and angulation of the aneurysm neck in relation to the aorta, to optimize the landing of the proximal stent-graft edge under the renal artery. Another consideration is the perceived ease of cannulating the "main body gate" (opening to the shorter limb) from the contralateral access site to facilitate the contralateral iliac limb insertion. Many times, the final decision is made after an aortoiliac arteriogram is obtained. Once bilateral access is obtained, a digital subtraction aortogram is performed to confirm craniocaudal distance and define aortic landmarks as well as aneurysmal sac extent using a calibrated multihole angiographic catheter (in the case of renal insufficiency, limited arteriograms are obtained, or intravascular ultrasound is used). Key measurements include distance from the lower edge of the lower renal artery to the ipsilateral hypogastric artery, distance from the lowest renal artery to the aortic bifurcation, diameter of the proximal aortic neck, and diameters of both CIA. The device is introduced over a stiff guidewire and positioned for either suprarenal or infrarenal fixation with the fabric-covered portion just distal to the lowest renal artery, and the device is carefully deployed to expose the contralateral gate.[24,33,38]

Thereafter, using the contralateral common femoral artery, a guidewire and catheter are advanced in a retrograde fashion and used to carefully cannulate the gate. Extreme care is taken to ensure that this contralateral access did indeed occur through the gate and not posterior to the gate. A curved catheter is advanced and rotated in the aorta once through the gate. Free rotation confirms intra-graft placement. At this stage, an angiogram may be obtained to determine the length of the contralateral limb from the gate to the distal attachment site (usually just proximal to the origin of the contralateral hypogastric artery). The contralateral iliac limb is then deployed over a stiff guidewire. Care is taken to ensure that there is adequate overlap between the main body at the gate and the contralateral limb (usually about 2–3 cm). An iliac extension limb can be used as needed for tall

patients, or an iliac bell-bottomed extension limb (**Fig. 5**) can be used if the CIA is ectatic. Using a compliant low-pressure balloon, the points of overlap and attachment sites are balloon dilated after stent-graft deployment. Occasionally, high-pressure inflation with noncompliant balloons is needed to adequately expand the endograft, especially in the iliac arteries, in the presence of iliac artery stenosis or calcification. A completion angiogram is performed at the end of the procedure to confirm patency of renal arteries, internal and external iliac arteries, to rule out any proximal aortic dissection and to detect endoleak.

STRATEGIES TO MANAGE COMMON ILIAC ARTERY ANEURYSM

EVAR devices are designed to seal distally in the CIA. However, dilatation and aneurysm of CIA pose a technical challenge by preventing adequate distal seal and fixation. Various endovascular techniques are used in the contemporary era to overcome this challenge.[44] Two commonly used methods are discussed here.

Internal Iliac Artery Embolization

If the common iliac is too large to seal with an iliac limb, extension into the external iliac with a limb extender can be performed (**Fig. 6**). However, this results in an endoleak from the retrograde flow from a patent internal iliac artery (IIA). In order to prevent this, the IIA can be occluded with either placement of coils or a vascular plug, and then the iliac limb extender is placed into the external iliac. IIA exclusion can result in buttock claudication, erectile

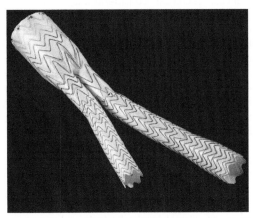

Fig. 5. Gore Excluder bifurcated stent graft with bell-bottomed iliac limb. (*Courtesy of* W.L. Gore and Associates, Inc., Newark, DE; with permission.)

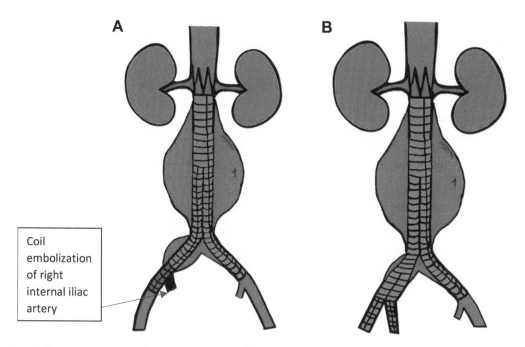

Fig. 6. Two common strategies to treat aneurysmal CIA during EVAR. (A) Occlusion of the IIA with coils (or plug) and extension of the iliac limb into the external iliac artery. (B) Preservation of the internal iliac flow and exclusion of the iliac aneurysm by use of a bifurcated iliac stent graft.

dysfunction, and rarely, symptoms of pelvic ischemia, such as pelvic or gluteal necrosis, colon ischemia, and spinal ischemia.[24,45,46] The complication rate is higher with bilateral than unilateral IIA occlusion.[24,45,47] Unilateral embolization of the IIA carries a reported 26% to 41% risk of buttock claudication; however, symptoms tend to improve with time.[25,48] Guidelines recommend preservation of at least one IIA if at all possible; however, certain situations demand bilateral IIA occlusion. In such circumstances, technical considerations, such as a staged approach, embolization of only the proximal main trunk of IIA, preservation of collateral branches from the femoral arteries, and use of dedicated iliac branched endoprostheses to maintain ipsilateral IIA perfusion, should be considered.[25] Hybrid approaches to preserve IIA circulation on 1 side, such as bypass of IIA to the ipsilateral external iliac artery, can also be considered in select cases.[49]

Iliac Branched Devices
Branch endoprostheses have demonstrated high rates of technical success and excellent early patency (see Fig. 6; Fig. 7).[24,50,51] Multiple versions of iliac branched devices have been developed, including straight-branch, helical-branch, and bifurcated-bifurcated.[52] The Gore Iliac Branch Endoprosthesis (Gore Medical,

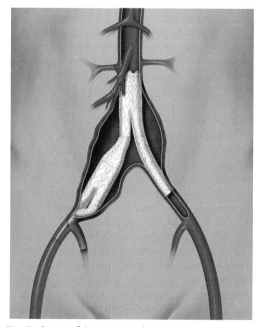

Fig. 7. Successful exclusion of an aortic and right common iliac aneurysm with a Gore Excluder Bifurcated stent graft with use of a Gore Excluder iliac branched endoprosthesis attached to a bell-bottomed right iliac limb of the aortic stent graft. (*Courtesy of* W.L. Gore and Associates, Inc., Newark, DE; with permission.)

Flagstaff, AZ, USA) is currently the only iliac branch device on the market and was approved for commercial use in 2016 (see Fig. 7).[24] Bell-bottomed (flared) iliac endograft limbs (see Fig. 5), parallel endografting, and proximal endograft have been used to preserve antegrade IIA perfusion.[48,53,54] The branched devices preserve the antegrade flow to the IIA; however, the addition of an iliac branch limb to standard EVAR results in longer procedure time and increases the complexity of the procedure.[48]

FOLLOW-UP

Long-term clinical and radiologic follow up is essential after EVAR to ensure continued successful exclusion of the AAA sac and to detect any problems, such as graft limb kinking and thrombosis. Contrast-enhanced computed tomographic (CT) imaging is currently the preferred initial follow-up modality. CT allows for adequate visualization of the device location, limb patency, and endoleaks. However, CT use is associated with contrast use and radiation. If no endoleak is detected, then subsequent follow-ups can be performed with noncontrast CT scan (to monitor sac size) or with duplex ultrasound. Ultrasonic contrast-enhanced ultrasound is also being used in some centers to detect endoleaks.[55,56]

Current recommendations on postprocedure follow-up include CTA imaging at 1 month.[25] If any concerning findings are present (such as type 1 endoleak), the same imaging modality should be repeated at 6 months. If 1-month imaging does not reveal endoleak (especially type I or III) or aneurysmal sac expansion, 6-month follow-up imaging can be omitted for a 1-year scan. If 1-year imaging confirms absence of endoleak and stable aneurysmal sac size, further imaging with duplex ultrasound can be considered to avoid contrast and radiation exposure.[25] If the patient had good anatomic features (Table 2) for EVAR, then it is reasonable to perform imaging every 5 years. However, if adverse features were present (such as shorter neck) or if any endoleak is present, then annual imaging should be considered. Prompt CT should be obtained for any new findings on surveillance duplex ultrasound.[25] The entire aorta should be imaged with CT every 5 years.

Patients should undergo complete lower-extremity pulse examination and ankle-brachial index (ABI) at their follow-up.[25] Patients with new-onset lower-extremity symptoms, such as claudication or resting pain, or reduction in

Table 2 Favorable anatomic features for endovascular aneurysm repair	
Location of Aneurysm	Infrarenal
Aortoiliac vessels	Distal aortic diameter >20 mm
	Iliac diameter >6 mm
	CIA length >3 cm
	Absence of significant tortuosity or calcification
Aneurysm morphology	Absence of branching vessels, tortuosity, intramural thrombus, or significant calcification
Aneurysm neck	Aortic neck diameter <32 mm
	Aneurysm neck angulation of <60°
	Proximal sealing zone of at least 15 mm in length
	Absence of reverse-tapered neck

ABIs should undergo a prompt evaluation to exclude graft limb occlusion.[25]

COMPLICATIONS

Detailed guidance on the management of various EVAR-related complications is beyond the scope of this review.[25] Early complications are most often related to contrast use or access site complications. Access site complications after surgical cutdown include arterial dissection, perforation, arterial thrombosis, hematoma, lymphocele, embolization, infection, and pseudoaneurysm formation. The incidence has ranged from 1% to 2% (with a higher rate in earlier experience).[43,57,58] Access site complications appear to be significantly lower with use of percutaneous access and closure.[58–60] Early graft limb thrombosis may occur infrequently and usually presents with critical or acute limb ischemia. It is more likely to occur in patients with smaller, tortuous iliac arteries or with external iliac stenosis that may result in limb kinking or poor outflow owing to distal arterial occlusive disease.[12,61] Inadequate, high-pressure balloon angioplasty of narrowed iliac limbs are also thought to be a factor. A self-limited inflammatory state commonly referred to as postimplantation syndrome may occur and manifests as fever, flulike symptoms, and leukocytosis. This presentation must be differentiated from graft infection, which is a serious condition.[62,63] Endovascular graft infection is, fortunately, less common and occurs in only 1% of patients in most studies.[64,65] Ischemic colitis owing to occlusion of the inferior mesenteric artery or hypogastric artery is a rare event with an incidence of less than 1% and usually occurs in the presence of preexisting visceral occlusive disease.[66–69]

ENDOLEAKS

Endoleak refers to the persistence of blood flow in the aneurysmal sac after EVAR (Fig. 8).[24,25] Endoleaks are categorized based on the source of the blood flow into the sac. Four types of endoleaks have been identified, and there are few instances where the cause of aneurysmal

sac expansion is indeterminate, sometimes referred to as type V[2,25,70,71]:

a. Type I: Occurs at endovascular graft attachment site because of loss of seal with the aortic wall.
   i. Type IA: proximal end
   ii. Type IB: distal end
b. Type II: Results from retrograde flow from the branch vessels arising from the AAA sac behind the stent graft (inferior mesenteric artery, lumbar arteries, median sacral artery). It is further subclassified into IIA (if from a single vessel) and IIB (if from multiple vessels).
c. Type III: Results from lack of seal between stent-graft components (IIIA) or because of a defect/tear in the graft (IIIB).

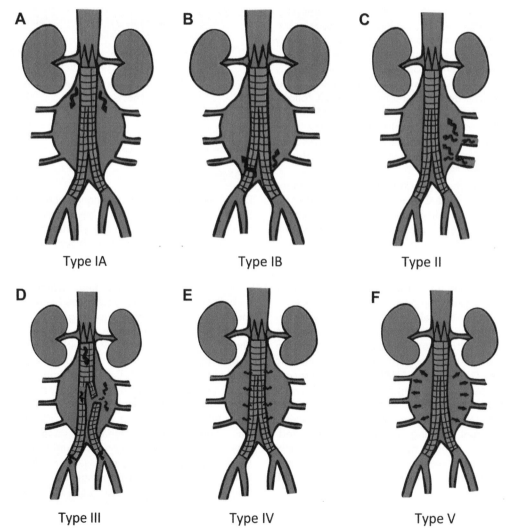

Fig. 8. Different subtypes of endoleaks. (A) Type IA endoleak, (B) type IB endoleak, (C) type II endoleak, (D) type III endoleak, (E) type IV endoleak, (F) type V endoleaks. Direction of blood flow (*curved arrow*). Direction of pressure transmission (*straight arrows*).

d. Type IV: Results from porosity of graft material (uncommon with most current generation devices).
e. Type V: AAA sac growth without contrast material seen in the sac on imaging.

Endoleak is the most common complication following EVAR. Overall, the combined incidence of endoleaks has been variably reported in the literature. Endoleaks can occur in up to 25% of the patients at the time of the repair.[25,72] The OVER trial reported the combined incidence of endoleaks at 30.5% (type I 12.3%, type II: 75.9%, type III: 3.2%, type IV: 2.7%, and type V: 5.9%).[73]

Buth and colleagues[74] evaluated the significance of type I and type III endoleaks from the EUROSTAR project, which included the data from 110 European institutes. They showed that more aneurysmal expansion was noted in patients with either type I or type III endoleaks with an average increase of 8 mm in aneurysm diameter in patients with endoleak compared with patients without endoleak. However, patients with type II endoleaks were excluded. They also showed that significant infrarenal neck angulation, aneurysmal thrombus, and less center experience adversely affected the endoleak incidence.

Abularrage and colleagues[75] evaluated the incidence and predictors of persistent type II endoleaks. They identified the presence of a patent inferior mesenteric artery, multiple lumbar branches, and a larger AAA sac size to be the most significant predictors of persistent type II endoleak with sac growth. Increasing age and warfarin use were other additional risk factors.

Management of Endoleaks

Most endoleaks are asymptomatic and are diagnosed on routine follow-up imaging. Type I and III are considered the most dangerous because these are relatively high-pressure endoleaks and can lead to rapid expansion of the aneurysm and subsequent rupture.

Traditionally, type I endoleaks were treated immediately after detection, but recent evidence suggests that select early type IA endoleaks (detected on 1-month follow-up CTA) may resolve spontaneously on follow-up imaging.[76] Persistent type I endoleaks require treatment that results in adequate apposition of the graft material to the aortic wall. The initial approach is to perform reangioplasty of the proximal aortic graft at the aortic neck at higher pressures using an appropriately sized aortic balloon.[77] If this does not resolve the endoleak,

then other options include placement of an aortic extension cuff (carefully avoiding covering the renal arteries) or a Palmaz-type stent across the renal arteries.[78,79] More advanced techniques include use of endostaples (Heli-FX EndoAnchor system) (see **Fig. 2**), proximal extension with the use of chimney grafts, insertion of coils or glue (into the crevice between the graft material and aortic wall), and conversion to fenestrated grafts or to open repair.[29,80–85] A type IB endoleak (which commonly occurs because of lack of apposition at the CIA level) is managed most often with the use of iliac extension limbs if angioplasty fails. In case there is no "landing zone" in the CIA, the IIA may need to be coiled and the iliac limb extended or a bifurcated iliac endoprosthesis may be used (see Procedure section above).

Type II endoleaks are the most common of all endoleaks (seen in about 25% at the time of EVAR) but are usually benign with low risk of rupture. Most (at least 50%) of these spontaneously resolve with expectant management.[86,87] The intervention is considered if there is a persistent leak with evidence of aneurysm sac enlargement of ≥5 mm. The goal of type II endoleak treatment is the elimination of aneurysm perfusing branch vessels. Both open and laparoscopic techniques have been described to eliminate side branch perfusion; however, endovascular methods are generally preferred. Endovascular methods for side branch embolization include transarterial embolization, CT-guided translumbar embolization (TLE), and transcaval embolization (TCE). Each of these methods involves embolization of the feeding vessel (inferior mesenteric artery or lumbar arteries) using coils, thrombin, gel foam, or onyx glue.[75,88] In many cases in which the feeding vessel cannot be successfully accessed, the embolic material is placed in the sac at the origin of the feeding vessels. The transarterial approach is the most commonly used method whereby the involved vessel is reached via a transfemoral or transbrachial approach and subsequently embolized (**Fig. 9**). When this approach is not feasible (eg, inaccessible inferior mesenteric, IIA, or prior failed transarterial approach due to vessel tortuosity), the alternative endovascular techniques, such as TLE or TCE, have been used to achieve successful embolization of the feeding vessels (**Fig. 10**).[89,90] A more recently described technique is laser-assisted transgraft embolization.[91] Regardless of the technique used, the long-term recurrence rate is relatively high with need for reintervention.[92] In cases

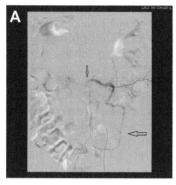
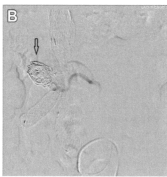

Fig. 9. Angiographic images of transarterial coil embolization of a type II endoleak from the left lumbar branch. (*A*) Microcatheter advanced via the iliolumbar artery into the lumbar branch (*horizontal arrow*). The region where the lumbar branch is emptying into the aneurysm sac (*vertical arrow*). The bifurcated stent graft can be seen in both images. (*B*) The microcatheter is now advanced all the way into the aneurysm sac. The coils that have been inserted into the aneurysm (*arrow*).

whereby none of the catheter-based techniques work, open surgical sac resection with oversewing of bleeding vessels and elimination of sac space generally work without the need for endograft explant.[93]

Type III endoleak is treated by closing the graft defect and is usually achieved by relining the disrupted zone with an extension limb. Type IV endoleaks occur because of the porosity

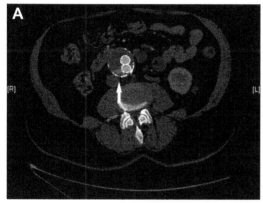
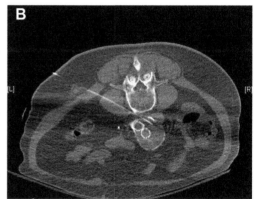
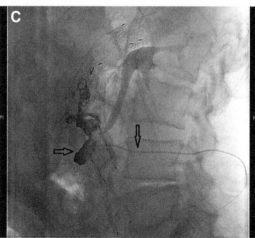

Fig. 10. Percutaneous translumbar embolization of a type II endoleak from lumbar branches. (*A*) Contrast-enhanced, delayed phase, axial CT image showing the aneurysm sac with bifurcated stent graft in place. The endoleak with contrast in the sac (*arrow*). (*B*) Intraprocedural image of a CT-guided placement of a needle into the aneurysm sac via the translumbar approach in the same patient. The patient is in the prone position. (*C*) Fluoroscopic image of the same patient during the embolization procedure. The microcatheter entering the aneurysm sac from the translumbar access position (*vertical arrow*). The embolic glue (*arrow*) that has been injected into the aneurysm sac. Superiorly some coils can also be seen.

in the graft material and are uncommonly seen with most current devices.

Type V endoleaks are thought to result from either transmission of pressure to the AAA sac through the graft material or from the persistent flow not visible by current imaging modalities. Although the natural history is less clear, most can be managed with observation (unless there is progressive sac growth). Some have reported success with relining the previous endograft with another graft or rarely with open repair.[94]

SUMMARY

EVAR is the preferred modality of AAA repair in current practice. It has a lower rate of perioperative mortality and morbidity compared with OSR. Endoleaks are a frequent cause of persistent flow into the excluded AAA sac. Type II endoleak is the most common, and most can be observed without intervention, unless the sac is growing. Most type I and III endoleaks require early treatment. Most endoleaks can be managed with transcatheter or endovascular means with only a minority requiring open repair. Anatomic factors, such as proximal aortic neck anatomy and iliac artery anatomy, are strong predictors of endoleaks and other complications. Technological improvements in endograft design and other ancillary devices are increasing the proportion of patients who may undergo successful EVAR. Regular, long-term follow-up with imaging is a requirement for anyone who has undergone EVAR, and inability to do so should be a strong contraindication for an EVAR procedure.

DISCLOSURE

The authors have no financial conflicts of interest to disclose.

REFERENCES

1. Eliason JL, Upchurch GR Jr. Endovascular abdominal aortic aneurysm repair. Circulation 2008; 117(13):1738–44.
2. Hirsch AT, Haskal ZJ, Hertzer NR, et al. ACC/AHA 2005 Practice Guidelines for the management of patients with peripheral arterial disease (lower extremity, renal, mesenteric, and abdominal aortic): a collaborative report from the American Association for Vascular Surgery/Society for Vascular Surgery, Society for Cardiovascular Angiography and Interventions, Society for Vascular Medicine and Biology, Society of Interventional Radiology, and the ACC/AHA Task Force on Practice Guidelines (Writing Committee to Develop Guidelines for the Management of Patients With Peripheral Arterial Disease): endorsed by the American Association of Cardiovascular and Pulmonary Rehabilitation; National Heart, Lung, and Blood Institute; Society for Vascular Nursing; TransAtlantic Inter-Society Consensus; and Vascular Disease Foundation. Circulation 2006;113(11):e463–654.
3. Volodos NL, Shekhanin VE, Karpovich IP, et al. A self-fixing synthetic blood vessel endoprosthesis. Vestn Khir Im I I Grek 1986;137(11):123–5 [in Russian].
4. Dua A, Kuy S, Lee CJ, et al. Epidemiology of aortic aneurysm repair in the United States from 2000 to 2010. J Vasc Surg 2014;59(6):1512–7.
5. Heikkinen M, Salenius JP, Auvinen O. Ruptured abdominal aortic aneurysm in a well-defined geographic area. J Vasc Surg 2002;36(2):291–6.
6. Naylor AR, Forbes TL. Trans-Atlantic debate: whether evidence supports reducing the threshold diameter to 5 cm for elective interventions in women with abdominal aortic aneurysms. Eur J Vasc Endovasc Surg 2014;48(6):611.
7. Medical Advisory Secretariat. Endovascular repair of abdominal aortic aneurysm: an evidence-based analysis. Ont Health Technol Assess Ser 2002;2(1):1–46.
8. von Segesser LK, Marty B, Ruchat P, et al. Routine use of intravascular ultrasound for endovascular aneurysm repair: angiography is not necessary. Eur J Vasc Endovasc Surg 2002;23(6):537–42.
9. Pecoraro F, Bracale UM, Farina A, et al. Single-center experience and preliminary results of intravascular ultrasound in endovascular aneurysm repair. Ann Vasc Surg 2019;56:209–15.
10. Wald R, Waikar SS, Liangos O, et al. Acute renal failure after endovascular vs open repair of abdominal aortic aneurysm. J Vasc Surg 2006;43(3):460–6 [discussion: 466].
11. Saratzis A, Sarafidis P, Melas N, et al. Comparison of the impact of open and endovascular abdominal aortic aneurysm repair on renal function. J Vasc Surg 2014;60(3):597–603.
12. De Bruin JL, Baas AF, Buth J, et al. Long-term outcome of open or endovascular repair of abdominal aortic aneurysm. N Engl J Med 2010;362(20):1881–9.
13. Prinssen M, Verhoeven EL, Buth J, et al. A randomized trial comparing conventional and endovascular repair of abdominal aortic aneurysms. N Engl J Med 2004;351(16):1607–18.
14. Greenhalgh RM, Brown LC, Powell JT, et al. Endovascular versus open repair of abdominal aortic aneurysm. N Engl J Med 2010;362(20):1863–71.
15. Lederle FA, Freischlag JA, Kyriakides TC, et al. Long-term comparison of endovascular and open repair of abdominal aortic aneurysm. N Engl J Med 2012;367(21):1988–97.

16. Becquemin JP, Pillet JC, Lescalie F, et al. A randomized controlled trial of endovascular aneurysm repair versus open surgery for abdominal aortic aneurysms in low- to moderate-risk patients. J Vasc Surg 2011;53(5):1167–73.e1.

17. Paravastu SC, Jayarajasingam R, Cottam R, et al. Endovascular repair of abdominal aortic aneurysm. Cochrane Database Syst Rev 2014;(1):CD004178.

18. Doonan RJ, Girsowicz E, Dubois L, et al. A systematic review and meta-analysis of endovascular juxtarenal aortic aneurysm repair demonstrates lower perioperative mortality compared with open repair. J Vasc Surg 2019;70(6):2054–64.e3.

19. Li B, Khan S, Salata K, et al. A systematic review and meta-analysis of the long-term outcomes of endovascular versus open repair of abdominal aortic aneurysm. J Vasc Surg 2019;70(3):954–69.e30.

20. Bulder RMA, Bastiaannet E, Hamming JF, et al. Meta-analysis of long-term survival after elective endovascular or open repair of abdominal aortic aneurysm. Br J Surg 2019;106(5):523–33.

21. Stather PW, Sidloff D, Dattani N, et al. Systematic review and meta-analysis of the early and late outcomes of open and endovascular repair of abdominal aortic aneurysm. Br J Surg 2013;100(7):863–72.

22. Kontopodis N, Antoniou SA, Georgakarakos E, et al. Endovascular vs open aneurysm repair in the young: systematic review and meta-analysis. J Endovasc Ther 2015;22(6):897–904.

23. de Vries JP. The proximal neck: the remaining barrier to a complete EVAR world. Semin Vasc Surg 2012;25(4):182–6.

24. Swerdlow NJ, Wu WW, Schermerhorn ML. Open and endovascular management of aortic aneurysms. Circ Res 2019;124(4):647–61.

25. Chaikof EL, Dalman RL, Eskandari MK, et al. The Society for Vascular Surgery practice guidelines on the care of patients with an abdominal aortic aneurysm. J Vasc Surg 2018;67(1):2–77.e2.

26. O'Donnell ME, Sun Z, Winder RJ, et al. Suprarenal fixation of endovascular aortic stent grafts: assessment of medium-term to long-term renal function by analysis of juxtarenal stent morphology. J Vasc Surg 2007;45(4):694–700.

27. Antonello M, Menegolo M, Piazza M, et al. Outcomes of endovascular aneurysm repair on renal function compared with open repair. J Vasc Surg 2013;58(4):886–93.

28. Miller LE, Razavi MK, Lal BK. Suprarenal versus infrarenal stent graft fixation on renal complications after endovascular aneurysm repair. J Vasc Surg 2015;61(5):1340–9.e1.

29. Jordan WD Jr, Mehta M, Varnagy D, et al. Results of the ANCHOR prospective, multicenter registry of EndoAnchors for type Ia endoleaks and endograft migration in patients with challenging anatomy. J Vasc Surg 2014;60(4):885–92.e2.

30. Muhs BE, Jordan W, Ouriel K, et al. Matched cohort comparison of endovascular abdominal aortic aneurysm repair with and without EndoAnchors. J Vasc Surg 2018;67(6):1699–707.

31. Masoomi R, Lancaster E, Robinson A, et al. Safety of EndoaNchors in real-world use: a report from the manufacturer and user facility device experience database. Vascular 2019;27(5):495–9.

32. Antoniou GA, Georgiadis GS, Antoniou SA, et al. A meta-analysis of outcomes of endovascular abdominal aortic aneurysm repair in patients with hostile and friendly neck anatomy. J Vasc Surg 2013;57(2):527–38.

33. Bryce Y, Rogoff P, Romanelli D, et al. Endovascular repair of abdominal aortic aneurysms: vascular anatomy, device selection, procedure, and procedure-specific complications. Radiographics 2015;35(2):593–615.

34. Ziegler P, Avgerinos ED, Umscheid T, et al. Fenestrated endografting for aortic aneurysm repair: a 7-year experience. J Endovasc Ther 2007;14(5):609–18.

35. Verhoeven EL, Katsargyris A, Oikonomou K, et al. Fenestrated endovascular aortic aneurysm repair as a first line treatment option to treat short necked, juxtarenal, and suprarenal aneurysms. Eur J Vasc Endovasc Surg 2016;51(6):775–81.

36. Roy IN, Millen AM, Jones SM, et al. Long-term follow-up of fenestrated endovascular repair for juxtarenal aortic aneurysm. Br J Surg 2017;104(8):1020–7.

37. Scali ST, Feezor RJ, Chang CK, et al. Critical analysis of results after chimney endovascular aortic aneurysm repair raises cause for concern. J Vasc Surg 2014;60(4):865–73 [discussion: 873–5].

38. Kim HO, Yim NY, Kim JK, et al. Endovascular aneurysm repair for abdominal aortic aneurysm: a comprehensive review. Korean J Radiol 2019;20(8):1247–65.

39. Wyss TR, Dick F, Brown LC, et al. The influence of thrombus, calcification, angulation, and tortuosity of attachment sites on the time to the first graft-related complication after endovascular aneurysm repair. J Vasc Surg 2011;54(4):965–71.

40. Aburahma AF, Campbell JE, Mousa AY, et al. Clinical outcomes for hostile versus favorable aortic neck anatomy in endovascular aortic aneurysm repair using modular devices. J Vasc Surg 2011;54(1):13–21.

41. AbuRahma AF, Yacoub M, Mousa AY, et al. Aortic neck anatomic features and predictors of outcomes in endovascular repair of abdominal aortic aneurysms following vs not following instructions for use. J Am Coll Surg 2016;222(4):579–89.

42. Kouvelos GN, Antoniou G, Spanos K, et al. Endovascular aneurysm repair in patients with a wide proximal aortic neck: a systematic review and meta-analysis of comparative studies. J Cardiovasc Surg (Torino) 2019;60(2):167–74.

43. Nelson PR, Kracjer Z, Kansal N, et al. A multicenter, randomized, controlled trial of totally percutaneous access versus open femoral exposure for endovascular aortic aneurysm repair (the PEVAR trial). J Vasc Surg 2014;59(5):1181–93.

44. Bekdache K, Dietzek AM, Cha A, et al. Endovascular hypogastric artery preservation during endovascular aneurysm repair: a review of current techniques and devices. Ann Vasc Surg 2015;29(2):367–76.

45. Bosanquet DC, Wilcox C, Whitehurst L, et al. Systematic review and meta-analysis of the effect of internal iliac artery exclusion for patients undergoing EVAR. Eur J Vasc Endovasc Surg 2017;53(4):534–48.

46. McGarry JG, Alenezi AO, McGrath FP, et al. How safe is internal iliac artery embolisation prior to EVAR? A 10-year retrospective review. Ir J Med Sci 2016;185(4):865–9.

47. Kouvelos GN, Katsargyris A, Antoniou GA, et al. Outcome after interruption or preservation of internal iliac artery flow during endovascular repair of abdominal aorto-iliac aneurysms. Eur J Vasc Endovasc Surg 2016;52(5):621–34.

48. Farivar BS, Abbasi MN, Dias AP, et al. Durability of iliac artery preservation associated with endovascular repair of infrarenal aortoiliac aneurysms. J Vasc Surg 2017;66(4):1028–36.e18.

49. Hosaka A, Kato M, Kato I, et al. Outcome after concomitant unilateral embolization of the internal iliac artery and contralateral external-to-internal iliac artery bypass grafting during endovascular aneurysm repair. J Vasc Surg 2011;54(4):960–4.

50. Karthikesalingam A, Hinchliffe RJ, Holt PJ, et al. Endovascular aneurysm repair with preservation of the internal iliac artery using the iliac branch graft device. Eur J Vasc Endovasc Surg 2010;39(3):285–94.

51. Serracino-Inglott F, Bray AE, Myers P. Endovascular abdominal aortic aneurysm repair in patients with common iliac artery aneurysms–initial experience with the Zenith bifurcated iliac side branch device. J Vasc Surg 2007;46(2):211–7.

52. Wong S, Greenberg RK, Brown CR, et al. Endovascular repair of aortoiliac aneurysmal disease with the helical iliac bifurcation device and the bifurcated-bifurcated iliac bifurcation device. J Vasc Surg 2013;58(4):861–9.

53. Malina M, Dirven M, Sonesson B, et al. Feasibility of a branched stent-graft in common iliac artery aneurysms. J Endovasc Ther 2006;13(4):496–500.

54. Ziegler P, Avgerinos ED, Umscheid T, et al. Branched iliac bifurcation: 6 years experience with endovascular preservation of internal iliac artery flow. J Vasc Surg 2007;46(2):204–10.

55. Kapetanios D, Kontopodis N, Mavridis D, et al. Meta-analysis of the accuracy of contrast-enhanced ultrasound for the detection of endoleak after endovascular aneurysm repair. J Vasc Surg 2019;69(1):280–94.e6.

56. Jawad N, Parker P, Lakshminarayan R. The role of contrast-enhanced ultrasound imaging in the follow-up of patients post-endovascular aneurysm repair. Ultrasound 2016;24(1):50–9.

57. Cuypers P, Buth J, Harris PL, et al. Realistic expectations for patients with stent-graft treatment of abdominal aortic aneurysms. Results of a European multicentre registry. Eur J Vasc Endovasc Surg 1999;17(6):507–16.

58. Buck DB, Karthaus EG, Soden PA, et al. Percutaneous versus femoral cutdown access for endovascular aneurysm repair. J Vasc Surg 2015;62(1):16–21.

59. Malkawi AH, Hinchliffe RJ, Holt PJ, et al. Percutaneous access for endovascular aneurysm repair: a systematic review. Eur J Vasc Endovasc Surg 2010;39(6):676–82.

60. Lee WA, Brown MP, Nelson PR, et al. Midterm outcomes of femoral arteries after percutaneous endovascular aortic repair using the Preclose technique. J Vasc Surg 2008;47(5):919–23.

61. Mehta M, Sternbach Y, Taggert JB, et al. Long-term outcomes of secondary procedures after endovascular aneurysm repair. J Vasc Surg 2010;52(6):1442–9.

62. Arnaoutoglou E, Kouvelos G, Papa N, et al. Prospective evaluation of post-implantation inflammatory response after EVAR for AAA: influence on patients' 30 day outcome. Eur J Vasc Endovasc Surg 2015;49(2):175–83.

63. Moulakakis KG, Alepaki M, Sfyroeras GS, et al. The impact of endograft type on inflammatory response after endovascular treatment of abdominal aortic aneurysm. J Vasc Surg 2013;57(3):668–77.

64. Schermerhorn ML, O'Malley AJ, Jhaveri A, et al. Endovascular vs. open repair of abdominal aortic aneurysms in the Medicare population. N Engl J Med 2008;358(5):464–74.

65. Vogel TR, Symons R, Flum DR. The incidence and factors associated with graft infection after aortic aneurysm repair. J Vasc Surg 2008;47(2):264–9.

66. Dadian N, Ohki T, Veith FJ, et al. Overt colon ischemia after endovascular aneurysm repair: the importance of microembolization as an etiology. J Vasc Surg 2001;34(6):986–96.

67. Maldonado TS, Rockman CB, Riles E, et al. Ischemic complications after endovascular abdominal aortic aneurysm repair. J Vasc Surg 2004;40(4):703–9 [discussion: 709–10].

68. Miller A, Marotta M, Scordi-Bello I, et al. Ischemic colitis after endovascular aortoiliac aneurysm repair: a 10-year retrospective study. Arch Surg 2009;144(10):900–3.

69. Becquemin JP, Majewski M, Fermani N, et al. Colon ischemia following abdominal aortic aneurysm repair in the era of endovascular abdominal aortic repair. J Vasc Surg 2008;47(2):258–63 [discussion: 263].

70. Rooke TW, Hirsch AT, Misra S, et al. 2011 ACCF/AHA Focused Update of the Guideline for the Management of Patients With Peripheral Artery Disease (updating the 2005 guideline): a report of the American College of Cardiology Foundation/American Heart Association Task Force on Practice Guidelines. J Am Coll Cardiol 2011;58(19):2020–45.

71. Erbel R, Aboyans V, Boileau C, et al. 2014 ESC Guidelines on the diagnosis and treatment of aortic diseases: document covering acute and chronic aortic diseases of the thoracic and abdominal aorta of the adult. The Task Force for the Diagnosis and Treatment of Aortic Diseases of the European Society of Cardiology (ESC). Eur Heart J 2014;35(41): 2873–926.

72. Abularrage CJ, Patel VI, Conrad MF, et al. Improved results using Onyx glue for the treatment of persistent type 2 endoleak after endovascular aneurysm repair. J Vasc Surg 2012;56(3):630–6.

73. Lal BK, Zhou W, Li Z, et al. Predictors and outcomes of endoleaks in the Veterans Affairs Open Versus Endovascular Repair (OVER) trial of abdominal aortic aneurysms. J Vasc Surg 2015;62(6):1394–404.

74. Buth J, Harris PL, van Marrewijk C, et al. The significance and management of different types of endoleaks. Semin Vasc Surg 2003;16(2):95–102.

75. Abularrage CJ, Crawford RS, Conrad MF, et al. Preoperative variables predict persistent type 2 endoleak after endovascular aneurysm repair. J Vasc Surg 2010;52(1):19–24.

76. O'Donnell TFX, Corey MR, Deery SE, et al. Select early type IA endoleaks after endovascular aneurysm repair will resolve without secondary intervention. J Vasc Surg 2018;67(1):119–25.

77. Thomas BG, Sanchez LA, Geraghty PJ, et al. A comparative analysis of the outcomes of aortic cuffs and converters for endovascular graft migration. J Vasc Surg 2010;51(6):1373–80.

78. Arthurs ZM, Lyden SP, Rajani RR, et al. Long-term outcomes of Palmaz stent placement for intraoperative type Ia endoleak during endovascular aneurysm repair. Ann Vasc Surg 2011;25(1):120–6.

79. Rajani RR, Arthurs ZM, Srivastava SD, et al. Repairing immediate proximal endoleaks during abdominal aortic aneurysm repair. J Vasc Surg 2011;53(5): 1174–7.

80. de Vries JP, Ouriel K, Mehta M, et al. Analysis of EndoAnchors for endovascular aneurysm repair by indications for use. J Vasc Surg 2014;60(6):1460–7.e1.

81. Sheehan MK, Barbato J, Compton CN, et al. Effectiveness of coiling in the treatment of endoleaks after endovascular repair. J Vasc Surg 2004;40(3):430–4.

82. Maldonado TS, Rosen RJ, Rockman CB, et al. Initial successful management of type I endoleak after endovascular aortic aneurysm repair with n-butyl cyanoacrylate adhesive. J Vasc Surg 2003;38(4): 664–70.

83. Kelso RL, Lyden SP, Butler B, et al. Late conversion of aortic stent grafts. J Vasc Surg 2009;49(3):589–95.

84. Martin Z, Greenberg RK, Mastracci TM, et al. Late rescue of proximal endograft failure using fenestrated and branched devices. J Vasc Surg 2014; 59(6):1479–87.

85. Montelione N, Pecoraro F, Puippe G, et al. A 12-year experience with chimney and periscope grafts for treatment of type I endoleaks. J Endovasc Ther 2015;22(4):568–74.

86. Makaroun M, Zajko A, Sugimoto H, et al. Fate of endoleaks after endoluminal repair of abdominal aortic aneurysms with the EVT device. Eur J Vasc Endovasc Surg 1999;18(3):185–90.

87. Kray J, Kirk S, Franko J, et al. Role of type II endoleak in sac regression after endovascular repair of infrarenal abdominal aortic aneurysms. J Vasc Surg 2015;61(4):869–74.

88. Chen J, Stavropoulos SW. Management of endoleaks. Semin Intervent Radiol 2015;32(3):259–64.

89. Uthoff H, Katzen BT, Gandhi R, et al. Direct percutaneous sac injection for postoperative endoleak treatment after endovascular aortic aneurysm repair. J Vasc Surg 2012;56(4):965–72.

90. Giles KA, Fillinger MF, De Martino RR, et al. Results of transcaval embolization for sac expansion from type II endoleaks after endovascular aneurysm repair. J Vasc Surg 2015;61(5):1129–36.

91. Mewissen MW, Jan MF, Kuten D, et al. Laser-assisted transgraft embolization: a technique for the treatment of type II endoleaks. J Vasc Interv Radiol 2017;28(11):1600–3.

92. Ultee KHJ, Buttner S, Huurman R, et al. Editor's choice–systematic review and meta-analysis of the outcome of treatment for type II endoleak following endovascular aneurysm repair. Eur J Vasc Endovasc Surg 2018;56(6):794–807.

93. Maitrias P, Belhomme D, Molin V, et al. Obliterative endoaneurysmorrhaphy with stent graft preservation for treatment of type II progressive endoleak. Eur J Vasc Endovasc Surg 2016;51(1):38–42.

94. Kougias P, Lin PH, Dardik A, et al. Successful treatment of endotension and aneurysm sac enlargement with endovascular stent graft reinforcement. J Vasc Surg 2007;46(1):124–7.

Renal and Mesenteric Artery Intervention

Tamunoinemi Bob-Manuel, MD[a], Christopher J. White, MD, MACC, MSCAI, FESC[a,b],*

KEYWORDS

- Renal artery stent • Mesenteric artery stent • Renal artery stenosis • Chronic mesenteric ischemia
- Renovascular hypertension

KEY POINTS

- Uncontrolled hypertension on 3 maximally tolerated antihypertensive medications (including a diuretic), ischemic nephropathy, and cardiac destabilization syndromes (flash pulmonary edema and acute coronary syndromes) with hemodynamically significant renal artery stenosis are likely to benefit from renal artery stenting.
- Use of radial access, embolic protection devices, special catheter techniques, and intravascular ultrasound–guided stenting may increase the safety and success rate of renal and mesenteric artery interventions.
- Symptomatic chronic mesenteric ischemia (CMI) usually results from significant stenosis affecting 2 or more vessels. Endovascular revascularization has largely replaced open surgery as the initial treatment.
- Endovascular therapy of CMI has greater than 90% success rate but a 12-month angiographic restenosis rate of 30% to 40%, so careful clinical and noninvasive follow-up is warranted.

INTRODUCTION

Percutaneous renal artery stenting is safe and effective for atherosclerotic renal artery stenosis (ARAS); however, randomized controlled trials (RCTs) have not shown superior outcomes compared with guideline-directed medical therapy (GDMT) alone.[1–3] Additionally, meta-analyses demonstrate that a high technical success rate (>95%) for renal stenting is accompanied by a surprisingly modest clinical improvement (approximately 70%). This discrepancy in procedural success and clinical effectiveness likely exists due to suboptimal patient selection by stenting nonhemodynamically significant lesions or patients with essential hypertension (HTN).

For chronic mesenteric ischemia (CMI), open surgical repair (OSR) historically was the standard of treatment. OSR has been largely supplanted by endovascular therapy (EVT), due to the significant morbidity and mortality associated with OSR in these frail undernourished patients. EVT is associated with a high technical success rate, with a low rate of complications in properly selected patients. Mesenteric artery stenting is associated, however, with 1-year restenosis rates of 30% to 40%.[4]

This article reviews the current literature and supporting evidence base, indications, contraindications, procedural technique, complications, and follow-up for renal and mesenteric artery interventions.

RENAL ARTERY INTERVENTIONS
Supporting Evidence Base
Renovascular hypertension
The safety and efficacy of renal stenting have been demonstrated in clinical trials, which have

[a] Department of Cardiovascular Diseases, John Ochsner Heart and Vascular Center, Ochsner Medical Center, The Ochsner Clinical School, University of Queensland, 1514 Jefferson Highway, New Orleans, LA 70121, USA;
[b] Department of Cardiology, Ochsner Medical Center, 3rd Floor, 1514 Jefferson Highway, New Orleans, LA 70121, USA
* Corresponding author. Department of Cardiology, Ochsner Medical Center, 1514 Jefferson Highway, New Orleans, LA 70121.
E-mail address: cwhite@ochsner.org

Intervent Cardiol Clin 9 (2020) 169–185
https://doi.org/10.1016/j.iccl.2019.11.002

shown significant decrease in systolic and diastolic blood pressure (BP). Renal stents have excellent long-term patency rates, with cumulative primary patency of 79% to 85% and a secondary patency of 92% to 98% at 5 years.[5,6] Secondary interventions for renal in-stent restenosis (ISR) have higher target lesion revascularization rates versus de novo renal stents (21% vs 11%; $P = .003$).[7]

Several RCTs over the past decade have failed to demonstrate a superiority of endovascular revascularization over GDMT in patients with mild to moderate ARAS. Three recent RCTs have failed to demonstrate superiority of renal stents with GDMT over GDMT alone in patients with mild to moderate ARAS (Table 1).[1–3] The Stent Placement in Patients with Atherosclerotic Renal Artery Stenosis and Impaired Renal Function: A Randomized Trial (STAR) enrolled patients with ARAS stenoses greater than 50% and a creatinine clearance less than 80 mL/min per 1.73 m[2].[2] GDMT alone compared with GDMT with renal artery stenting had no effect on progression of chronic kidney disease (CKD). A major limitation of this study was that 30% of the patients randomized to the renal stenting arm had ARAS less than 50% and as such would not be candidates for revascularization.

The Angioplasty and Stenting for Renal Artery Lesions (ASTRAL) trial reported no benefit of revascularization over medical therapy in regard to BP, renal function, cardiovascular events, or mortality.[1] The revascularization group were on fewer antihypertensive medications than the medical group (2.77 vs 2.97; $P = .03$). The major criticisms include that only 60% of the patients had a greater than 70% ARAS (by ultrasound, not angiographic measurement), so that many of the patients in the trial may not have been candidates for revascularization, and the complication rate by these operators was very high (9%).

The Cardiovascular Outcomes in Renal Atherosclerotic Lesions (CORAL) trial enrolled patients with HTN, defined as a systolic BP of greater than or equal to 155 mm Hg despite taking greater than or equal to 2 antihypertensive medications, which, by definition, included patients without refractory HTN.[3] Because the hemodynamic severity of moderate (50%–70% diameter stenosis) lesions was not hemodynamically confirmed, it is likely that patients with nonobstructive ARAS were enrolled in the trial and would be unlikely to benefit from revascularization.

Because a requirement for randomization was clinical equipoise for GDMT, patients with severe ARAS and severe clinical symptoms were not well represented in these trials. This paradox is best illustrated by the parachute RCT, which proved that parachutes, compared with empty backpacks, were not more effective in preventing death and/or major trauma when jumping from aircraft.[8] The article humorously illustrates the limitations of RCTs. The investigators were able to ethically randomize 2 treatments, parachutes versus empty backpacks, when jumping from aircraft, because the study cohort only jumped from the wing of a parked aircraft, approximately 2 m above the ground. Because of little risk of harm from a fall at this height, the investigators believed there was equipoise for the 2 treatments (parachutes vs empty backpacks).

Had the trial been conducted from an aircraft flying at 10,000 m above the ground, there clearly would have been no equipoise, and the authors' bias would have prevented enrollment into the empty backpack cohort. The conclusion, "that there was no difference in outcomes between parachutes and empty backpacks," only applied to the conditions tested, that is, a very small distance to fall. The investigators did not test the hypothesis that parachutes were superior to empty backpacks from 10,000 m above the ground, and therefore there is no "evidence" that parachutes are superior to empty backpacks from 10,000 ft above ground, other than compelling observational data.

The 3 RCTs, discussed previously, all enrolled patients with mild to moderate ARAS, in whom the benefit of renal stents was uncertain, and with equipoise, allowing the investigators to enroll low-risk patients to justify the option of GDMT alone. These trials failed to document the hemodynamic significance of the mild to moderate ARAS (ie, translesional gradient). They did not include patients with the most severe ARAS, in whom observational data would justify renal stenting and in whom investigators would be unwilling to randomize to GDMT alone. The population tested in the 3 RCTs, similar to the parachute trial, were at low risk for adverse events with mild to moderate ARAS, and therefore it was safe to withhold renal stenting.

Unfortunately, the conclusion of the 3 trials, that renal stenting with GDMT was not more effective than GDMT alone, has been generalized to all ARAS patients and not limited to the mild to moderate ARAS patients studied. The implication that there is little, if any, role for renal stenting in severe ARAS patients has not been proved.

Table 1
Summary of recent renal stent trials

Trial	STAR[2]	ASTRAL[1]	CORAL[3]
Year	2009	2009	2014
Number of patients	140	806	947
Inclusion criteria	• Impaired renal function (CrCl <80 mL/min) • Ostial ARAS of 50% or more (CTA, MRA, DSA) • Controlled BP <140/90 mm Hg	• Renal artery atherosclerotic disease in ≥1 renal artery amenable to revascularization • Clinician unsure if revascularization would provide clear benefit	• Severe RAS (angiographically defined as >60% but <100% AND • HTN with systolic BP ≥155 mm Hg on 2 or more agents OR • CKD defined as GFR <60
Exclusion criteria	• Renal size <8 cm • Renal artery <4 mm • CrCl <15 mL/min • Diabetes with proteinuria >3 g/d • Malignant HTN	• Disease needing surgical revascularization • High likelihood of needing revascularization in 6 mo • Nonatheromatous disease • Prior ARAS revascularization • Lack of informed consent	• FMD • CKD from causes other than ischemic nephropathy • Cr >4 mg/dL • Kidney size <7 cm • Lesions that could not be treated with 1 stent
Primary end point	• Worsening renal function >20% decrease of CrCl	• Slope of the reciprocal of Cr over 5 y	• Time to major renal or cardiovascular event (stroke, heart attack, CHF hospitalization, progressive renal insufficiency, need for dialysis)
Limitations	• Patients had controlled BP • Considerable number of patients had <50% stenoses	• Rate of complications much higher than reported • Lower number of antihypertensives used in intervention group • Diagnosis of ARAS made with noninvasive imaging without functional studies • Patients with kidney size <6 cm included in study • Patients with nonsignificant lesions included	• Patients were not optimized on antihypertensive therapy • Inclusion of patients with mild stenosis • Only moderate correlation between angiography and hemodynamically significant stenoses

Abbreviations: Cr, creatinine; CrCl, creatinine clearance.

In 2016, the Agency for Healthcare Research and Quality published a comparative effectiveness analysis that concluded that there was low strength of evidence for the relative benefits and harms of percutaneous transluminal renal artery balloon angioplasty and renal artery stenting versus GDMT alone in patients with ARAS.[9] Selection bias may have prevented enrollment of patients who would likely benefit from revascularization, that is, those with very severe stenoses and uncontrolled BP; recurrent sudden-onset, flash pulmonary edema; or refractory HTN. There may well have been equipoise for patients with borderline, uncertain ARAS permitting their randomization, but there may not have been equipoise for patients with the most severe ARAS. This is a common problem for many RCTs, which could have been addressed with a parallel registry but unfortunately was not.

In a meta-analysis of 678 patients, the renal artery stenting procedure success rate was 98%; however, clinical improvement in HTN was only approximately 70% and improvement in renal function occurred in 30% of patients, with stabilization in 38%.[10] These discrepant data suggest that either patients with non–flow-limiting ARAS lesions were treated or that their symptom of HTN or CKD was unrelated to their ARAS.

Ischemic nephropathy

Multiple observational studies have demonstrated that renal artery stent placement is associated with improvement or stabilization of renal function in patients with atherosclerotic renovascular renal insufficiency. Harden and coworkers[11] reported on a series of 32 patients (33 kidneys) with unexplained renal insufficiency and hemodynamically significant renal artery stenosis (RAS) treated with renal artery stent placement. The majority of patients had bilateral or solitary RASs, although unilateral disease was present in 7 patients. The investigators concluded that stent placement slows the progression of RAS.

A second study examined 33 patients undergoing successful renal artery stent placement for bilateral or solitary RAS ($\geq$70%) with a baseline serum creatinine between 1.5 mg/dL and

4.0 mg/dL.[12] Follow-up ($\geq$8 months) data were available in 25 patients, all of whom had either improvement or stabilization of renal function. One of the strongest predictors of improvement in renal function after intervention for RAS is rapidly progressing renal failure.[13] The slope of the reciprocal serum creatinine plot before renal intervention was associated with a favorable change in renal function. Three prospective trials have established renal function benefit after successful stent treatment of unilateral RAS.[14–16] They all consistently demonstrate that hyperfiltration of the normal kidney returns toward normal, and glomerular filtration rate (GFR) of the treated kidney increases with net stabilization of total GFR after successful revascularization.

Cardiac destabilization syndromes

Patients with ARAS can suffer acutely decompensated heart failure (ie, flash pulmonary edema), refractory heart failure, or exacerbations of acute coronary syndrome (ACS), the so-called cardiac destabilization syndromes. Often, patients with a solitary functioning kidney or bilateral RAS manifest volume overload as decompensated heart failure. This can result in increased myocardial oxygen consumption leading to unstable angina.

The importance of renal artery stent placement in the treatment of cardiac disturbance has been described in a series of patients with presenting with either congestive heart failure (CHF) or an ACS.[17] Successful renal stent placement was associated with a significant decrease in BP and control of symptoms in 88% (42 of 48) of the patients (Fig. 1). Some patients underwent both coronary and renal intervention, whereas others had only renal artery stent placement due to no coronary lesions suitable for

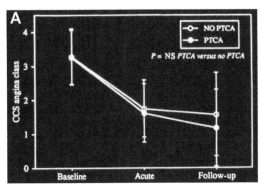
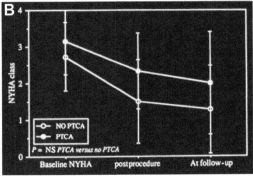

Fig. 1. (A) Graph demonstrating improvement in Canadian Cardiovascular Society (CCS) angina classification in patients with renal stenting showing no difference for those with and without coronary interventions. (B) Graph demonstrating improvement in New York Heart Association (NYHA) classification of heart failure in patients with renal stenting showing no difference for those with and without coronary interventions. NS, non-significant; PTCA, percutaneous transluminal coronary angioplasty.

revascularization. Assessment of the treatment effects acutely and at 8 months using the Canadian Cardiovascular Society angina classification and the New York Heart Association functional classification were not different between the combined coronary and renal revascularization group compared with those who had only renal stent placement, suggesting that renal revascularization was the most significant intervention.

In another study, 39 patients underwent renal artery stent implantation for control of heart failure, which represented 19% of the renal artery stent population.[18] Eighteen (46%) patients had bilateral RAS and 21 (54%) patients had stenosis of a solitary functioning kidney. Renal artery stent implantation was successful in all patients. HTN responded to the successful renal stent placement in 72% of the patients. Renal function improved in 51% and remained stable in an additional 26% of patients. The mean number of hospitalizations for heart failure prior to stenting was 2.37 ± 1.42 (range 1–6) and after renal stenting was $0.30 \pm .065$ (range 0–3) ($P<.001$). Three-quarters of their patients had no further hospitalizations after renal artery stenting over a 2-year follow-up.

In a literature review of 87 reported cases of bilateral RAS and flash pulmonary edema (ie, Pickering syndrome), 35% were treated with unilateral angioplasty and 22% with bilateral angioplasty.[19] In 43% of patients, in earlier reports, surgical revascularization was performed. Renal function improved in 81% of patients and the mean creatinine on follow-up was 1.6 mg/dL (141 mol/L) after the procedure. Importantly, in 92% of all patients there were no further episodes of flash pulmonary edema after revascularization. The American College of Cardiology (ACC)/American Heart Association (AHA) guidelines make renal stenting for hemodynamically significant RAS and recurrent, unexplained CHF or sudden unexplained pulmonary edema a class I, level of evidence (LOE) B indication. Renal stenting for unstable angina earned a class IIa, LOE B indication.[20]

Diagnostic Methods
Noninvasive
Renal Doppler ultrasound (DUS) imaging is an excellent tool for the diagnosis of ARAS. A peak systolic velocity (PSV) of greater than 200 cm/s is very sensitive and specific for greater than 50% stenosis. A ratio of renal artery PSV to the PSV of the aorta of greater than 3.5 has 92% sensitivity for greater than 60% diameter stenosis.[21] If DUS is unable to confirm the hemodynamic severity of ARAS,

then cross-sectional imaging with computed tomographic angiography (CTA) or magnetic resonance angiography (MRA) is the next option (Fig. 2). The sensitivity and specificity of CTA have been shown to be 90% to 100% and 97% for stenosis greater than 50%. The sensitivity of MRA is 92% to 97%, with a specificity of 73% to 93%; however, patients with acute or chronic renal dysfunction may not be candidates for these modalities.[22]

Split renal function (SRF) is a nuclear imaging technique to assess the impact of hemodynamically significant unilateral ARAS on overall renal function. SRF using [99m]technetium Tc-diethylene-triamine-pentaacetate (DTPA) renal scintigraphy was performed before and after renal stenting for unilateral ARAS. After successful stenting, ambulatory systolic BP and diastolic BP significantly decreased from 145 mm Hg to 138 mm Hg, diastolic BP decreased from 80 mm Hg to 77 mm Hg ($P = .005$), and estimated GFR increased in the stented kidney from 22 to 26 and normalized in the hyperfiltering, nonstenotic kidney from 37 to 34 ($P<.026$).[23] This technique may be helpful in determining who may benefit from revascularization when a significant unilateral stenosis is detected but GFR is normal.

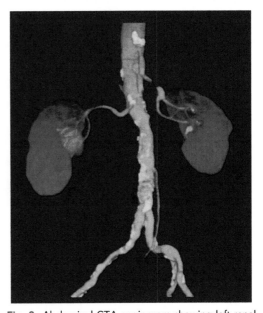

Fig. 2. Abdominal CTA angiogram showing left renal artery stenosis. (*From* Khosla S, White C, Collins T, Jenkins J, Shaw D, Ramee S. Effects of renal artery stent implantation in patients with renovascular HTN presenting with unstable angina or congestive heart failure. *American Journal of Cardiology*. 1997;80(3):363-366; with permission.)

Invasive

Digital subtraction angiography (DSA) is a 2-dimensional imaging modality that suffers from relatively poor discrimination of renal artery lesion severity because these stenoses are often located in tortuous, overlapping arteries. By consensus of experts, an angiographic ARAS greater than 70% diameter stenosis is severe/significant, and diameter stenoses of 50% to 69% are considered moderately severe, of uncertain hemodynamic significance.[20] For moderately severe stenoses (50% to 69%), confirmation of the hemodynamic severity of the RAS is recommended prior to stenting.[24,25]

A resting or hyperemic translesional systolic gradient of greater than or equal to 20 mm Hg, a resting or hyperemic mean translesional gradient of greater than or equal to 10 mm Hg, or a renal fractional flow reserve (RFFR) less than or equal to 0.8 confirms hemodynamically severe ARAS (Fig. 3).[24,25] The authors compared conventional angiography to RFFR and to translesional pressure gradients to determine ARAS stenosis severity. There was a poor correlation between the angiographic stenosis, and RFFR ($r = -0.18$; $P = .54$) as well as to the translesional pressure gradient ($r = 0.22$; $P = .44$). The correlation between RFFR and the translesional pressure gradient, however, was excellent ($r = 0.76$; $P = .0016$) (Fig. 4).[26]

The translesional pressure gradient should be measured with a nonobstructive catheter or with a 0.014-in pressure wire. Hyperemia may be induced with an intrarenal bolus of papaverine at a dose of 40 mg or an intrarenal bolus of 50 μg/kg dopamine.[26,27] Papaverine precipitates in heparinized saline solutions commonly used for catheterization laboratory flush solutions.

Indications and Contraindications

The ACC/AHA guidelines[20] and appropriate use criteria (AUC)[24,25] recommend that patients most likely to benefit from renal artery stenting have hemodynamically significant ARAS (moderate [50%−70%] ARAS with a resting/hyperemic translesional mean gradient of ≥10 mm Hg, systolic gradient ≥20 mm Hg, or angiographically severe [>70%] ARAS) and (1) recurrent CHF, or sudden-onset, flash, pulmonary edema; patients with hemodynamically significant ARAS with refractory ACS, (2) those with refractory HTN who fail or are intolerant of GDMT, and (3) patients with progressive CKD, due to bilateral/solitary ARAS, or with unilateral ARAS (Table 2).

There is no indication for the treatment of ARAS in asymptomatic patients.[24,25] The initial treatment of symptomatic ARAS, as demonstrated in the CORAL trial, is GDMT.[3] When evaluating patients with ARAS, it is important to determine whether their symptoms are caused by renal hypoperfusion or if ARAS is an innocent bystander. ARAS may be found on routine abdominal imaging when evaluating a patient for other problems. If ARAS is not causing a clinical problem, however, there is no role for revascularization. Also, not likely to benefit from renal artery stenting are patients who have uncontrolled BP but are not on maximally tolerated GDMT, including a total of 3 antihypertensives with

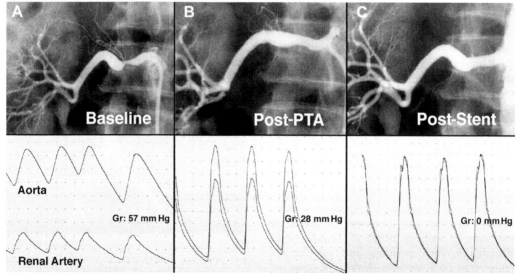

Fig. 3. Angiogram and proximal and distal pressure tracing. (*A*) Baseline angiogram with 57 mm Hg translesional gradient. (*B*) After balloon angioplasty with improvement in stenosis but residual 28 mm Hg gradient. (*C*) After renal stent with slight angiographic improvement but no residual translesional gradient. Gr, gradient; PTA, percutaneous transluminal angioplasty.

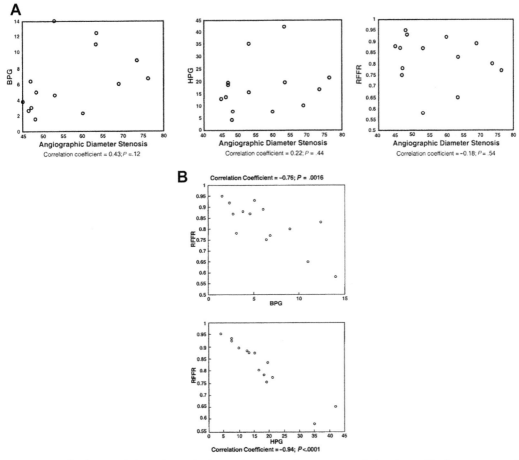

Fig. 4. (A) (Left) The correlation of quantitative angiographic diameter stenosis (angiographic diameter stenosis) with baseline mean translesional pressure gradient (BPG); (center) hyperemic mean translesional pressure gradient (HPG); and (right) RFFR. (B) The correlation of RFFR with the (top) baseline mean translesional pressure gradient (BPG) and (bottom) hyperemic mean translesional pressure gradient (HPG). (From Subramanian R, White C, Rosenfield K, et al. Renal fractional flow reserve: A hemodynamic evaluation of moderate renal artery stenoses. Catheterization and Cardiovascular Interventions. 2005;64(4):480-486; with permission.)

a diuretic. Lastly, ischemic nephropathy patients unlikely to benefit from revascularization include those with chronic CKD stage III to stage IV and a pole-to-pole kidney size of less than or equal to 7 cm or patients on hemodialysis greater than or equal to 3 months.[20,24,25]

Procedural Technique
Preprocedural imaging
A nonselective renal angiogram should be performed prior to renal intervention unless prior noninvasive imaging is available (CTA or MRA) to delineate the curvature of the aorta and renal arteries (Fig. 5).

The catheter-in-catheter or no-touch techniques
The catheter-in-catheter or no-touch techniques should be used to minimize contact with the aortic wall and prevent injury to the renal ostium during guiding catheter manipulation (Fig. 6). The no-touch technique requires a 0.035-in J-wire resting on the suprarenal wall of the aorta during engagement of the renal artery. This 0.035-in J-wire prevents the tip of the guide catheter from scraping the wall of the aorta during maneuvering. Once the artery is engaged, a 0.014-in guide wire is advanced into the renal artery.[28]

Radial access
Radial artery access with a 6F sheath or sheathless with a 6F guiding catheter is the preferred route for percutaneous diagnostic and interventional renal artery procedures to reduce access site bleeding complications, improve postprocedural patient comfort, and facilitate renal artery ostial engagement.

Table 2
Renal artery stenting and appropriate use criteria and guidelines

Scenario	Appropriate Use Criteria[24,25]	American Heart Association/ American College of Cardiology Guideline[20]
Cardiac disturbance syndromes (flash pulmonary edema, unstable angina, or ACS) with HTN and significant ARAS[a]	Appropriate	Class I, LOE B (CHF) Class IIa, LOE B (unstable angina)
CKD stage IV with bilateral significant ARAS with a with a kidney size >7 cm in pole-to-pole length	Appropriate	Class IIa, LOE B
CKD stage IV and global renal ischemia (unilateral significant ARAS with a solitary kidney or bilateral significant ARAS) without another explanation	Appropriate	Class IIb, LOE B
Resistant HTN (uncontrolled HTN having failed maximally tolerated doses of at least 3 antihypertensive agents, 1 of which a diuretic) and bilateral or solitary significant ARAS	Appropriate	Class IIa, LOE B
Recurrent CHF with unilateral significant ARAS	May be appropriate	Class IIa, LOE B
Resistant HTN (uncontrolled HTN having failed maximally tolerated doses of at least 3 antihypertensive agents, one of which a diuretic) and unilateral significant ARAS	May be appropriate	Class IIa, LOE B
Asymptomatic, unilateral, bilateral, or solitary kidney with hemodynamically significant ARAS	Rarely appropriate	Class III, LOE C

[a] Significant ARAS = moderate (50%–70%) ARAS with a resting/hyperemic translesional mean gradient of greater than or equal to 10 mm Hg, systolic gradient greater than or equal to 20 mm Hg, or severe (>70%) ARAS.

For renal interventions, there is an operator learning curve for catheter manipulation, catheter guide selection, and stent placement. The left radial artery may provide a shorter route to the renal arteries. The use of longer guiding catheters (125 cm to 135 cm) and balloon shafts (150 cm) in taller patients often is necessary with the radial technique.

Embolic protection devices
Atheroembolism likely plays a role in postprocedural deterioration of renal function, after successful stent placement seen in approximately one-quarter of renal artery stent patients. Embolic protection devices (EPDs) may prevent embolic injury during renal stenting and have been shown to be safe.[29,30] A small randomized study (100 patients) looking at patients with CKD undergoing renal artery stenting suggested there was preservation of renal function with embolic protection when combined with antiplatelet therapy.[31]

More data are needed to evaluate the impact of EPDs in patients with normal and abnormal renal function undergoing renal stenting. EPDs may be considered in high-risk patients with baseline renal insufficiency as a strategy to prevent worsening renal function related to atheroembolism resulting from stent placement.

Stent sizing with intravascular ultrasound
In renal interventions, it is harder to visually estimate vessel diameter in these larger arteries (5 mm to 8 mm). Intravascular ultrasound (IVUS) can help operators with better lesion measurement, appropriate stent sizing, appropriate stent expansion, and achieving better outcomes measured by decrease in BP and a lower incidence of angiographic restenosis. Restenosis in renal artery stenting with bare metal stents (BMSs) is largely driven by the acute gain in lumen area, placing a premium on delivery the largest stent that is safely possible. Although

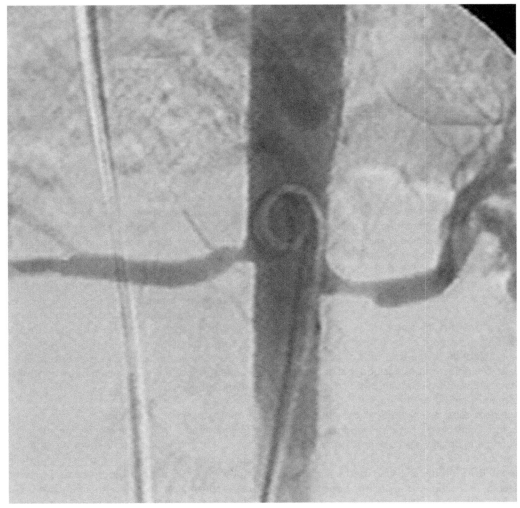

Fig. 5. Abdominal aortogram showing mild to moderate RAS of uncertain hemodynamic significance.

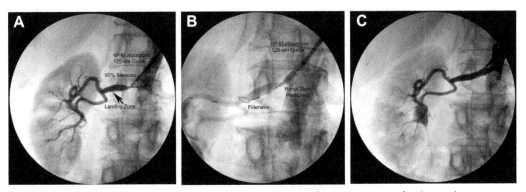

Fig. 6. (A) Baseline angiography using right radial artery access of a 90% stenosis of right renal artery using a 6F multipurpose (125-cm) guide catheter. Note the landing zone prior to the bifurcation, suitable for a filter device (off-label use). (B) The filter device has been deployed and the undeployed stent is being positioned across the lesion. (C) Final angiography after stent deployment and filter retrieval. (From White CJ. Optimizing outcomes for renal artery intervention. Circulation Cardiovascular interventions. 2010;3(2):184-192; with permission.)

undersizing renal stents is safe, it is associated with significantly higher restenosis rates.[32] The judicious use of IVUS can assist the operator to safely place optimally sized stents.

Drug-eluting stents versus bare metal stents

A prospective trial that compared BMSs to drug-eluting stents (DESs) in ARAS found no difference in the restenosis rate for sirolimus-eluting stents compared with the BMSs.[33] At 6 months and 1 year, the target lesion revascularization rate was not different between the 2 types of stents. There are data favoring the DESs in renal stenting in the setting of a hybrid technique of placing a BMS within a DES.[34] These results are hypothesis generating and need to be more rigorously studied. A major problem with coronary DESs in the renal arteries is their lack of radial strength due to their thin struts, resulting in stent recoil due to the bulky renal plaque exerting external compression.

In-stent restenosis lesions

The best treatment of renal artery ISR has not been established due to a lack of comparative trials. Multiple options include balloon angioplasty, DES-in-BMS, BMS-in-BMS, covered stent placement, and brachytherapy.

Repeat renal artery BMS placement demonstrated improved patency compared with balloon angioplasty alone, with a 58% reduction in recurrent ISR (29.4% vs 71.4%; $P = .02$).[35] The repeat BMS group also had better secondary patency ($P = .05$) and a greater freedom from repeat ISR ($P = .01$) when compared with balloon angioplasty alone. There was a trend favoring repeat BMS placement for cumulative freedom from target vessel revascularization ($P = .08$). In a small series of patients having at least their second ISR after BMS, covered stents had 17% (1/6) ISR at a mean follow-up of 36 months whereas coronary DESs were free of ISR (0/10).[36] There is no evidence supporting a role for the use of debulking devices or cutting balloons in the management of renal artery ISR.

Complications and Their Management

Vascular access

The most common complications in renal artery interventions are related to femoral access (hematoma, pseudoaneurysm, arteriovenous fistula, and retroperitoneal bleed).[37,38] All are minimized or eliminated if radial artery access is utilized. Management of femoral access complications include use of covered stent placement, thrombin injection for pseudoaneurysms, and vascular surgical repair when necessary.

Vessel rupture and dissections

Fortunately, catastrophic complications during renal artery stenting are uncommon. The overall incidence of major complications with renal artery stenting is near 2%.[38] The cause for significant dissection of the renal artery is typically the subintimal passage of the guide wire, excess catheter manipulations, overdilation prior to stent deployment, oversizing the stent, or aggressive balloon dilatation of the stent. The use of coated glide wires is discouraged because of the higher risk of vessel perforation.

It is critical to maintain guide wire access across the lesion. With a guide wire in place, the dissection flap may be sealed with prolonged balloon inflation or the placement of an additional stent. If complete arterial thrombosis occurs, this can be managed with a local infusion of a thrombolytic agent, but reestablishing a patent lumen is essential for lytics to be successful.

If vessel perforation occurs, reversal of anticoagulation and prolonged balloon inflation are the first steps to control the hemorrhage. Covered stents have been used for intraprocedural complications, such as perforation or vessel rupture. If bleeding cannot be controlled, nephrectomy may be required.

Follow-up and Surveillance

The current AUC recommendations for DUS follow-up after renal intervention are that it is appropriate to perform a post-stent baseline study within 30 days of the procedure.[39] It may be appropriate to perform additional DUS studies at 6 months and/or 9 months. It is appropriate to perform a follow-up DUS at 12 months and annually thereafter.

When duplex imaging is performed after renal stent placement, it is important to make adjustments to the velocity parameters post-stenting compared with a native vessel, because decreased compliance due to the stent results in higher velocities.[21] Therefore, obtaining a post-procedure DUS is reasonable to establish a new baseline PSV. If anatomic renal ISR is detected with surveillance, the patient still must meet the clinical requirements for reintervention, that is, refractory HTN despite GDMT, progressive CKD, or developing a cardiac destabilization syndrome. Many patients can be followed with serial DUS and GDMT with stable ISR for years.

MESENTERIC ARTERY INTERVENTIONS

Supporting Evidence Base

There are no large randomized clinical trials comparing EVT to OSR for CMI. There are multiple retrospective studies,[40–49] however, supporting EVT for CMI, especially in older, higher-risk OSR patients.

Using the National Inpatient Sample data from 1998 to 2006, there were 6,342 cases of EVT compared to 16,071 of OSR for patients with CMI. In 2002, EVT cases surpassed OSR for annual volume.[50] The mortality rate was lower after EVT than after OSR for CMI (3.7% vs 13%; *P*<.01) and AMI (16% vs 28%; *P*<.01) (Fig. 7). Bowel resection was more common after OSR than EVT for CMI (7% vs 3%; *P*<.01).

A more modern sample of the National Inpatient Sample was used to retrospectively examine 4150 patients treated for CMI between 2007 and 2014 comparing OSR to EVT.[51] In this propensity-matched cohort, major adverse cardiovascular and cerebrovascular events and composite in-hospital complications occurred significantly less often after EVT than after OSR (8.6% vs 15.9%, respectively; *P*<.001 and 15.3% vs 20.3%, respectively; *P*<.006). EVT also was associated with lower median hospital costs ($20,807.00 vs $31,137.00, than was OSR respectively; *P*<.001) and a shorter length of stay (5 days vs 10 days, respectively; *P*<.001) compared with OSR.

A 2015 meta-analysis of 8 CMI studies compared EVT to OSR and found no difference in 30-day mortality or 3-year cumulative survival rate. Compared with OSR, EVT resulted in a significantly lower rate of in-hospital complications (*P* = .002), whereas the recurrence rate within 3 years after revascularization was significantly greater for EVT (*P*<.00001).[47] A listing of studies reporting outcomes for CME treatment by EVT and/or OSR is available in Table 3.[4,45,52–55] A comparative effectiveness and cost-effectiveness comparison of EVT versus OSR demonstrated that EVT was the preferred treatment of CMI patients despite more reinterventions.[56]

Diagnosis of Chronic Mesenteric Ischemia

CMI is defined as insufficient blood supply to the gastrointestinal tract resulting in ischemic symptoms with a duration of at least 3 months. The diagnosis of CMI is a clinical one, based on symptoms and consistent anatomic findings.[57] The clinical presentation often is vague and nonspecific: chronic abdominal pain (often postprandial and described as crampy), diarrhea, fear of eating, and significant weight loss/malnutrition (Fig. 8). A majority of the patients are female, have a history of cardiovascular disease, and have had prior revascularization. A broad differential diagnosis is necessary for nonatherosclerotic etiologies, such as fibromuscular dysplasia (FMD), median arcuate ligament syndrome, vasculitis, malignancy and postradiation stenoses.[58]

Once clinical suspicion for CMI is high, imaging with DUS is the first choice, followed by cross-sectional noninvasive imaging with CTA or MRA.[59] The reported accuracy for DUS in identifying significant stenoses of the celiac and superior mesenteric artery approaches 90% with the caveat that ultrasound velocities are higher for stented arteries than native arteries, making a diagnosis of ISR more difficult. DUS success is heavily influenced by technician expertise, patient body habitus, and presence of bowel gas.

CTA is the favored cross-sectional noninvasive angiographic imaging modality of choice due to its higher resolution compared with MRA.[60] MRA has the advantage of better imaging in heavily calcified vessels without exposure to radiation or iodinated contrast.[61]

Selective mesenteric DSA remains the gold standard for diagnosing CMI, especially for

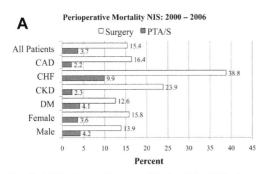
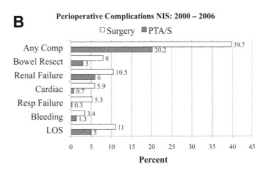

Fig. 7. (*A*) Perioperative mortality for CMI. (*B*) Perioperative complications for CMI. CAD, coronary artery disease; Comp, complications; DM, diabetes mellitus; LOS, length of stay; NIS, national inpatient sample; PTA/S, percutaneous transluminal angioplasty/stent; Resect, resection; Resp, respiratory. (*Data from* Schermerhorn ML, Giles KA, Hamdan AD et al. Mesenteric revascularization: management and outcomes in the United States, 1988-2006. Journal of Vascular Surgery 2009;50:341-348.)

Table 3
Results of revascularization for chronic mesenteric ischemia

Study	N	Study Details	Technical Success	Outcomes	Primary Patency
Matsumoto et al,[52] 2002	33 EVT	Retrospective	81.3	Complications = 13.8%	89% at 2 y
Sharafuddin et al,[53] 2003	25 EVT	Retrospective	96%	Major complication = 12%	85% at 11 mo
Landis et al,[45] 2005	29 EVT	Retrospective	97%	Major complication = 3.4%	70% 1 y
Silva et al,[4] 2006	59 EVT	Retrospective	96%	81% 3-y survival	71% at 14
Oderich et al,[54] 2009	229 (OSR = 146 vs EVT = 83)	Retrospective	95%	OSR patients had more complications (36% vs 18%; P<.001)	3 y: OSR 93% vs EVT 52% (P<.05).
Oderich et al,[55] 2013	225 EVT (164 BMSs 61 CS)	Retrospective	CS = 95% BMS = 98%	Complications: BMS = 21% vs CS = 12%	3 y: CS = 92% vs BMT = 52% (P = .003)

Abbreviation: CS, covered stent.

detection of distal vessel disease, or when a concurrent intervention is planned. It is important to perform both anteroposterior and lateral views to delineate the visceral vessels that arise anteriorly from the aorta (**Fig. 9**).

Indications and Contraindications for Revascularization

Percutaneous EVT of intestinal arterial stenosis is indicated in patients with symptomatic CMI not amenable to conservative therapy (class I, LOE B).[20] The reported recurrence rates mandate careful follow-up of patients treated with EVT.

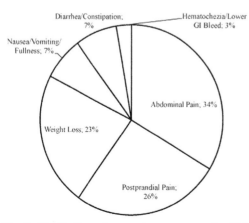

Fig. 8. Distribution of presenting symptoms for CMI. GI, gastrointestinal.

Revascularization of intestinal arterial stenosis that is discovered incidentally in an asymptomatic patient is rarely appropriate (class III harm).[20]

Procedural Technique

Stenting atherosclerotic aorto-ostial obstructions of the visceral vessels is similar to that of the renal arteries, and the technical skills necessary for EVT are similar to those for renal stenting (**Fig. 10**). Some considerations before EVT include adequate operator experience and surgical backup to rescue acute treatment failure. Meticulous case selection and procedure planning are necessary because some lesion(s) may not be amenable to an endovascular approach and may be better surgical candidates due to calcification, angulation of vessel or lesion, and number or recurrence of stenoses. The patient and physician must make a joint and informed decision to proceed with EVT, knowing that despite high initial success rates (88%–100%), patency rates at 1 year may decrease to 60% to 70%.[62]

Technical Aspects of Endovascular Intervention

Vascular access

In the past, EVT for CMI patients were performed using a femoral approach but the current preferred access for these cases should

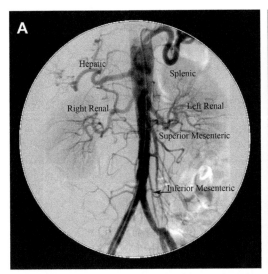 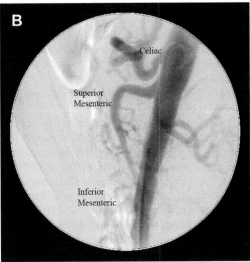

Fig. 9. (*A*) Anteroposterior abdominal angiogram. (*B*) Lateral abdominal angiogram.

be radial artery access, when possible. Radial access reduces the difficulty of coaxial alignment of the guiding catheter for stent delivery because these vessels typically arise in a caudal direction, making delivery of stents from the femoral access more difficult. The delivery of covered stents may require larger equipment (7F–8F) and thus necessitate femoral access.

Recommended equipment for endovascular therapy
Equipment choices for CMI EVT parallels renal stent placement. From the radial artery, a multipurpose shaped guide is ideal. From the femoral artery, a shepherd's crook shape (ie, Simmons) often is helpful. The use of 6F guides requires a 0.014-in platform, whereas larger catheters from the femoral access may

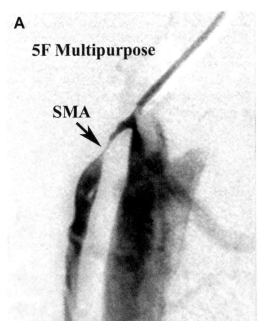 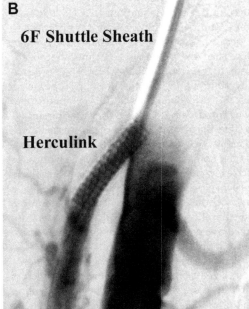

Fig. 10. (*A*) Baseline selective angiogram of the superior mesenteric artery (SMA) with a 5F multipurpose catheter from right radial access. (*B*) Stent delivery to the SMA using a 6F shuttle sheath over a 0.014-in guide wire (Herculink, Abbott, Santa Clara, CA).

accommodate 0.018-in or 0.035-in systems. As in the case for renal stenting, the authors strongly discourage the use of coated glide wires, because the risk of vessel perforation is increased.

Periprocedural Issues, Complications, and Their Management

In a series of 156 patients reported from the Mayo Clinic, serious complications occurred in 7% of cases, including branch perforation, distal embolization, vessel dissection, and stent embolization.[46] The use of antiplatelet therapy reduced the risk of embolization, and smaller platform equipment (0.014-in vs 0.035-in) reduced the risk of vessel complications.[46]

The Achilles heel of mesenteric EVT has been restenosis. Recently, a nonrandomized 225-patient CMI case series suggested a possible advantage for balloon-expandable covered stents compared with BMSs.[55] Significant reduction in restenosis was seen in both de novo lesions and restenosis lesions. No increased risk of stent thrombosis was observed. The disadvantage of the balloon-expandable covered stents is the requirement for a larger, 0.035-in platform, rather than the smaller 0.014-in stent platform. These encouraging data need confirmation in controlled trials as well as exploration of the benefits of drug-coated balloons, which have improved patency in other vascular beds.

Follow-up

The current recommendations for DUS follow-up after CMI intervention are that it is appropriate to perform a post-stent baseline study within 30 days of the procedure.[39] It may be appropriate to perform additional DUS surveillance at 6 months or 9 months. It is appropriate to perform a follow-up DUS at 12 months and annually thereafter. When DUS is performed after stent placement, it is important to make adjustments to the velocity parameters post-stenting compared with a native vessel, because decreased compliance due to the stent results in higher velocities.[63,64] Therefore, obtaining a postprocedure DUS is reasonable to establish a new baseline PSV. Clinical symptoms are required even in the setting of ISR before repeat intervention.

ISR can be seen in 30% to 40% of EVT patients within 2 years after EVT. Independent predictors of restenosis after mesenteric revascularization are prior mesenteric intervention, female gender, and small (<6 mm) diameter.[65] Severe mesenteric calcification, occlusions, longer lesions, and small vessel diameter are associated with an increased risk of distal embolization, restenosis and reinterventions after endovascular revascularization.

SUMMARY
Renal Stenting

Significant ARAS is caused by the narrowing of arteries transporting blood to the kidney(s) most often caused by atherosclerosis and increases the risk of developing resistant HTN or ischemic nephropathy as well as cardiac destabilization syndromes (acute decompensated heart failure, specifically flash pulmonary edema, and ACS).

Patients with refractory, uncontrolled renovascular HTN despite maximally tolerated GDMT, progressive ischemic nephropathy, and cardiac destabilization syndromes who have hemodynamically severe ARAS are likely to benefit from renal stenting. Radial access is preferred to avoid access-related complications and to facilitate stent delivery. Use of IVUS, EPDs, and hydration may reduce the risk of complications. Surveillance post-stenting can be done with periodic clinic visits, laboratory testing, and DUS.

Mesenteric Artery Stenting

CMI is an unusual but serious condition. A high index of clinical suspicion is necessary for the diagnosis. In most cases, the cause is atherosclerotic stenosis or occlusion involving the mesenteric arteries. Because there is significant mesenteric collateral circulation, multivessel visceral stenosis usually is present in symptomatic patients. The limited comparative evidence available suggests that EVT is the preferred cost-effective choice in selected patients over OSR. The current treatment recommendation is that patients who are candidates for either OSR or EVT should receive percutaneous therapy with stent placement.

DISCLOSURE

The authors have no financial disclosures.

REFERENCES

1. Investigators A, Wheatley K, Ives N, et al. Revascularization versus medical therapy for renal-artery stenosis. N Engl J Med 2009;361:1953–62.
2. Bax L, Woittiez AJ, Kouwenberg HJ, et al. Stent placement in patients with atherosclerotic renal artery stenosis and impaired renal function: a randomized trial. Ann Intern Med 2009;150:840–8. W150–1.
3. Cooper CJ, Murphy TP, Cutlip DE, et al. Stenting and medical therapy for atherosclerotic renal-artery stenosis. N Engl J Med 2014;370:13–22.

4. Silva JA, White CJ, Collins TJ, et al. Endovascular therapy for chronic mesenteric ischemia. J Am Coll Cardiol 2006;47:944–50.

5. Blum U, Krumme B, Flugel P, et al. Treatment of ostial renal-artery stenoses with vascular endoprostheses after unsuccessful balloon angioplasty. N Engl J Med 1997;336:459–65.

6. Henry M, Amor M, Henry I, et al. Stents in the treatment of renal artery stenosis: long-term follow-up. J Endovasc Surg 1999;6:42–51.

7. Stone PA, Campbell JE, Aburahma AF, et al. Ten-year experience with renal artery in-stent stenosis. J Vasc Surg 2011;53:1026–31.

8. Yeh RW, Valsdottir LR, Yeh MW, et al. Parachute use to prevent death and major trauma when jumping from aircraft: randomized controlled trial. BMJ 2018;363:k5094.

9. Raman G, Adam GP, Halladay CW, et al. Comparative effectiveness of management strategies for renal artery stenosis: an updated systematic review. Ann Intern Med 2016;165:635–49.

10. Leertouwer TC, Gussenhoven EJ, Bosch JL, et al. Stent placement for renal arterial stenosis: where do we stand? A meta-analysis. Radiology 2000; 216:78–85.

11. Harden PN, MacLeod MJ, Rodger RS, et al. Effect of renal-artery stenting on progression of renovascular renal failure. Lancet 1997;349:1133–6.

12. Watson P, Hadjipetrou P, Cox S, et al. Effect of renal artery stenting on renal function and size in patients with atherosclerotic renovascular disease. Circulation 2000;102:1671–7.

13. Muray S, Martin M, Amoedo ML, et al. Rapid decline in renal function reflects reversibility and predicts the outcome after angioplasty in renal artery stenosis. Am J Kidney Dis 2002;39:60–6.

14. La Batide-Alanore A, Azizi M, Froissart M, et al. Split renal function outcome after renal angioplasty in patients with unilateral renal artery stenosis. J Am Soc Nephrol 2001;12:1235–41.

15. Leertouwer TC, Derkx FH, Pattynama PM, et al. Functional effects of renal artery stent placement on treated and contralateral kidneys. Kidney Int 2002;62:574–9.

16. Coen G, Moscaritolo E, Catalano C, et al. Atherosclerotic renal artery stenosis: one year outcome of total and separate kidney function following stenting. BMC Nephrol 2004;5:15.

17. Khosla S, White CJ, Collins TJ, et al. Effects of renal artery stent implantation in patients with renovascular hypertension presenting with unstable angina or congestive heart failure. Am J Cardiol 1997;80: 363–6.

18. Gray BH, Olin JW, Childs MB, et al. Clinical benefit of renal artery angioplasty with stenting for the control of recurrent and refractory congestive heart failure. Vasc Med 2002;7:275–9.

19. Messerli FH, Bangalore S. The Pickering Syndrome—a pebble in the mosaic of the cardiorenal syndrome. Blood Press 2011;20:1–2.

20. Hirsch AT, Haskal ZJ, Hertzer NR, et al. ACC/AHA 2005 guidelines for the management of patients with peripheral arterial disease (lower extremity, renal, mesenteric, and abdominal aortic): executive summary a collaborative report from the American Association for Vascular Surgery/Society for Vascular Surgery, Society for Cardiovascular Angiography and Interventions, Society for Vascular Medicine and Biology, Society of Interventional Radiology, and the ACC/AHA Task Force on Practice Guidelines (Writing Committee to Develop Guidelines for the Management of Patients With Peripheral Arterial Disease) endorsed by the American Association of Cardiovascular and Pulmonary Rehabilitation; National Heart, Lung, and Blood Institute; Society for Vascular Nursing; TransAtlantic Inter-Society Consensus; and Vascular Disease Foundation. J Am Coll Cardiol 2006;47:1239–312.

21. Chi YW, White CJ, Thornton S, et al. Ultrasound velocity criteria for renal in-stent restenosis. J Vasc Surg 2009;50:119–23.

22. Tan KT, van Beek EJ, Brown PW, et al. Magnetic resonance angiography for the diagnosis of renal artery stenosis: a meta-analysis. Clin Radiol 2002; 57:617–24.

23. Saeed A, Fortuna EN, Jensen G. Split renal function in patients with unilateral atherosclerotic renal artery stenosis-effect of renal angioplasty. Clin Kidney J 2017;10:496–502.

24. Klein AJ, Jaff MR, Gray BH, et al. SCAI appropriate use criteria for peripheral arterial interventions: an update. Catheter Cardiovasc Interv 2017;90:E90–110.

25. Bailey SR, Beckman JA, Dao TD, et al. ACC/AHA/SCAI/SIR/SVM 2018 appropriate use criteria for peripheral artery intervention: a report of the American College of Cardiology appropriate use criteria task force, American Heart Association, Society for Cardiovascular Angiography and Interventions, Society of Interventional Radiology, and Society for Vascular Medicine. J Am Coll Cardiol 2019;73:214–37.

26. Subramanian R, White CJ, Rosenfield K, et al. Renal fractional flow reserve: a hemodynamic evaluation of moderate renal artery stenoses. Catheter Cardiovasc Interv 2005;64:480–6.

27. Mangiacapra F, Trana C, Sarno G, et al. Translesional pressure gradients to predict blood pressure response after renal artery stenting in patients with renovascular hypertension. Circ Cardiovasc Interv 2010;3:537–42.

28. Safian RD, Madder RD. Refining the approach to renal artery revascularization. JACC Cardiovasc Interv 2009;2:161–74.

29. Holden A, Hill A, Jaff MR, et al. Renal artery stent revascularization with embolic protection in patients with ischemic nephropathy. Kidney Int 2006; 70:948–55.

30. Laird JR, Tehrani F, Soukas P, et al. Feasibility of FiberNet(R) embolic protection system in patients undergoing angioplasty for atherosclerotic renal artery stenosis. Catheter Cardiovasc Interv 2012; 79:430–6.

31. Cooper CJ, Haller ST, Colyer W, et al. Embolic protection and platelet inhibition during renal artery stenting. Circulation 2008;117:2752–60.

32. Lederman RJ, Mendelsohn FO, Santos R, et al. Primary renal artery stenting: characteristics and outcomes after 363 procedures. Am Heart J 2001; 142:314–23.

33. Zahringer M, Sapoval M, Pattynama PM, et al. Sirolimus-eluting versus bare-metal low-profile stent for renal artery treatment (GREAT Trial): angiographic follow-up after 6 months and clinical outcome up to 2 years. J Endovasc Ther 2007;14:460–8.

34. Bradaric C, Eser K, Preuss S, et al. Drug-eluting stents versus bare metal stents for the prevention of restenosis in patients with renovascular disease. EuroIntervention 2017;13:e248–55.

35. N'Dandu ZM, Badawi RA, White CJ, et al. Optimal treatment of renal artery in-stent restenosis: repeat stent placement versus angioplasty alone. Catheter Cardiovasc Interv 2008;71:701–5.

36. Patel PM, Eisenberg J, Islam MA, et al. Percutaneous revascularization of persistent renal artery in-stent restenosis. Vasc Med 2009;14:259–64.

37. Ivanovic V, McKusick MA, Johnson CM 3rd, et al. Renal artery stent placement: complications at a single tertiary care center. J Vasc Interv Radiol 2003;14:217–25.

38. Rocha-Singh K, Jaff MR, Rosenfield K, et al. Evaluation of the safety and effectiveness of renal artery stenting after unsuccessful balloon angioplasty: the ASPIRE-2 study. J Am Coll Cardiol 2005;46: 776–83.

39. Mohler ER 3rd, Gornik HL, Gerhard-Herman M, et al. ACCF/ACR/AIUM/ASE/ASN/ICAVL/SCAI/ SCCT/SIR/SVM/SVS/SVU [corrected] 2012 appropriate use criteria for peripheral vascular ultrasound and physiological testing part I: arterial ultrasound and physiological testing: a report of the American College of Cardiology Foundation Appropriate Use Criteria Task Force, American College of Radiology, American Institute of Ultrasound in Medicine, American Society of Echocardiography, American Society of Nephrology, Intersocietal Commission for the Accreditation of Vascular Laboratories, Society for Cardiovascular Angiography and Interventions, Society of Cardiovascular Computed Tomography, Society for Interventional Radiology, Society for Vascular Medicine, Society

for Vascular Surgery, [corrected] and Society for Vascular Ultrasound. [corrected]. J Am Coll Cardiol 2012;60:242–76.

40. Kihara TK, Blebea J, Anderson KM, et al. Risk factors and outcomes following revascularization for chronic mesenteric ischemia. Ann Vasc Surg 1999; 13:37–44.

41. Cho JS, Carr JA, Jacobsen G, et al. Long-term outcome after mesenteric artery reconstruction: a 37-year experience. J Vasc Surg 2002;35: 453–60.

42. Park WM, Cherry KJ Jr, Chua HK, et al. Current results of open revascularization for chronic mesenteric ischemia: a standard for comparison. J Vasc Surg 2002;35:853–9.

43. Silva J, White C, Collins T, et al. Endovascular stenting for the treatment of chronic mesenteric ischaemia. Eur Heart J 2004;25:204–5.

44. Brown DJ, Schermerhorn ML, Powell RJ, et al. Mesenteric stenting for chronic mesenteric ischemia. J Vasc Surg 2005;42:268–74.

45. Landis MS, Rajan DK, Simons ME, et al. Percutaneous management of chronic mesenteric ischemia: outcomes after intervention. J Vasc Interv Radiol 2005;16:1319–25.

46. Oderich GS, Bower TC, Sullivan TM, et al. Open versus endovascular revascularization for chronic mesenteric ischemia: risk-stratified outcomes. J Vasc Surg 2009;49:1472–9.e3.

47. Cai W, Li X, Shu C, et al. Comparison of clinical outcomes of endovascular versus open revascularization for chronic mesenteric ischemia: a meta-analysis. Ann Vasc Surg 2015;29:934–40.

48. Erben Y, Jean RA, Protack CD, et al. Improved mortality in treatment of patients with endovascular interventions for chronic mesenteric ischemia. J Vasc Surg 2018;67:1805–12.

49. Erben Y, Protack CD, Jean RA, et al. Endovascular interventions decrease length of hospitalization and are cost-effective in acute mesenteric ischemia. J Vasc Surg 2018;68:459–69.

50. Schermerhorn ML, Giles KA, Hamdan AD, et al. Mesenteric revascularization: management and outcomes in the United States, 1988-2006. J Vasc Surg 2009;50:341–8.e1.

51. Lima FV, Kolte D, Kennedy KF, et al. Endovascular versus surgical revascularization for chronic mesenteric ischemia: insights from the national inpatient sample database. JACC Cardiovasc Interv 2017; 10:2440–7.

52. Matsumoto AH, Angle JF, Spinosa DJ, et al. Percutaneous transluminal angioplasty and stenting in the treatment of chronic mesenteric ischemia: results and longterm followup. J Am Coll Surg 2002;194:S22–31.

53. Sharafuddin MJ, Olson CH, Sun S, et al. Endovascular treatment of celiac and mesenteric arteries

stenoses: applications and results. J Vasc Surg 2003;38:692–8.

54. Oderich GS, Malgor RD, Ricotta JJ 2nd. Open and endovascular revascularization for chronic mesenteric ischemia: tabular review of the literature. Ann Vasc Surg 2009;23:700–12.

55. Oderich GS, Erdoes LS, Lesar C, et al. Comparison of covered stents versus bare metal stents for treatment of chronic atherosclerotic mesenteric arterial disease. J Vasc Surg 2013;58:1316–23.

56. Hogendoorn W, Hunink MG, Schlosser FJ, et al. A comparison of open and endovascular revascularization for chronic mesenteric ischemia in a clinical decision model. J Vasc Surg 2014;60:715–725 e2.

57. Clair DG, Beach JM. Mesenteric ischemia. N Engl J Med 2016;374:959–68.

58. Escarcega RO, Mathur M, Franco JJ, et al. Nonatherosclerotic obstructive vascular diseases of the mesenteric and renal arteries. Clin Cardiol 2014; 37:700–6.

59. Biri S, Biri I, Gultekin Y, et al. Doppler ultrasonography criteria of superior mesenteric artery stenosis. J Clin Ultrasound 2019;47:267–71.

60. Schaefer PJ, Pfarr J, Trentmann J, et al. Comparison of noninvasive imaging modalities for stenosis grading in mesenteric arteries. Rofo 2013;185: 628–34.

61. Hohenwalter EJ. Chronic mesenteric ischemia: diagnosis and treatment. Semin Intervent Radiol 2009;26:345–51.

62. Rawat N, Gibbons CP, Joint Vascular Research G. Surgical or endovascular treatment for chronic mesenteric ischemia: a multicenter study. Ann Vasc Surg 2010;24:935–45.

63. AbuRahma AF, Scott Dean L. Duplex ultrasound interpretation criteria for inferior mesenteric arteries. Vascular 2012;20:145–9.

64. AbuRahma AF, Stone PA, Srivastava M, et al. Mesenteric/celiac duplex ultrasound interpretation criteria revisited. J Vasc Surg 2012;55:428–36.e6 [discussion: 435–6].

65. Sivamurthy N, Rhodes JM, Lee D, et al. Endovascular versus open mesenteric revascularization: immediate benefits do not equate with short-term functional outcomes. J Am Coll Surg 2006;202: 859–67.

Iliac Artery Intervention

Andrew J. Klein, MD, FSCAI[a],*, Ammar Nasir, MD, FSCAI[b]

KEYWORDS

- Iliac artery • Endovascular intervention • Aortoiliac intervention • Covered stents

KEY POINTS

- Endovascular intervention to obstructive aortoiliac disease is first-line therapy for patients with symptoms or in whom large-bore access is required.
- Balloon-expandable stents are most often chosen for kissing stents and/or isolated common iliac arterial intervention. Self-expanding stents are typically used in the external iliac artery. Covered stents in the aortoiliac bed have demonstrated enhanced patency over noncovered stents in more complex anatomy. Further studies are required to definitively determine optimal device choices.
- Iliac perforation and distal embolization are the most serious complications associated with endovascular intervention in this vascular bed. The full array of bail-out tools to manage these complications and a familiarity with their use are essential.

INTRODUCTION

Lower-extremity peripheral artery disease (PAD) affects between 8 and 12 million people in the United States.[1] Aortoiliac occlusive arterial disease (AIOD) may be present in upward of 50% of these patients.[2] Endovascular therapy (EVT) for this vascular bed has evolved over time and is now considered the optimal treatment strategy for most patients with AIOD.[3–5] The indications for revascularization have expanded beyond claudication and critical limb ischemia to include facilitation of large-bore access for other interventional procedures (transcatheter aortic valve replacement [TAVR], mechanical circulatory support) and appropriate use criteria support EVT for these expanded indications.[5] Consequently, structural interventionalists must become familiar with the treatment and management of AIOD or work closely with endovascular colleagues with expertise in this bed. All cardiovascular physicians performing procedures via a transfemoral approach should become familiar with AIOD and its treatment. In this article, the authors review the evidence for available endovascular treatment strategies for AIOD, indications, contraindications, procedural technique, prevention and management of complications and detail appropriate postprocedure follow-up.

AORTOILIAC OCCLUSIVE ARTERIAL DISEASE TREATMENT OPTIONS

EVT, exercise, and medical therapy have been evaluated for AIOD. Claudication: Exercise Versus Endoluminal Revascularization (CLEVER) was a randomized controlled trial (RCT) comparing EVT, supervised exercise therapy (SET), and optimal medical therapy (OMT).[6] This trial demonstrated an improvement in peak walking distance and quality of life (QOL) for SET and EVT compared with OMT at 18 months. This trial firmly demonstrated that SET is an alternative to EVT for patients with AIOD and helped move the Centers for Medicare and Medicaid Services to approve reimbursement for SET. Endovascular Revascularization and Supervised Exercise for Peripheral Artery Disease and Intermittent Claudication (ERASE)[7] randomized patients with aortoiliac and femoropopliteal disease to EVT + SET versus SET alone. The greatest improvement in walking distance and QOL occurred in patients treated with

[a] Piedmont Heart Interventional Cardiology, 95 Collier Road, Suite 2065, Atlanta, GA 30309, USA; [b] John Cochran VA Medical Center, Section 2B Cardiology, 915 N. Grand Boulevard, St Louis, MO 63106, USA
* Corresponding author.
E-mail address: Andrew.Klein@piedmont.org

Intervent Cardiol Clin 9 (2020) 187–196
https://doi.org/10.1016/j.iccl.2019.12.009
2211-7458/20/© 2020 Elsevier Inc. All rights reserved.

EVT + SET. The benefits of EVT + SET were also seen in 2 other studies, including the MIMIC and OBACT trials. In the MIMIC trial,[8] patients with both femoropopliteal and aortoiliac disease were randomized to percutaneous transluminal angioplasty (PTA) while receiving SET. Those who received PTA showed better walking distance and an improvement in their ankle-brachial index (ABI). The OBACT trial[9] further confirmed these findings and demonstrated that PTA enhanced not only walking distance but also QOL. Collectively, these trials demonstrated that SET is a valid treatment modality for AIOD. CLEVER, ERASE, MIMIC, and OBACT suggest that the combination of SET plus EVT provides the greatest improvement in walking disease and QOL score, underscoring that a combination of EVT and exercise therapy may be the best treatment.

Surgical therapy for AIOD with bypass (either aortobifemoral,[10] ax-femoral, or femoral-femoral) was previously considered the treatment of choice for severely symptomatic patients. The now outdated 2007 TASC-II document,[4] which described the anatomic characteristics of lower-extremity PAD in relation to therapeutic options relegated more complex disease (TASC C/D) to surgery and more simple lesions (TASC A/B) to EVT. However, given the significantly increased risks with open surgery in these patients,[11] and given concomitant improvements in equipment, technique, and operator experience, an "endovascular first" approach is now considered the care standard. The multispecialty 2016 American College of Cardiology/American Heart Association (ACC/AHA) Peripheral Arterial Disease Guidelines[12] support EVT, with primary or provisional stenting as first-line therapy for patients with AIOD on the basis of its high success rates and lower morbidity and mortality compared with surgical intervention.

ENDOVASCULAR THERAPY INDICATIONS

The traditional indication for EVT for AIOD is claudication and/or critical limb ischemia (CLI). A complete history and physical examination are essential to determine if AIOD is present. Patients with AIOD may complain of claudication symptoms at any level of the leg, including buttocks and hip, in the case of common iliac (CIA) or internal iliac stenosis/occlusion. On physical examination, patients with AIOD may have decreased femoral pulses, but given the large caliber of these vessels, the pulse examination can also be normal. The resting ABI is often normal in this setting, and the ABI should be performed following exercise when AIOD is suspected. Patients with isolated internal iliac stenosis may present with hip/buttock claudication and/or vasculogenic erectile dysfunction with normal resting and exercise ABIs. The main objectives of EVT for AIOD are to augment blood flow for resolution of symptoms and/or limb salvage and to improve functional status and QOL.[5] Additional indications for AIOD EVT include facilitation of large-bore access for other interventional procedures to prevent acute limb ischemia and/or iatrogenic vessel injury. These indications include patients requiring hemodynamic support (eg, IABP, percutaneous left ventricular assist devices, or extracorporeal membrane oxygenation), those undergoing structural heart procedures (eg, TAVR), and/or vascular interventions in other beds (eg, endovascular aortic repair [EVAR]).

The assessment of lesion severity in this vascular bed can be challenging with 2-dimensional angiography given the propensity of these lesions to be eccentric and calcified. It has been recommended that physicians consider assessing the severity of intermediate lesions (50%–70% diameter stenosis) by measuring translesional gradients with pressure wires or microcatheters.[5] The use of sheaths to determine gradients is not recommended because it can falsely induce a gradient. A translesional gradient of 10 mm Hg at rest or with hyperemia (induced by papaverine or nitroglycerin) is considered significant in the aortoiliac vascular bed given the caliber of these vessels and the peak flows that occur with exercise.[5,12,13]

ENDOVASCULAR THERAPY CONTRAINDICATIONS

Patients should not undergo EVT to the aortoiliac bed for asymptomatic lesions absent other clinical indications (eg, need for large-bore access). In patients with concomitant aneurysms who may be candidates for EVAR, lesion treatment should be generally deferred until the time of the EVAR procedure because the implantation of aortoiliac stents may complicate the EVAR procedure. AIOD revascularization is relatively contraindicated in patients who cannot take aspirin or other antiplatelet agents, although this has not been well studied. The large caliber of these vessels and the high flow are thought to be protective against stent thrombosis, although this complication has been reported.[14]

ENDOVASCULAR THERAPY PROCEDURAL TECHNIQUES

The treatment strategy for AIOD is highly dependent on anatomy and vessel characteristics. The CIA arteries may present a challenge when heavily calcified or tortuous and include ostial disease, which may require a kissing stent strategy even when only 1 side is affected. The external iliac arteries (EIA) may be highly tortuous, posing challenges in the assessment of lesion severity. The internal iliac artery (IIA), although frequently ignored, may be important. Significant buttock claudication, vasculogenic erectile dysfunction, and symptoms resulting from impairment of collateral flow must be considered when evaluating patients with IIA AIOD.

Vascular Access

The optimal access choice is dependent on (a) location of the lesion; (b) presence/absence of contralateral iliac artery lesions; (c) presence of common femoral artery disease; (d) aortoiliac bifurcation angulation; (e) severity of the lesion (stenosis vs occlusion); and (f) availability of alternative access, such as the brachial and/or radial arteries.[15] An ipsilateral retrograde approach is often used for ipsilateral CIA and mid EIA lesions and contralateral CIA, internal iliac (IIA), and EIA lesions. In cases of bilateral ostial CIA disease, bilateral common femoral access is ideal to permit "kissing" (simultaneous inflation) balloon angioplasty and/or stenting. This approach also may be needed for isolated ostial CIA artery disease to prevent plaque shift to the contralateral iliac artery and to insure adequate lesion coverage (Fig. 1). For iliac occlusions, 2 access sites are often required to permit safe traversal of the occlusion and provide adequate support to cross the proximal cap. For EIA occlusions, a crossover approach with use of the IIA to wire and anchor a crossover sheath (Fig. 2) is often required. One can then cross from the ipsilateral common femoral artery (CFA) access retrograde using the controlled antegrade retrograde technique (CART) or reverse-CART technique. Placing a sheath in the CFA downstream from an occlusion can be challenging and, in these cases, a patent lateral femoral circumflex is helpful to provide enough wire support for sheath insertion to facilitate retrograde crossing. For CIA occlusions or CIA lesions with severe calcification, a contralateral antegrade approach may be possible, but inadequate support may prompt the operator to choose a retrograde ipsilateral or brachial approach instead (Fig. 3).

In these situations, visualization of the target vessel downstream from the occlusion is often helpful. Visualization of the downstream segment is particularly helpful when crossing a CIA occlusion to visualize the aortoiliac bifurcation and may involve the advancement of a diagnostic catheter from the radial and/or brachial artery.

The most common access for treating AIOD is the common femoral artery. This approach allows for shorter transit distance to the iliacs, compared with the radial or brachial approach, and also allows for larger-bore access. However, as operator experience increases and technology continues to evolve, use of the radial and brachial approaches has become more common. Several device manufacturers have developed and tailored equipment specifically for radial and/or brachial access. Many have developed self-expanding stents (SES) on long shafts, enabling treatment from radial or brachial access sites. A metaanalysis of 19 trials and 638 patients demonstrated a high degree of procedural success and safety for transradial treatment of aorto-iliac and femoral disease.[16]

Periprocedural Anticoagulation

Most studies of peripheral vascular intervention (PVI) for AIOD have used unfractionated heparin (UFH) as a periprocedural anticoagulant. UFH is an ideal choice given its potential reversal with protamine and its low cost. It is particularly prudent to use heparin in cases of heavily calcified lesions and/or chronic total occlusions, whereby the risk of perforation is higher. The ideal activated clotting time (ACT) for PVI has not been established. However, heparin doses greater than 60 units/kg and ACT greater than 250 seconds have both been associated with increased need for postprocedural transfusion following PVI.[17] Direct thrombin inhibitors (eg, bivalirudin) have been used for AIOD EVT, but pose issues with irreversibility and higher procedural cost compared with UFH. Despite this cost difference and issues with reversibility, there have been several recent publications demonstrating the safety and effectiveness of bivalirudin for PVI. In a propensity analyzed study, Kimmelstiel and colleagues[18] observed superior outcomes associated with bivalirudin than with UFH. More recent metaanalyses[19–22] have also demonstrated superior outcomes with bivalirudin compared with UFH for PVI, with less bleeding and shorter length of stay associated with the former. The ENDOMAX RCT (NCT01913483) intended to shed light on this issue but was terminated prematurely because of lack of enrollment. Further RCTs are needed to

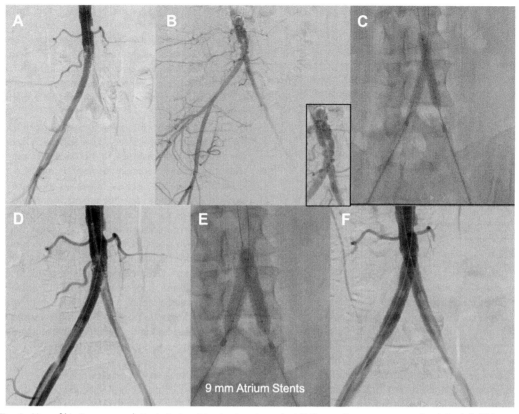

Fig. 1. Use of kissing covered stents to treat in-stent restenosis. (A) Severe in-stent restenosis of the left CIA stent with undersizing of the stents (original stents were 6 mm), leading to reoccurrence of symptoms. (B) Angiography after predilatation of the left CIA lesion showing diffuse distal abdominal aortic disease (inset). (C) Predilitation with 8-mm balloons in a kissing fashion. (D) Angiography after predilition. (E) Deployment of two 9-mm covered stents. (E) Final angiography after postdilitation using kissing 10-mm balloons.

determine which agent is more cost-effective in this setting.

Lesion Wiring
Lesion wiring is similar to that for other interventional procedures and can be performed with any size wire (0.014 in, 0.018 in, and 0.035 in). Steerable hydrophilic wires are often used given the tortuosity in this vascular bed, but dissection risk is higher with these. Transit catheters can be used to exchange wires and can be helpful to cross and obtain

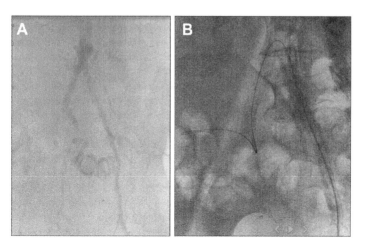

Fig. 2. Internal iliac anchoring technique. (A) Complex external iliac occlusion with a patent IIA. (B) Wiring of the IIA with a softer wire followed by exchange using a transit catheter for a stiff wire to facilitate successful advancement of a contralateral sheath to address the occlusion.

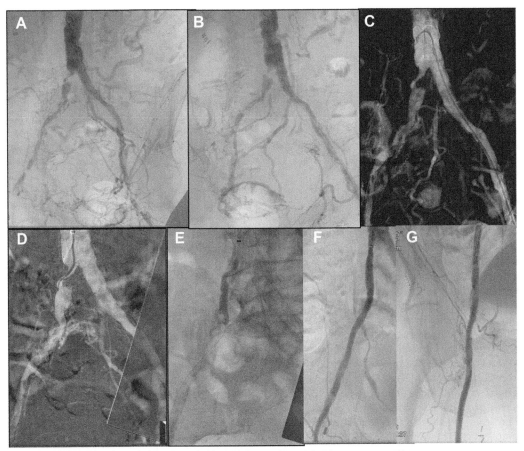

Fig. 3. Use of the brachial approach for complex disease. (*A, B*) Oblique angiography of the aortoiliac vasculature showing marked angulation and heavy calcification. (*C*) Withdrawal of an RIM catheter after attempting to wire this lesion from the contralateral approach. (*D*) Roadmapping showing a 6F multipurpose catheter telescoped through a brachial sheath engaging the complex CIA lesion to wire the lesions and occlusion. (*E*) Balloon predilitation of the CIA lesion demonstrated a marked waist consistent with severe restrictive calcific disease through an advanced brachial sheath. (*F, G*) Completion angiography via the brachial sheath.

adequate support when treating complex lesions. Although many smaller profile systems exist (4-6F) for iliac intervention, these small sheaths often cannot accommodate covered stents in the event of perforation. Operators must have a full array of bail-out supplies (covered stents, balloons, coils) and a thorough knowledge of this equipment before aortoiliac intervention is undertaken because iliac perforation can be rapidly catastrophic if not fatal.

Indeed, the highest risk for perforation is with revascularization of chronic total occlusions. Several devices exist for crossing chronic total occlusions in addition to the wire/catheter subintimal looping technique. The device and technique choice are dependent on anatomy and operator experience. Using a variety of techniques, the overall success rate of crossing even the most complex lesions is 85% to 95% for experienced operators.[15,23–25]

Stenting: Provisional Versus Primary

Although most operators choose a primary stenting strategy for AIOD to limit recoil, shorten procedural time, and prevent abrupt occlusion, this practice remains debatable. The Dutch Iliac Stent Trial[13] demonstrated that PTA with provisional stenting (for residual gradient of 10 mm Hg) had similar results to primary stenting, although this study enrolled low-risk lesions (no chronic total occlusions). At 5 years, for these less-complex lesions, there was no difference in patency rates, ABI, and QOL scores between provisional and primary stenting, highlighting that stents are not always required in this vascular bed.[26]

For more complex lesions (TASC C/D), primary stenting is often performed and is supported by data from a 2000 patient metaanalysis whereby primary stenting led to a

43% reduction in procedural failure at 4 years compared with balloon alone.[27] Of interest, the Stents versus Angioplasty (STAG) trial,[28] which randomized iliac chronic total occlusions (CTO) to primary stenting versus PTA demonstrated stents to be superior with respect to technical success with a lower rate of major procedural complications, although there was no difference in 1- or 2-year primary or secondary patency rates. The trial was stopped early secondary to higher distal embolization (DE) in the PTA group.

Patency

The immediate success rate of EVT for AIOD exceeds 90% with 4- to 5-year patency rates of 60% to 86%, secondary patency rates of 80% to 98%, and limb salvage rates of 98%.[24,25,29] Although EVT success rates are high for AIOD, there is a decrease in procedural success and an increase in periprocedural complications with more complex lesions. The variability in patency and outcomes was demonstrated in a recent large retrospective study of more than 2000 patients from Japan. In this study, when procedures involving TASC D lesions were compared with those involving TASC A-C lesions, procedural success rates were lower (91.6% vs 99.3%; $P<.01$) and periprocedural complications more frequent (11.1% vs 5.2%, $P\leq0.01$) with the former, more complex lesions.[29] In contrast, the BRAVISSIMO[30] (Belgiane Italian tRial investigating Abbott Vascular Iliac StentS in the Treatment of TASC A, B, C, and D iliac lesions) registry, which included experienced operators using advanced techniques, found no difference in outcome according to TASC lesion classification. This registry of 325 patients with aortoiliac lesions had a procedural technical success rate of 100% with a 24-month primary patency rate of 87.9% (88.0% for TASC A, 88.5% for TASC B, 91.9% for TASC C, and 84.8% for TASC D, P = NS) and concluded that neither lesion length nor TASC category was predictive of restenosis. These results will require confirmation.

Long-term (10-year) patency rates of aortoiliac revascularization exceed 86%.[31] Lesion location is a factor in patency, with higher rates in the CIA versus the EIA.[28] Other risk factors predictive of late restenosis and occlusion include occlusion versus stenosis, longer versus shorter lesions, and smaller diameter arteries, especially those with circumferential calcification. Female sex may also be a risk factor but could be secondary to smaller vessel diameter.[5,32,33]

Stent Type

Stents used for treatment of AIOD include balloon-expandable (BES) and SES. Covered versions of these stents are also available for use in perforations, in aneurysms, or as primary treatment of more complex lesions. There is much debate regarding optimal stent choice. The advantages of BES are the enhanced radial strength of this stent, precision in deployment, and the ability to expand 1 to 2 mm after deployment with larger balloons. The disadvantages of BES include the need for larger sheaths for deployment, lack of flexibility in tortuous vessels, and inability to taper in vessels of varying diameters. BES are most often used in aortoiliac lesions and CIA lesions with or without calcification (need for precision and radial strength). SES are more flexible, can conform to vessels of varying diameters, and are available in lower-profile delivery systems and in longer lengths. SES are limited by their radial strength, especially in calcified vessels, as well as have a propensity to move during stent deployment. In the ICE (Iliac Artery Stents for Common or External Iliac Artery Occlusive Disease) trial, a multicenter RCT of 660 patients with aortoiliac disease, patients were randomized to BES or SES. The primary patency at 12 months favored SES over BES with an SES restenosis rate of 6.1% versus a BES restenosis rate of 14.9% ($P<.006$).[34] Although the results were surprising to many operators, issues with trial design were highlighted in an accompanying editorial,[35] and there remains no consensus on the optimal stent type.

Covered Stents

Covered versions of BES and SES are also available, usually containing expanded polytetrafluoroethylene (ePTFE) or a similar material. Traditionally, covered stents were reserved for limited applications, including iatrogenic perforations, iliac aneurysms, and AV-fistulae. In recent years, however, additional studies have emerged using covered stents for primary stenting or for the treatment of in-stent restenosis (see Fig. 1). The comparison of covered versus bare expandable stents (COBEST) for the treatment of aorto-iliac occlusive disease[36] randomized 168 TASC B-D iliac lesions to ePTFE or bare metal stents. Although early results favored ePTFE over their uncovered counterparts, at 18 months there was no difference between the 2 stents for binary restenosis and freedom from occlusion.[37] Interestingly, TASC C/D lesions fared better with ePTFE stents (hazard ratio 0.036 [95% confidence interval 0.042–0.442]) with no difference observed in TASC B lesions. The challenge with ePTFE stents is their deliverability, need for large-bore sheaths (7 or 8F) as well as their stiffness, which makes navigation through tortuous vessels often challenging and can lead to the stent dislodgement from the delivery balloon. One technique to obviate this is to use a long sheath for delivery placed just at or beyond the desired lesion location; withdrawal can then "unsheathe" the stent at the correct location. Finally, covered stents by their nature exclude arterial side branches, which could include vessels that supply critical collateral flow. Operators should be careful to assess baseline collateral flow before the stent deployment and potential occlusion of side branches.

There are 2 currently available balloon-expandable covered stents in the United States, the Advanta V12 balloon-expandable stent (Atrium-Maquet, Hudson, NH, USA) and the Gore VBX stent (W.L. Gore and Associates, Flagstaff, AZ, USA). The COBEST trial involved the Advanta V12 balloon-expandable stent. The VBX stent graft was recently evaluated in the treatment of AIOD in a prospective, multicenter, single-arm safety and efficacy study.[38] In 134 patients with 213 iliac lesions (32.1% TASC C/D), the patency at 9 months was excellent with only 3 patients requiring target lesion revascularization (TLR). The VIABAHN (W.L. Gore and Associates) is the only commercially available covered SES. This stent has been extensively studied in the femoropopliteal vascular bed with no large studies for AIOD. It is not unusual for covered stents to be used in combination. In a recent small study[39] of 39 patients with complete CIA-EIA occlusions treated with both Advanta V12 and Viabahn stents, there was reported primary, assisted, and secondary patency rates of such an approach at 24 months of 96.8% despite most of these patients having CLI.

ENDOVASCULAR THERAPY COMPLICATIONS

Complications with EVT of the aortoiliac vascular bed include access site issues (bleeding/dissection), iliac and aortic dissections, perforations, DE, and contrast-related reactions (allergic reaction and contrast induced nephropathy). Aortoiliac arterial perforation is the most serious complication that can occur during EVT for AIOD. With the large-caliber nature of these vessels, patients can bleed quickly into the large retroperitoneal space and expire in minutes if the perforation is not recognized and treated (**Fig. 4**). It is imperative for operators to be prepared with adequate vascular access to deliver covered stents, adequate intravenous (IV) access (2 IVs of 20 gauge or larger), type, and screen for blood products and to be constantly vigilant during balloon inflation for pain (indicative of adventitial stretch and possible rupture) and hypotension after balloon inflation. The incidence of this potentially fatal complication ranges from 0.5% to 3% and can occur from guidewire or device-mediated rupture.[15,24] The immediate treatment of perforation is balloon tamponade proximal to the perforation while readying the supplies for definitive therapy. In most cases of device-mediated rupture, attempts at prolonged balloon tamponade is not recommended given the propensity for rapid bleeding if this fails after the procedure. Operators must have a full array of bailout devices and an intimate knowledge of how to quickly deploy them if needed. Covered stents, for example, are available in various sizes with varying wire demands (0.018 and 0.035 in) and access sheath requirements (6–10F).

DE is another potential complication that requires preprocedural and postprocedural runoff angiography to detect. Its incidence ranges from 0.4% to 9%[40–43] and demands operator vigilance and careful angiography both before and after intervention. DE may be treated with aspiration thrombectomy, low-pressure PTA, or stent placement.[15] Readers should recall that the STAG trial was terminated prematurely because of a higher incidence of DE in the PTA arm.

ENDOVASCULAR THERAPY PERIPROCEDURAL ISSUES

ACC/AHA guidelines recommend that before undergoing EVT, patients should be on aspirin (81–325 mg).[12] The role of dual antiplatelet therapy (DAPT: clopidogrel, prasugrel, or ticagrelor) in the setting of aortoiliac intervention has not been well studied. The role of extended DAPT is even more unclear; however, common convention is for DAPT for at least 1 to 3 months after intervention. In some cases, operators may prefer life-long DAPT, especially in the setting of kissing iliac stents extending into the distal aorta. To date, no randomized trials have examined the results of DAPT versus aspirin alone after iliac intervention. In the setting of bare metal stent usage, generally 1 month of DAPT is acceptable, because endothelialization occurs typically within 2 to 3 weeks of stent implantation. In the setting of covered stent usage, intimal hyperplasia at the edges of the stent can result in stenosis or reocclusion, and duplex

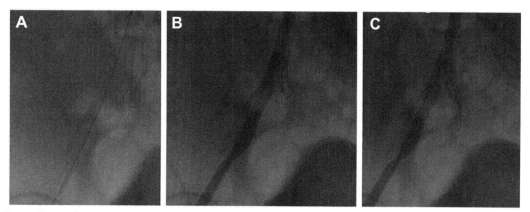

Fig. 4. Iliac perforation: (A) a stent expanded in the right EIA; (B, C) large EIA perforation. Note the crescent indentation of the bladder from blood in the retroperitoneal space.

angiography should be considered to monitor for this complication. Operators should consider peak systolic velocities greater than 250 seconds significant for restenosis and consider repeat imaging or intervention to maintain secondary patency.

LONG-TERM FOLLOW-UP AFTER ENDOVASCULAR THERAPY

Patients with AIOD after EVT should be followed in a comprehensive vascular clinic for monitoring of patency, but also for optimization of medical therapy to preclude cardiovascular morbidity and mortality. Postprocedure follow-up should include assessment for symptomatic improvement and changes in physical examination findings. The strength of the common femoral pulse may provide an indication of the patency of the aortoiliac bed. In experienced vascular laboratories, duplex ultrasound can be used to follow the patency of aortoiliac stents. The ABI following exercise can detect (although is not specific to) aortoiliac restenosis as well. Careful clinical follow-up of all patients is required to monitor for any evidence of clinically significant restenosis.

SUMMARY

Endovascular intervention for obstructive aortoiliac disease is first-line therapy for patients with symptoms or in whom large-bore access is required. There are numerous trials supporting an endovascular-first approach to AIOD given its low morbidity and mortality. Although there is a debate regarding provisional vs primary stenting for less complex lesions, most operators choose stenting to preclude abrupt vessel closure, optimize luminal gain, and expedite the procedure.

There are 2 main types of stents available for treatment of AIOD. Most operators choose BES for kissing stents and/or isolated CIA arterial intervention and SES for the EIA. Covered stents in the aortoiliac bed have shown enhanced patency over standard stents when chronic total occlusions are revascularized, although further studies are required to definitively determine the optimal treatment strategy. Iliac perforation and DE are the most feared complications of endovascular intervention in this vascular bed. Any operator performing revascularization in this territory must have the full array of bail-out tools for these complications along with an intimate knowledge of their use.

DISCLOSURE

None.

REFERENCES

1. Hirsch AT, Criqui MH, Treat-Jacobson D, et al. Peripheral arterial disease detection, awareness, and treatment in primary care. JAMA 2001;286:1317–24.
2. Aboyans V, Desormais I, Lacroix P, et al. The general prognosis of patients with peripheral arterial disease differs according to the disease localization. J Am Coll Cardiol 2010;55:898–903.
3. Dotter CT, Judkins MP. Transluminal treatment of arteriosclerotic obstruction. Description of a new technic and a preliminary report of its application. Circulation 1964;30:654–70.
4. Norgren L, Hiatt WR, Dormandy JA, et al. Inter-society consensus for the management of peripheral arterial disease (TASC II). J Vasc Surg 2007; 45(Suppl S):S5–67.
5. Klein AJ, Jaff MR, Gray BH, et al. SCAI appropriate use criteria for peripheral arterial interventions: an

update. Catheter Cardiovasc Interv 2017;90:E90–110.

6. Murphy TP, Cutlip DE, Regensteiner JG, et al. Supervised exercise versus primary stenting for claudication resulting from aortoiliac peripheral artery disease: six-month outcomes from the claudication: exercise versus endoluminal revascularization (CLEVER) study. Circulation 2011;125:130–9.

7. Fakhry F, Spronk S, van der Laan L, et al. Endovascular revascularization and supervised exercise for peripheral artery disease and intermittent claudication: a randomized clinical trial. JAMA 2015;314:1936–44.

8. Greenhalgh RM, Belch JJ, Brown LC, et al. The adjuvant benefit of angioplasty in patients with mild to moderate intermittent claudication (MIMIC) managed by supervised exercise, smoking cessation advice and best medical therapy: results from two randomised trials for stenotic femoropopliteal and aortoiliac arterial disease. Eur J Vasc Endovasc Surg 2008;36:680–8.

9. Nylaende M, Abdelnoor M, Stranden E, et al. The Oslo balloon angioplasty versus conservative treatment study (OBACT)–the 2-years results of a single centre, prospective, randomised study in patients with intermittent claudication. Eur J Vasc Endovasc Surg 2007;33:3–12.

10. Chiu KW, Davies RS, Nightingale PG, et al. Review of direct anatomical open surgical management of atherosclerotic aorto-iliac occlusive disease. Eur J Vasc Endovasc Surg 2010;39:460–71.

11. Sutzko DC, Andraska EA, Obi AT, et al. Risk factors associated with perioperative myocardial infarction in major open vascular surgery. Ann Vasc Surg 2018;47:24–30.

12. Gerhard-Herman MD, Gornik HL, Barrett C, et al. 2016 AHA/ACC guideline on the management of patients with lower extremity peripheral artery disease: executive summary: a report of the American College of Cardiology/American Heart Association task force on clinical practice guidelines. J Am Coll Cardiol 2016;69:1465–508.

13. Tetteroo E, van der Graaf Y, Bosch JL, et al. Randomised comparison of primary stent placement versus primary angioplasty followed by selective stent placement in patients with iliac-artery occlusive disease. Dutch Iliac Stent Trial Study Group. Lancet 1998;351:1153–9.

14. Katsanos K, Al-Lamki SA, Parthipun A, et al. Peripheral stent thrombosis leading to acute limb ischemia and major amputation: incidence and risk factors in the aortoiliac and femoropopliteal arteries. Cardiovasc Intervent Radiol 2017;40:351–9.

15. Klein AJ, Feldman DN, Aronow HD, et al. SCAI expert consensus statement for aorto-iliac arterial intervention appropriate use. Catheter Cardiovasc Interv 2014;84:520–8.

16. Meertens MM, Ng E, Loh SEK, et al. Transradial approach for aortoiliac and femoropopliteal interventions: a systematic review and meta-analysis. J Endovasc Ther 2018;25:599–607.

17. Kasapis C, Gurm HS, Chetcuti SJ, et al. Defining the optimal degree of heparin anticoagulation for peripheral vascular interventions: insight from a large, regional, multicenter registry. Circ Cardiovasc Interv 2010;3:593–601.

18. Kimmelstiel C, Pinto D, Aronow HD, et al. Bivalirudin is associated with improved in-hospital outcomes compared with heparin in percutaneous vascular interventions: observational, propensity-matched analysis from the premier hospital database. Circ Cardiovasc Interv 2016;9:e002823.

19. Olmedo W, Villablanca PA, Sanina C, et al. Bivalirudin versus heparin in patients undergoing percutaneous peripheral interventions: a systematic review and meta-analysis. Vascular 2019;27:78–89.

20. Omran J, Enezate T, Abdullah O, et al. Bivalirudin versus unfractionated heparin in peripheral vascular interventions. Cardiovasc Revasc Med 2018;19:695–9.

21. Ortiz D, Singh M, Jahangir A, et al. Bivalirudin versus unfractionated heparin during peripheral vascular interventions: a propensity-matched study. Catheter Cardiovasc Interv 2017;89:408–13.

22. Hu Y, Liu AY, Zhang L, et al. A systematic review and meta-analysis of bivalirudin application in peripheral endovascular procedures. J Vasc Surg 2019;70:274–84.e5.

23. Kashyap VS, Pavkov ML, Bena JF, et al. The management of severe aortoiliac occlusive disease: endovascular therapy rivals open reconstruction. J Vasc Surg 2008;48:1451–7, 1457.e1-3.

24. Jongkind V, Akkersdijk GJ, Yeung KK, et al. A systematic review of endovascular treatment of extensive aortoiliac occlusive disease. J Vasc Surg 2010;52:1376–83.

25. Ye W, Liu CW, Ricco JB, et al. Early and late outcomes of percutaneous treatment of TransAtlantic Inter-Society Consensus class C and D aorto-iliac lesions. J Vasc Surg 2011;53:1728–37.

26. Klein WM, van der Graaf Y, Seegers J, et al. Long-term cardiovascular morbidity, mortality, and reintervention after endovascular treatment in patients with iliac artery disease: the Dutch Iliac Stent Trial Study. Radiology 2004;232:491–8.

27. Bosch JL, Hunink MG. Meta-analysis of the results of percutaneous transluminal angioplasty and stent placement for aortoiliac occlusive disease. Radiology 1997;204:87–96.

28. Goode SD, Cleveland TJ, Gaines PA, et al. Randomized clinical trial of stents versus angioplasty

for the treatment of iliac artery occlusions (STAG trial). Br J Surg 2013;100:1148–53.

29. Suzuki K, Mizutani Y, Soga Y, et al. Efficacy and safety of endovascular therapy for aortoiliac TASC D lesions. Angiology 2017;68:67–73.

30. de Donato G, Bosiers M, Setacci F, et al. 24-month data from the BRAVISSIMO: a large-scale prospective registry on Iliac stenting for TASC A & B and TASC C & D lesions. Ann Vasc Surg 2015;29: 738–50.

31. Houston JG, Bhat R, Ross R, et al. Long-term results after placement of aortic bifurcation self-expanding stents: 10 year mortality, stent restenosis, and distal disease progression. Cardiovasc Intervent Radiol 2007;30:42–7.

32. Galaria II, Davies MG. Percutaneous transluminal revascularization for iliac occlusive disease: long-term outcomes in TransAtlantic Inter-Society Consensus A and B lesions. Ann Vasc Surg 2005; 19:352–60.

33. Galyfos G, Zografos G, Filis K. Regarding "The influence of gender on patency rates after iliac artery stenting. J Vasc Surg 2014;60:269.

34. Krankenberg H, Zeller T, Ingwersen M, et al. Self-expanding versus balloon-expandable stents for iliac artery occlusive disease: the Randomized ICE Trial. JACC Cardiovasc Interv 2017;10:1694–704.

35. Feldman DN, Klein AJP. Stent selection in the iliac arteries: don't fall through the ICE! JACC Cardiovasc Interv 2017;10:1705–7.

36. Mwipatayi BP, Thomas S, Wong J, et al. A comparison of covered vs bare expandable stents for the treatment of aortoiliac occlusive disease. J Vasc Surg 2011;54:1561–70.

37. Mwipatayi BP, Sharma S, Daneshmand A, et al. Durability of the balloon-expandable covered versus bare-metal stents in the Covered versus Balloon Expandable Stent Trial (COBEST) for the treatment of aortoiliac occlusive disease. J Vasc Surg 2016;64:83–94.e1.

38. Bismuth J, Gray BH, Holden A, et al. Pivotal study of a next-generation balloon-expandable stent-graft for treatment of Iliac occlusive disease. J Endovasc Ther 2017;24:629–37.

39. Zanabili Al-Sibbai AA, Camblor Santervas LA, Marcos FA, et al. Midterm results of endovascular treatment for complete iliac axis occlusions using covered stents. Ann Vasc Surg 2019. [Epub ahead of print].

40. Scheinert D, Schroder M, Ludwig J, et al. Stent-supported recanalization of chronic iliac artery occlusions. Am J Med 2001;110:708–15.

41. Dyet JF, Gaines PA, Nicholson AA, et al. Treatment of chronic iliac artery occlusions by means of percutaneous endovascular stent placement. J Vasc Interv Radiol 1997;8:349–53.

42. Henry M, Amor M, Ethevenot G, et al. Percutaneous endoluminal treatment of iliac occlusions: long-term follow-up in 105 patients. J Endovasc Surg 1998;5:228–35.

43. Vorwerk D, Guenther RW, Schurmann K, et al. Primary stent placement for chronic iliac artery occlusions: follow-up results in 103 patients. Radiology 1995;194:745–9.

Device Selection in Femoral-Popliteal Arterial Interventions

Samuel M. Kim, MD, MS*, Luke K. Kim, MD,
Dmitriy N. Feldman, MD

KEYWORDS

- Peripheral artery disease • Femoral-popliteal artery • Superficial femoral artery
- Drug-coated balloon • Drug-eluting stent • Percutaneous transluminal angioplasty

KEY POINTS

- Supervised exercise and medical and endovascular therapies remain mainstays in the management of symptomatic femoral-popliteal arterial disease.
- Recent randomized controlled trials demonstrated that drug-eluting stents and drug-coated balloons resulted in improved short- and mid-term patency over uncoated balloon angioplasty.
- Adjunctive technologies for lesion preparation including atherectomy are available to treat complex and calcified lesions, but comparative studies are still needed.

INTRODUCTION

Lower extremity peripheral artery disease (PAD) consists of atherosclerotic occlusive disease of the aortoiliac, femoral-popliteal (FP), and infra-popliteal arterial beds. Annually, more than $3 billion is spent on management of PAD and its complications.[1] It is estimated that nearly 6% of Americans over 40 years of age have PAD.[2] Patients with PAD have an approximately 3-fold higher risk of cardiovascular events and for developing critical limb ischemia (CLI).[1,2] Furthermore, patients with CLI represent a particularly high-risk population, with approximately a 25% mortality and major amputation rate at 1 year.[2,3] Two major risk factors for PAD are smoking and diabetes mellitus; other risk factors include age, hyperlipidemia, family history, chronic kidney disease, and hypertension.[1]

The current American College of Cardiology/American Heart Association 2016 and European Society of Cardiology 2017 guidelines recommend supervised walking exercise (typically 12-week program) as a class I recommendation and unsupervised exercise if supervised therapy is not available.[4,5] Additionally, lifestyle modifications such as smoking cessation and medical therapy with antiplatelet agents and statins have been emphasized in the guidelines. However, despite advances in medical therapy that help to prevent future cardiovascular events, there are few evidence-based therapies available for the treatment of claudication and prevention of amputation in patients with CLI.

In symptomatic patients with claudication with inadequate clinical response to a supervised exercise program or in those with CLI, revascularization should be considered. The Claudication: Exercise versus Endoluminal Revascularization (CLEVER) trial, in 111 symptomatic PAD patients, demonstrated that both exercise and stenting were superior to medical therapy with respect to its primary endpoint, change in peak walking time at 6 and 18 months.[6] The peak walking time improved at 18 months for exercise of 5.0 ± 5.4 minutes and revascularization of 3.2 ± 4.7 minutes (P<.001) compared with medical therapy of

Greenberg Division of Cardiology, Weill Cornell Medical College, New York Presbyterian Hospital, 520 East 70th Street, Starr-434 Pavilion, New York, NY 10021, USA
* Corresponding author.
E-mail address: smk9018@nyp.org

Intervent Cardiol Clin 9 (2020) 197–206
https://doi.org/10.1016/j.iccl.2019.12.001
2211-7458/20/© 2019 Elsevier Inc. All rights reserved.

0.2 $\pm$ 2.1 minutes ($P = .16$).[7] The Endovascular Revascularization and Supervised Exercise for Peripheral Artery Disease and Intermittent Claudication (ERASE) trial evaluated 212 patients in the Netherlands allocated to either endovascular intervention with supervised exercise or supervised exercise only. At the 1-year follow-up, the combination therapy group had significantly greater improvement in walking distance (285 m vs 1240 m; $P = .001$) and in quality life scores such as the Vascular Quality of Life and Short Form-36 metrics.[8] Additionally, a recent meta-analysis demonstrated that combination treatment with endovascular revascularization followed by supervised exercised therapy showed greater improvement in walking distance and quality of life at 12 months compared with endovascular therapy or exercise alone. Endovascular therapy with supervised exercise demonstrated improvement in walking distance of 290 m (95% confidence interval, 180–390 m; $P<.001$) compared with medical therapy and 110 m compared with exercise therapy (95% confidence interval, 16–200 m; $P<.001$).[9]

ANATOMIC LESION CONSIDERATIONS

Lower extremity PAD can be divided into aortoiliac, FP, and below-the-knee infrapopliteal or infrageniculate vascular territories. The FP segment consists of the common femoral artery (CFA), profunda femoris artery, superficial femoral artery (SFA), and popliteal artery. The CFA bifurcation includes the common femoral bifurcation and ostial SFA/popliteal artery. The above-the-knee popliteal artery includes the P1 (intercondylar fossa to proximal edge of patella) and P2 (proximal part of patella to center of knee joint space).[10,11]

The FP vascular segment is long and endovascular interventions in this segment are subject to multiple mechanical forces. including extension, flexion, torsion, and elongation.[2,11] FP disease can be classified based on length of lesions, stenosis versus occlusion, severity of calcification, and whether there is presence of in-stent restenosis (ISR).[10,11] In general, stenosis of 70% or more by angiography or stenosis of 50% or more and a translesional pressure gradient of 10 or more to 20 mm Hg is considered physiologically significant disease in symptomatic patients.[4] Lesion length can be grouped into focal (<10 cm), intermediate (10–20 cm), and diffuse (>20 cm) based on existing trial data and consensus document recommendations.[10] Traditionally, the Inter-Society Consensus for the Management of Peripheral Artery Disease (TASC II) classification

has been used to divide FP disease into 4 anatomic categories based on length of disease and whether chronic total occlusions (CTOs) are present. The TASC II system classifies lesions into type A (single stenosis ≤10 cm in length, single occlusion ≤5 cm in length), type B (multiple lesions each ≤5 cm, single stenosis ≤15 cm not involving the infrageniculate popliteal artery, single or multiple lesions in the absence of continuous tibial vessels, heavily calcified occlusions, and single popliteal stenosis), type C (multiple stenoses >15 cm or recurrent stenosis that needs treatment after 2 interventions), or type D (CTOs).[12,13] Although TASC A and B lesions were traditionally considered ideal candidates for catheter-based intervention, TASC C and D lesions are now commonly amenable to endovascular therapy given advances in reentry and crossing techniques and devices.[12–14]

COMMON FEMORAL ARTERY DISEASE: SPECIAL CONSIDERATIONS

Historically, surgical endarterectomy has been the treatment of choice for CFA disease. However, recent studies have shown comparable success rates, safety, and midterm patency rates with endovascular intervention compared with surgery.[15–17] The Vascular Quality Initiative showed low procedural morbidity with CFA interventions from a pooled analysis of 1014 patients, with 87.2% survival rate at 3 years and 93.5% amputation-free survival at 1 year.[16] Additionally, the TECCO (The Endovascular vs Open Repair of the Common Femoral Artery) trial randomized 117 patients with de novo CFA disease to endarterectomy or stent placement and showed no significant difference in patency, clinical improvement, or target lesion recurrence (TLR) at 2 years.[17] Importantly, the surgical group had a higher rate of perioperative complications (26% vs 12.5%; $P = .05$) and longer duration of hospitalization (6.3 days vs 3.2 days; $P<.0001$).[17] The National Surgical Quality Improvement Program database from 2005 to 2010 showed approximately a 15% combined mortality and morbidity rate associated with endarterectomy.[18] Endarterectomy carries a higher risk of periprocedural complications, including delayed wound healing and wound infections, making endovascular intervention a viable alternative for anatomically and clinically appropriate patients.[15]

UNCOATED BALLOON PERCUTANEOUS TRANSLUMINAL ANGIOPLASTY

Traditionally, an uncoated percutaneous transluminal angioplasty (PTA)-first approach had been used for FP disease. However, recent trials have challenged this approach given the benefit for drug-eluting stents (DES) and drug-coated balloon (DCB) devices in FP intervention over stand-alone PTA with uncoated balloons. The STAR registry demonstrated that even for short lesions (<5 cm), uncoated balloon angioplasty had poor patency rates of approximately 70% after 3 years. Additionally, as lesion length increases, particularly for longer lesions (>10 cm), stenting is associated with better patency compared with uncoated balloon angioplasty.[19] Furthermore, uncoated balloon angioplasty has limited procedural success and poor long-term patency in calcified lesions. Outcomes in CTOs in FP lesions also remain suboptimal. Uncoated balloon PTA has less than 80% patency at 5 months and approximately 50% patency at 3 years in CTOs and ISR lesions.[20]

A number of specialty balloons (ie, the Angiosculpt scoring balloon [Royal Philips, Amsterdam, the Netherlands], the peripheral cutting balloon [Boston Scientific, Inc, Marlborough, MA], the Chocolate PTA balloon [TriReme Medical, LLC, Pleasanton, CA], the VascuTrak [Bard Peripheral Vascular, Inc, Tempe, AZ]) are currently available to aid in treatment of severely calcified and undilatable lesions, but the data for these devices remain limited and primarily based on small, observational trials. Given the associated cost and risk of complications (eg, distal embolization), these devices are reserved for use as adjunctive therapy for vessel preparation when uncoated PTA therapy alone would be suboptimal.[10,21,22]

BARE METAL STENTS

BMS were initially designed to address procedural complications of balloon angioplasty (ie, dissection, acute closure) as well as to prevent restenosis. Three major randomized clinical trials have shown modest short-term (<2 years) benefits of self-expanding BMS in moderate length FP lesions, including the Vienna Absolute, The Balloon Angioplasty vs Stenting with Nitinol Stents in Intermediate Length Superficial Femoral Artery Lesions (ASTRON), and Randomized Study Comparing the Edwards Self-Expanding Lifestent vs Angioplasty Alone in Lesions Involving the SFA and/or Proximal Popliteal Artery (RESILIENT).[23] A meta-analysis of 11 randomized controlled studies of symptomatic patients with FP disease showed an improved 1-year patency with BMS when compared with uncoated PTA (odds ratio, 1.78; 95% confidence interval, 1.02–3.10; P = .04).[23]

Earlier studies have shown no significant difference in patency between PTA and self-expanding BMS in short lesions, but in longer lesions (>6 cm) self-expanding stents have shown improved 1- and 2-year patency.[24] However, few data exist regarding the use of BMS in very long FP lesions (>30 cm) and concerns remain about the high risk of ISR and future therapeutic challenges of ISR.[11] More studies are needed to understand the effectiveness of newer generation BMS, particularly in comparison to commercially available DES and DCB. Adjunctive pharmacologic approaches to reduce BMS ISR have been investigated as well. One trial suggested that the addition of cilostazol might decrease ISR in intermediate-length lesions treated with self-expanding BMS.[25] In that study, the cilostazol group had a lower restenosis rate at 12 months (20% vs 49%; P = .02).[25]

DRUG-ELUTING STENTS

Initial trials of DES with sirolimus-eluting self-expanding stents did not show significant benefit when compared with uncoated PTA. However, the next generation of paclitaxel-eluting stents has shown clinical superiority in short- and long-term outcomes over PTA alone in FP bed.[26,27] The Zilver PTX paclitaxel-eluting self-expanding DES (Cook Medical, Bloomington, IN) is a paclitaxel-coated nitinol stent that provides a scaffold and drug coating designed to limit neointimal hyperplasia.[10] In patients with SFA or proximal popliteal artery disease, the Zilver PTX randomized trial has shown that paclitaxel-coated DES is superior to uncoated PTA, with a patency rate at 1-year of 83.1% versus 32.8%, a 3-year patency of 70.7% versus 49.1%, and a 5-year patency of 67.6% versus 45.5%.[27–29] Additionally, provisional DES after failed PTA in a secondary randomization showed an improved 1-, 2-, and 5-year patency rates compared with provisional BMS.[27–30] To date, there are 3 multicenter DES observational studies that have shown similar outcomes, including the Zilver PTX single arm study, Japanese ZEPHYR registry, and Japanese postmarket surveillance study.[14,31,32] Most recently, the IMPERIAL trial compared the safety and efficacy of a new polymer-coated paclitaxel-eluting Eluvia stent (Boston Scientific) with a traditional polymer-fee, paclitaxel-coated Zilver PTX stent in a randomized, single blind, noninferiority study of 465 patients with SFA or proximal popliteal artery disease. The study demonstrated overall noninferiority of efficacy and safety end points for the Eluvia and Zilver stents at

12 months, respectively, for primary patency (86.8% vs 81.5%; P<.0001) and for major adverse events (94.9% vs 91.0%; P<.0001).[33]

Currently, there are few head-to-head comparative studies of DES versus either BMS or DCB. The REAL PTX pilot trial, a small prospective randomized controlled trial of 150 patients with symptomatic FP disease, examined a primary DES strategy versus DCB angioplasty strategy and demonstrated similar primary patency results at 12 months (78.3% vs 79.3%; P = .96).[34] The 2018 Society for Cardiovascular Angiography and Interventions consensus guidelines document gave DES devices a class I recommendation for most FP lesions, class IIa recommendation for CFA bifurcation lesions and intermediate to diffuse ISR lesions, and class IIb recommendation for focal ISR lesions.[10]

DRUG-COATED BALLOONS

Several recent trials have demonstrated superiority of DCB over uncoated PTA in terms of patency and clinically driven TLR.[35–37] There are currently 3 DCBs that have received approval from the US Food and Drug Administration for the treatment of FP disease including, Lutonix (Bard Lutonix, New Hope, MN), IN.PACT (Medtronic Vascular, Santa Rosa, CA), and Stellarex (Royal Phillips, Amsterdam, the Netherlands).[10] These DCBs have varying paclitaxel dose from 2 to 3.5 µg/mm^2, the carrier (excipient), balloon material, and coating technology.

The Lutonix Paclitaxel-Coated Balloon for the Prevention of Femoropopliteal Restenosis (LEVANT) 1 and 2 studies were multicenter randomized controlled trials that showed improved patency compared with uncoated PTA. The first feasibility trial enrolled 101 patients and randomized them to DCB versus uncoated PTA, with reduced late lumen loss favoring the former but no significant difference in TLR at the 2-year follow-up.[38] The second trial examined 476 patients and higher rates of 12-month primary patency were seen in the DCB arm (65% vs 53%; P = .02), with lower rates of thrombotic and embolic events.[39] The IN.PACT Admiral Drug-Coated Balloon vs Standard Balloon Angioplasty for the Treatment of Superficial Femoral Artery and Proximal Popliteal Artery (IN.PACT SFA) trial also showed that 1- and 2-year patency rates were higher in DCB versus uncoated balloon PTA (82.2% vs 52.4% [P<.001] at 1 year; 78.9% vs 50.1% [P<.001] at 2 years).[40] The ILLUMENATE trial examined the Stellarex DCB; among nearly 300 patients in the European trial arm, this DCB showed improved primary

patency (83.9% vs 60.6%; P<.001) and TLR rates (5.9% vs 16.7%; P = .014) at the 1-year follow-up.[41] The US-based trial showed similar lower restenosis rates (23.7% vs 42.2%; P = .003) and TLR rates (7.9% and 16.8%; P = .023) at the 1-year follow-up.[41]

A number of studies have examined the use of DCBs in ISR and CTOs. The Paclitaxel-Eluting Balloon vs Conventional Balloon Angioplasty for In-Stent Restenosis of Superficial Femora Artery (ISAR-PEBIS) was a randomized German trial of patients with symptomatic SFA ISR that examined DCB versus uncoated PTA. At the 2-year follow-up there was a significant decrease in TLR (19% vs 50%; P = .007) with DCBs.[42] The IN.PACT Global observational study showed that the use of DCB in long lesions (>15 cm), ISR, and CTOs greater than 5 cm was associated with a greater than 85% primary patency at 1 year in each of these subsets of lesions.[43] The initial concerns about fibrosis and aneurysm formation at the sites of DCB therapy have not been seen in clinical studies.[44] Based on these studies, the 2018 Society for Cardiovascular Angiography and Interventions consensus guidelines afforded DCBs a class I recommendation for most FP lesions, with the exception of those at the CFA bifurcation.

COVERED STENTS

Covered stents for FP disease are self-expanding nitinol stent platforms covered with polytetrafluroethylene.[10] Currently, covered stents are not recommended as first-line therapy for most FP lesions, particularly for ostial SFA or lesions with major side branches. There have been data suggestive of improved patency using covered stents compared with BMS, especially in more complex, longer lesions and ISR. The Viabahn endoprosthesis with PROPATEN bioactive surface vs bare nitinol stent in the treatment of long lesions in SFA occlusive disease (VIASTAR) trial showed that covered stents had improved primary patency at 12 months compared with BMS, particularly in long lesions more than 20 cm in length.[45] The VIBRANT trial showed that patency rates were not significantly different between covered stents and BMS in symptomatic occlusive SFA disease at the 1-, 2-, and 3-year follow-ups.[46] The RELINE trial randomized patients with FP ISR to either PTA or PTA with covered stents. At the 1-year follow-up, the stent graft group had a higher rate of patency (74.8% vs 37.0%; P<.001).[47] Currently, covered stents have limited usefulness as a first-line treatment given the concerns regarding stent thrombosis, which can result in limb ischemia.[4,11,48,49] The 2018 Society for Cardiovascular Angiography and Interventions consensus guidelines endorsed a class IIa recommendation for most diffuse lesions, including ISR and CTOs, and a class IIb recommendation for other lesions.[10]

ATHERECTOMY

Atherectomy refers to the removal of atheromatous tissue by cutting, shaving, or ablating it to enlarge the luminal area. They can be classified into 4 categories based on their mechanism of action: directional atherectomy, orbital or rotational atherectomy, excisional/aspiration atherectomy, and laser atherectomy. To date, there have been limited comparative data comparing atherectomy alone with either BMS, DES, or DCB.[50,51] Atherectomy devices are currently used as adjunctive therapy for lesion preparation rather than devices for intended definitive therapy.

Directional atherectomy removes or cuts the plaque from within the arterial walls, and the removed plaque is directly captured in the nose cone or other receptacle of the atherectomy device.[51,52] The current devices approved by the US Food and Drug Administration include the SilverHawk (Medtronic, MN, USA), TurboHawk (Medtronic, MN, USA), HawkOne (Medtronic, MN, USA), and optimal coherence tomography–guided Avinger Pantheris (Avinger, Redwood City, CA) devices.[50] The Determine of Effectiveness of the SilverHawk PerIpheral Plaque ExcisioN System for the Treatment of Infrainguinal VEssels/Lower Extremities (DEFINIVE LE) was a 47-center prospective study that examined 800 patients with infrainguinal disease using directional atherectomy. The overall 1-year patency was 78%, with no significant difference between diabetics and nondiabetics (77% vs 78%; P<.001). The major adverse events included distal embolization (3.8%), perforation (5.3%), abrupt closure (2.0%), and bail-out stenting (3.2%).[53] The DEFINITIVE AR trial compared use of directional atherectomy plus DCB versus DCB alone. In 100 patients with intermediate length lesions, there was no significant difference in patency and TLR after 1 year.[54] One study suggested that the SilverHawk device could be used as a first-line treatment for ISR with high procedural success rate of 86% with atherectomy alone and 97% with combined PTA at 1-year follow-;p, however, target lesion patency decreased from 86% at 3 months to 25% at 1 year.[55]

A number of noncomparative studies of orbital atherectomy and early single-center studies of rotational atherectomy in FP disease have been published.[56–58] Orbital atherectomy uses a diamond-coated crown that orbitally rotates 360° designed to preferentially cut or sand the plaque while avoiding the arterial wall. Currently, the Diamondback Orbital Atherectomy System (Cardiovascular Systems, Inc, St Paul, MN) is approved for use. The Orbital Atherectomy System for Treatment of Peripheral Vascular Stenosis (OASIS) study was a nonrandomized trial of 124 patients with infrapopliteal occlusive disease treated with orbital atherectomy that demonstrated 90% procedural success rate with low 30-day and 6-month major events, including death, myocardial infarction, repeat revascularization, or amputation.[56] Follow-up small randomized pilot studies, including the Prospective, Randomized Multi-Center Trial to Study Clinical Benefit of Alteration in Vessel Compliance by Comparing Balloon Angioplasty to Diamondback 360 Orbital Atherectomy System in Calcified Femoropopliteal Disease (COMPLIANCE 360) and Comparison of orbital atherectomy plus balloon angioplasty vs balloon angioplasty alone in patients with critical limb ischemia (CALCIUM 360), did not show significant difference in TLR or restenosis rates when compared with uncoated PTA at the 1-year follow-up.[57,58]

The currently approved rotational atherectomy devices include the Rotablator system (Boston Scientific), Pathway Jetstream PV atherectomy system (Boston Scientific), and the Phoenix atherectomy catheter (Volcano Corporation, San Diego, CA).[50,59–62] Rotational atherectomy uses a high-speed rotating tip that cuts the atheroma while preserving the tissue wall of the native vessel.[50] The Pathway is a catheter system with a reusable power source, front-cutting tip and continuous aspiration. In a multicenter study of 172 patients, the device had a 99% success rate and repeat revascularization rate of 15% and 26% at 6 months and 12 months, respectively.[61] The Phoenix device is an over-the-wire system that consists of a double-lumen catheter with a distal metal cutting element and handle. When turned on, the distal tip rotates and cuts the plaque, which is dispensed into the catheter. The Phoenix system was studied in the Endovascular Atherectomy Safety and Effectiveness (EASE) study, a prospective, single-center study of 105 patients that showed a technical success rate of 95.1% and major adverse event rate of 5.7% at the 30-day follow-up.[62]

Laser atherectomy uses ultraviolet laser light to dissolve plaque by delivering short bursts of energy. The device currently uses a fiber optic catheter (2.7F–7.5F) and can be used for infrainguinal de novo stenosis, CTOs, or restenosis.[50] The Peripheral Excimer Laser Angioplasty (PELA) trial compared laser-assisted PTA versus PTA alone in SFA CTOs and showed no significant difference in patency or success rates.[63] The Laser Angioplasty for Critical Limb Ischemic (LACI) prospective study examined 155 patients with CLI and showed that at the 2-year follow-up laser atherectomy with PTA versus PTA had significantly lower rates of TLR (14% vs 44%; $P = .05$).[64] The EXCImer Laser Randomized Controlled Study for Treatment of FemoropopliTEal In-Stent Restenosis (EXCITE-ISR) prospective trial randomized patients with FP ISR to laser atherectomy plus PTA versus PTA alone. At 6 months of follow-up, the excimer laser atherectomy PTA in lesions of average 19 cm (onethird were CTOs) showed superior TLR, but later follow-up was compromised by significant losses to follow-up.[65] A small trial comparing laser atherectomy plus DCB versus DCB alone in patients with CLI showed higher patency rates at 12 months (66.7% vs 37.5%; $P = .01$).[66] A large, prospective, randomized study, the Photoablative Atherectomy Followed by a Paclitaxel-Coated Balloon to Inhibit Restenosis in In-Stent Femoropopliteal Obstructions (PHOTOPAC) study, is currently in progress to examine the efficacy of laser therapy with DCB.[67]

EMERGING THERAPIES

Fractional flow reserve, which is a guide wirebased procedure that measures translesional pressure gradient, has not been commonly used in current management of PAD. Small studies suggest that fractional flow reserve might have a significant linear correlation with postexercise ankle brachial index and provide physiologic data to guide treatment decisions.[68]

Several adjunctive therapies, including external beam radiation, brachytherapy, and cryoplasty, have been evaluated. A small randomized trial examining the role of external beam radiation after SFA stenting failed to show a benefit of 14 Gy dose of radiation on in-stent stenosis.[69] The Vienna-2 trial examined the effectiveness of endovascular brachytherapy in patients with long FP lesions and at 5 years showed that time to recurrence was significantly delayed in PTA plus brachytherapy group (17.5 months vs 7.4 months; $P<.05$); however, after 5 years the rate of recurrence was similar in both groups (72.5% vs 72.5%; $P>.99$).[70] Cryoplasty, a procedure used to simultaneously dilate and treat stenosis by cooling via liquid nitrous oxide delivery, has also been studied. The Study Comparing Two Methods of Expanding Stents Placed in Legs of Diabetics with Peripheral Vascular Disease (COBRA) trial evaluated 74 patients with diabetes undergoing self-expanding stents assigned to cryoplasty versus conventional balloon PTA. At 12 months, binary restenosis was reduced in the cryoplasty group (29.3% vs 55.8%; $P = .01$); however, long-term data are needed.[71] Recently, lithoplasty PTA, which uses pulsatile sonic pressure waves to treat calcified disease, has become an emerging area of interest.[50] The DISRUPT PAD II was a small, nonrandomized study evaluating 60 patients with calcified, complex lesions and showed that lithotripsy could be used safely. The randomized DISRUPT PAD III study is currently underway to further assess the efficacy and safety of this novel technology.[72]

MORTALITY CONTROVERSY

In December 2018, a meta-analysis of 28 RCTs reported that paclitaxel-coated devices were associated with an increased risk of all-cause mortality at 2 to 5 years in patients with FP disease. At the 5-year follow-up, the relative risk of mortality was nearly doubled compared with uncoated devices (14.7% vs 8.1%).[44] This study caused significant controversy in the vascular community, leading to a temporary delay in patient enrollment of other randomized controlled studies such as BASIL-3 and SWEDEPAD.[73] There were several limitations of the metaanalysis: exclusion of intention-to-treat methods, simplistic mortality calculation by dividing the number of deaths by the total number enrolled, failure to control for loss to follow-up, and a lack of a mechanistic explanation for the long-term mortality finding. In contrast, a 2019 retrospective study of paclitaxel-coated versus uncoated devices among 51,546 Medicare beneficiaries undergoing FP revascularization demonstrated that mortality was slightly lower in the paclitaxel-eluting group over a 600-day followup (32.5% vs 34.4%; $P = .007$).[74] The US Food and Drug Administration convened a panel meeting in June of 2019 and concluded that a late mortality signal was present with paclitaxel-coated devices, with uncertainty regarding the signal magnitude, relationship between paclitaxel dose and mortality, whether a class effect was present, and inability to identify a particular cause of death to explain the late mortality signal in patients treated with paclitaxel-coated devices. "The panel unanimously agreed that the short-term benefits of paclitaxel-coated devices continue to outweigh the risks," and that the risks should be discussed with patients to support and informed consent. Furthermore, clinicians should continue diligent monitoring of patients who have been treated with paclitaxel-coated balloons and paclitaxel-eluting stents. Additional analyses of randomized trials and registry datasets are being planned to provide further insight into the magnitude and potential causes of the late mortality risk.[75]

SUMMARY

Uncoated balloon angioplasty has limited procedural success and poor long-term patency in most lesions. DES and DCB devices have shown superiority over uncoated PTA in terms of patency and clinically driven TLR. Adjunctive therapies such as atherectomy are available for lesion preparation in complex and calcified lesions. Prevention of long-term restenosis and management of complex CTOs and ISR lesions remains an ongoing challenge. Recent controversy regarding a potential increase in late mortality associated with paclitaxel-coated devices has brought attention to the importance of quality trial data.

DISCLOSURE

The authors have no disclosures.

REFERENCES

1. Fowkes FG, Rudan D, Rudan I, et al. Comparison of global estimates of prevalence and risk factors for peripheral artery disease in 2000 and 2010: a systematic review and analysis. Lancet 2013; 382(9901):1329–40.
2. Sampson UK, Fowkes FG, McDermott MM, et al. Global and regional burden of death and disability from peripheral artery disease: 21 world regions, 1990 to 2010. Glob Heart 2014;9(1):145–58.e21.
3. Olin JW, White CJ, Armstrong EJ, et al. Peripheral artery disease: evolving role of exercise, medical therapy, and endovascular options. J Am Coll Cardiol 2016;67(11):1338–57.
4. Gerhard-Herman MD, Gornik HL, Barrett C, et al. 2016 AHA/ACC guideline on the management of patients with lower extremity peripheral artery disease: executive summary: a report of the American College of Cardiology/American Heart Association Task Force on clinical practice guidelines. J Am Coll Cardiol 2017;69(11):1465–508.
5. Aboyans V, Ricco JB, Bartelink MEL, et al. 2017 ESC guidelines on the diagnosis and treatment of peripheral arterial diseases, in collaboration with the European Society for Vascular Surgery (ESVS): document covering atherosclerotic disease of extracranial carotid and vertebral, mesenteric, renal, upper and lower extremity arteries endorsed by: the European Stroke Organization (ESO)The Task Force for the Diagnosis and Treatment of Peripheral Arterial Diseases of the European Society of Cardiology (ESC) and of the European Society for Vascular Surgery (ESVS). Eur Heart J 2018; 39(9):763–816.
6. Murphy TP, Cutlip DE, Regensteiner JG, et al. Supervised exercise versus primary stenting for claudication resulting from aortoiliac peripheral artery disease: six-month outcomes from the claudication: exercise versus endoluminal revascularization (CLEVER) study. Circulation 2012;125(1):130–9.
7. Murphy TP, Cutlip DE, Regensteiner JG, et al. Supervised exercise, stent revascularization, or medical therapy for claudication due to aortoiliac peripheral artery disease: the CLEVER study. J Am Coll Cardiol 2015;65(10):999–1009.
8. Fakhry F, Spronk S, van der Laan L, et al. Endovascular revascularization and supervised exercise for peripheral artery disease and intermittent claudication: a randomized clinical trial. JAMA 2015;314(18): 1936–44.
9. Saratzis A, Paraskevopoulos I, Patel S, et al. Supervised exercise therapy and revascularization for intermittent claudication: network meta-analysis of randomized controlled trials. JACC Cardiovasc Interv 2019;12(12):1125–36.
10. Feldman DN, Armstrong EJ, Aronow HD, et al. SCAI consensus guidelines for device selection in femoral-popliteal arterial interventions. Catheter Cardiovasc Interv 2018;92(1):124–40.
11. Shishehbor MH, Jaff MR. Percutaneous therapies for peripheral artery disease. Circulation 2016; 134(24):2008–27.
12. Jaff MR, White CJ, Hiatt WR, et al. An update on methods for revascularization and expansion of the TASC lesion classification to include below-the-knee arteries: a supplement to the inter-society consensus for the management of peripheral arterial disease (TASC II): the TASC steering committee. Ann Vasc Dis 2015;8(4):343–57.
13. Norgren L, Hiatt WR, Dormandy JA, et al. Inter-society consensus for the management of peripheral arterial disease (TASC II). J Vasc Surg 2007; 45(Suppl S):S5–67.
14. Bosiers M, Peeters P, Tessarek J, et al, Single-Arm Study Investigators. The Zilver(R) PTX(R) single arm study: 12-month results from the TASC C/D lesion subgroup. J Cardiovasc Surg (Torino) 2013; 54(1):115–22.

15. Kang JL, Patel VI, Conrad MF, et al. Common femoral artery occlusive disease: contemporary results following surgical endarterectomy. J Vasc Surg 2008;48(4):872–7.

16. Siracuse JJ, Van Orden K, Kalish JA, et al. Endovascular treatment of the common femoral artery in the vascular quality initiative. J Vasc Surg 2017; 65(4):1039–46.

17. Goueffic Y, Della Schiava N, Thaveau F, et al. Stenting or surgery for De Novo common femoral artery stenosis. JACC Cardiovasc Interv 2017; 10(13):1344–54.

18. Nguyen BN, Amdur RL, Abugideiri M, et al. Postoperative complications after common femoral endarterectomy. J Vasc Surg 2015; 61(6):1489–94.e1.

19. Clark TW, Groffsky JL, Soulen MC. Predictors of long-term patency after femoropopliteal angioplasty: results from the STAR registry. J Vasc Interv Radiol 2001;12(8):923–33.

20. Nguyen BN, Conrad MF, Guest JM, et al. Late outcomes of balloon angioplasty and angioplasty with selective stenting for superficial femoral-popliteal disease are equivalent. J Vasc Surg 2011;54(4): 1051–7.e1.

21. Dick P, Sabeti S, Mlekusch W, et al. Conventional balloon angioplasty versus peripheral cutting balloon angioplasty for treatment of femoropopliteal artery in-stent restenosis: initial experience. Radiology 2008;248(1):297–302.

22. Poncyljusz W, Falkowski A, Safranow K, et al. Cutting-balloon angioplasty versus balloon angioplasty as treatment for short atherosclerotic lesions in the superficial femoral artery: randomized controlled trial. Cardiovasc Intervent Radiol 2013; 36(6):1500–7.

23. Chowdhury MM, McLain AD, Twine CP. Angioplasty versus bare metal stenting for superficial femoral artery lesions. Cochrane Database Syst Rev 2014;(6):CD006767.

24. Krankenberg H, Schluter M, Steinkamp HJ, et al. Nitinol stent implantation versus percutaneous transluminal angioplasty in superficial femoral artery lesions up to 10 cm in length: the femoral artery stenting trial (FAST). Circulation 2007;116(3):285–92.

25. Iida O, Yokoi H, Soga Y, et al. Cilostazol reduces angiographic restenosis after endovascular therapy for femoropopliteal lesions in the sufficient treatment of peripheral intervention by cilostazol study. Circulation 2013;127(23):2307–15.

26. Duda SH, Bosiers M, Lammer J, et al. Drug-eluting and bare nitinol stents for the treatment of atherosclerotic lesions in the superficial femoral artery: long-term results from the SIROCCO trial. J Endovasc Ther 2006;13(6):701–10.

27. Dake MD, Ansel GM, Jaff MR, et al. Durable clinical effectiveness with paclitaxel-eluting stents in the femoropopliteal artery: 5-year results of the zilver PTX randomized trial. Circulation 2016;133(15): 1472–83 [discussion: 1483].

28. Dake MD, Scheinert D, Tepe G, et al. Nitinol stents with polymer-free paclitaxel coating for lesions in the superficial femoral and popliteal arteries above the knee: twelve-month safety and effectiveness results from the Zilver PTX single-arm clinical study. J Endovasc Ther 2011;18(5):613–23.

29. Dake MD, Ansel GM, Jaff MR, et al. Sustained safety and effectiveness of paclitaxel-eluting stents for femoropopliteal lesions: 2-year follow-up from the Zilver PTX randomized and single-arm clinical studies. J Am Coll Cardiol 2013; 61(24):2417–27.

30. Zeller T, Dake MD, Tepe G, et al. Treatment of femoropopliteal in-stent restenosis with paclitaxel-eluting stents. JACC Cardiovasc Interv 2013;6(3): 274–81.

31. Iida O, Takahara M, Soga Y, et al. 1-year results of the ZEPHYR registry (zilver PTX for the femoral artery and proximal popliteal artery): predictors of restenosis. JACC Cardiovasc Interv 2015;8(8): 1105–12.

32. Kichikawa K, Ichihashi S, Yokoi H, et al. Zilver PTX post-market surveillance study of paclitaxel-eluting stents for treating femoropopliteal artery disease in Japan: 2-year results. Cardiovasc Intervent Radiol 2019;42(3):358–64.

33. Gray WA, Keirse K, Soga Y, et al. A polymer-coated, paclitaxel-eluting stent (Eluvia) versus a polymer-free, paclitaxel-coated stent (Zilver PTX) for endovascular femoropopliteal intervention (IMPERIAL): a randomised, non-inferiority trial. Lancet 2018;392(10157):1541–51.

34. Bausback Y, Wittig T, Schmidt A, et al. Drug-eluting stent versus drug-coated balloon revascularization in patients with femoropopliteal arterial disease. J Am Coll Cardiol 2019;73(6):667–79.

35. Tepe G, Zeller T, Albrecht T, et al. Local delivery of paclitaxel to inhibit restenosis during angioplasty of the leg. N Engl J Med 2008;358(7):689–99.

36. Werk M, Langner S, Reinkensmeier B, et al. Inhibition of restenosis in femoropopliteal arteries: paclitaxel-coated versus uncoated balloon: femoral paclitaxel randomized pilot trial. Circulation 2008; 118(13):1358–65.

37. Giacoppo D, Cassese S, Harada Y, et al. Drug-coated balloon versus plain balloon angioplasty for the treatment of femoropopliteal artery disease: an updated systematic review and meta-analysis of randomized clinical trials. JACC Cardiovasc Interv 2016;9(16):1731–42.

38. Scheinert D, Duda S, Zeller T, et al. The LEVANT I (Lutonix paclitaxel-coated balloon for the prevention of femoropopliteal restenosis) trial for femoropopliteal revascularization: first-in-human

randomized trial of low-dose drug-coated balloon versus uncoated balloon angioplasty. JACC Cardiovasc Interv 2014;7(1):10–9.

39. Rosenfield K, Jaff MR, White CJ, et al. Trial of a paclitaxel-coated balloon for femoropopliteal artery disease. N Engl J Med 2015;373(2):145–53.

40. Tepe G, Laird J, Schneider P, et al. Drug-coated balloon versus standard percutaneous transluminal angioplasty for the treatment of superficial femoral and popliteal peripheral artery disease: 12-month results from the IN.PACT SFA randomized trial. Circulation 2015;131(5):495–502.

41. Krishnan P, Faries P, Niazi K, et al. Stellarex drug-coated balloon for treatment of femoropopliteal disease: twelve-month outcomes from the randomized ILLUMENATE pivotal and pharmacokinetic studies. Circulation 2017;136(12):1102–13.

42. Ott I, Cassese S, Groha P, et al. ISAR-PEBIS (paclitaxel-eluting balloon versus conventional balloon angioplasty for in-stent restenosis of superficial femoral artery): a randomized trial. J Am Heart Assoc 2017;6(7) [pii:e006321].

43. Schmidt A, Piorkowski M, Gorner H, et al. Drug-coated balloons for complex femoropopliteal lesions: 2-year results of a real-world registry. JACC Cardiovasc Interv 2016;9(7):715–24.

44. Katsanos K, Spiliopoulos S, Kitrou P, et al. Risk of death following application of paclitaxel-coated balloons and stents in the femoropopliteal artery of the leg: a systematic review and meta-analysis of randomized controlled trials. J Am Heart Assoc 2018;7(24):e011245.

45. Lammer J, Zeller T, Hausegger KA, et al. Sustained benefit at 2 years for covered stents versus bare-metal stents in long SFA lesions: the VIASTAR trial. Cardiovasc Intervent Radiol 2015;38(1):25–32.

46. Geraghty PJ, Mewissen MW, Jaff MR, et al, VIBRANT Investigators. Three-year results of the VIBRANT trial of VIABAHN endoprosthesis versus bare nitinol stent implantation for complex superficial femoral artery occlusive disease. J Vasc Surg 2013;58(2):386–95.e4.

47. Bosiers M, Deloose K, Callaert J, et al. Superiority of stent-grafts for in-stent restenosis in the superficial femoral artery: twelve-month results from a multicenter randomized trial. J Endovasc Ther 2015;22(1):1–10.

48. Gorgani F, Telis A, Narakathu N, et al. Long-term outcomes of the Viabahn stent in the treatment of in-stent restenosis in the superficial femoral artery. J Invasive Cardiol 2013;25(12):670–4.

49. Saxon RR, Chervu A, Jones PA, et al. Heparin-bonded, expanded polytetrafluoroethylene-lined stent graft in the treatment of femoropopliteal artery disease: 1-year results of the VIPER (Viabahn Endoprosthesis with Heparin Bioactive Surface in the Treatment of Superficial Femoral Artery Obstructive Disease) trial. J Vasc Interv Radiol 2013;24(2):165–73.

50. Bhat TM, Afari ME, Garcia LA. Atherectomy in peripheral artery disease: a review. J Invasive Cardiol 2017;29(4):135–44.

51. Ramkumar N, Martinez-Camblor P, Columbo JA, et al. Adverse events after atherectomy: analyzing long-term outcomes of endovascular lower extremity revascularization techniques. J Am Heart Assoc 2019;8(12):e012081.

52. Mehta M, Zhou Y, Paty PS, et al. Percutaneous common femoral artery interventions using angioplasty, atherectomy, and stenting. J Vasc Surg 2016;64(2):369–79.

53. McKinsey JF, Zeller T, Rocha-Singh KJ, et al, DEFINITIVE LE Investigators. Lower extremity revascularization using directional atherectomy: 12-month prospective results of the DEFINITIVE LE study. JACC Cardiovasc Interv 2014;7(8):923–33.

54. Zeller T, Langhoff R, Rocha-Singh KJ, et al. Directional atherectomy followed by a paclitaxel-coated balloon to inhibit restenosis and maintain vessel patency: twelve-month results of the DEFINITIVE AR study. Circ Cardiovasc Interv 2017;10(9). https://doi.org/10.1161/CIRCINTERVENTIONS.116.004848.

55. Trentmann J, Charalambous N, Djawanscher M, et al. Safety and efficacy of directional atherectomy for the treatment of in-stent restenosis of the femoropopliteal artery. J Cardiovasc Surg (Torino) 2010;51(4):551–60.

56. Safian RD, Niazi K, Runyon JP, et al. Orbital atherectomy for infrapopliteal disease: device concept and outcome data for the OASIS trial. Catheter Cardiovasc Interv 2009;73(3):406–12.

57. Dattilo R, Himmelstein SI, Cuff RF. The COMPLIANCE 360 degrees trial: a randomized, prospective, multicenter, pilot study comparing acute and long-term results of orbital atherectomy to balloon angioplasty for calcified femoropopliteal disease. J Invasive Cardiol 2014;26(8):355–60.

58. Shammas NW, Lam R, Mustapha J, et al. Comparison of orbital atherectomy plus balloon angioplasty vs. balloon angioplasty alone in patients with critical limb ischemia: results of the CALCIUM 360 randomized pilot trial. J Endovasc Ther 2012;19(4):480–8.

59. Beschorner U, Krankenberg H, Scheinert D, et al. Rotational and aspiration atherectomy for infrainguinal in-stent restenosis. Vasa 2013;42(2):127–33.

60. Shammas NW, Shammas GA, Banerjee S, et al. Jet-Stream rotational and aspiration atherectomy in treating in-stent restenosis of the femoropopliteal arteries: results of the JETSTREAM feasibility study. J Endovasc Ther 2016;23:339–46.

61. Zeller T, Krankenberg H, Steinkamp H, et al. One-year outcome of percutaneous rotational atherectomy

with aspiration in infrainguinal peripheral arterial occlusive disease: the multicenter Pathway PVD trial. J Endovasc Ther 2009;16(6):653–62.

62. Davis T, Ramaiah V, Niazi K, et al. Safety and effectiveness of the Phoenix Atherectomy System in lower extremity arteries: early and midterm outcomes from the prospective multicenter EASE study. Vascular 2017;25(6):563–75.

63. Scheinert D, Laird JR Jr, Schroder M, et al. Excimer laser-assisted recanalization of long, chronic superficial femoral artery occlusions. J Endovasc Ther 2001;8(2):156–66.

64. Laird JR, Zeller T, Gray BH, et al. Limb salvage following laser-assisted angioplasty for critical limb ischemia: results of the LACI multicenter trial. J Endovasc Ther 2006;13(1):1–11.

65. Dippel EJ, Makam P, Kovach R, et al. Randomized controlled study of excimer laser atherectomy for treatment of femoropopliteal in-stent restenosis: initial results from the EXCITE ISR trial (EXCImer Laser Randomized Controlled Study for Treatment of FemoropopliTEal In-Stent Restenosis). JACC Cardiovasc Interv 2015;8(1 Pt A):92–101.

66. Gandini R, Del Giudice C, Merolla S, et al. Treatment of chronic SFA in-stent occlusion with combined laser atherectomy and drug-eluting balloon angioplasty in patients with critical limb ischemia: a single-center, prospective, randomized study. J Endovasc Ther 2013;20(6):805–14.

67. Photoablative atherectomy followed by a paclitaxel-coated balloon to inhibit restenosis in instent femoro-popliteal obstructions (PHOTO-PAC). Available at: https://clinicaltrials.gov/ct2/show/NCT01298947. Accessed August 27, 2019.

68. Hioki H, Miyashita Y, Miura T, et al. Diagnostic value of peripheral fractional flow reserve in isolated iliac artery stenosis: a comparison with the post-exercise ankle-brachial index. J Endovasc Ther 2014;21(5):625–32.

69. Therasse E, Donath D, Elkouri S, et al. Results of a randomized clinical trial of external beam radiation to prevent restenosis after superficial femoral artery stenting. J Vasc Surg 2016;63(6):1531–40.

70. Wolfram RM, Budinsky AC, Pokrajac B, et al. Endovascular brachytherapy for prophylaxis of restenosis after femoropopliteal angioplasty: five-year follow-up–prospective randomized study. Radiology 2006;240(3):878–84.

71. Banerjee S, Das TS, Abu-Fadel MS, et al. Pilot trial of cryoplasty or conventional balloon post-dilation of nitinol stents for revascularization of peripheral arterial segments: the COBRA trial. J Am Coll Cardiol 2012;60(15):1352–9.

72. Brodmann M, Werner M, Holden A, et al. Primary outcomes and mechanism of action of intravascular lithotripsy in calcified, femoropopliteal lesions: results of Disrupt PAD II. Catheter Cardiovasc Interv 2019;93(2):335–42.

73. BASIL-3 and SWEDEPAD trials paused for review of paclitaxel meta-analysis data. Interventional News; 2019. Available at: https://www.fda.gov/medical-devices/letters-health-care-providers/treatment-peripheral-arterial-disease-paclitaxel-coated-balloons-and-paclitaxel-eluting-stents. Accessed August 27, 2019.

74. Secemsky EA, Kundi H, Weinberg I, et al. Drug-eluting stent implantation and long-term survival following peripheral artery revascularization. J Am Coll Cardiol 2019;73(20):2636–8.

75. Treatment of peripheral arterial disease with paclitaxel-coated balloons and paclitaxel-eluting stents potentially associated with increased mortality - letter to health care providers. U.S. Food and Drug Administration; 2019. Available at: https://www.fda.gov/medical-devices/letters-health-care-providers/august-7-2019-update-treatment-peripheral-arterial-disease-paclitaxel-coated-balloons-and-paclitaxel. Accessed August 27, 2019.

Diagnostic and Therapeutic Approaches in the Management of Infrapopliteal Arterial Disease

Larry J. Díaz-Sandoval, MD[a,b],*

KEYWORDS

- Infrapopliteal • Chronic limb threatening ischemia (CLTI) • Ultrasound-guided access (access)
- Tibiopedal arterial minimally invasive retrograde revascularization (TAMI)
- Cap morphology (CTOP classification) • Angiosome directed therapy (ADT)
- Endovascular therapy (EVT) • Deep venous arterialization (DVA)

KEY POINTS

- The updated 2015 Inter-Society Consensus for the Management of Peripheral Arterial Disease document includes an anatomic classification for multivessel infrapopliteal atherosclerotic disease.
- Traditionally used noninvasive limb hemodynamics should be cautiously interpreted in patients with chronic limb-threatening ischemia, because they underestimate the severity of disease.
- An analysis of the cap morphology is easily reproducible and useful to plan access strategy and treatment approach of chronic total occlusions.
- CO2 angiography and duplex ultrasound allow significant decreases in contrast and radiation exposure, making it feasible to safely treat chronic limb-threatening ischemia patients with chronic kidney disease.
- The establishment of direct flow to the affected angiosome and drug-eluting stents are the most efficient therapies for infrapopliteal lesions in patients with chronic limb-threatening ischemia.

INTRODUCTION

Chronic limb-threatening ischemia (CLTI) is the most severe clinical presentation of peripheral artery disease (PAD), and its increasing incidence make it a global health concern.[1,2] CLTI has a prevalence between 1% and 2%, and as high as 11% among patients with known PAD. In the United States, among insured adults, the annual incidence of PAD and CLTI are 2.35% and 0.35%, and the prevalence is 10.69% and 1.33% respectively.[3] Over a 5-year period, 5% to 10% of patients with asymptomatic PAD or intermittent claudication will progress to CLTI.[4] Such

progression has been independently associated with advanced age, smoking, diabetes mellitus, and chronic kidney disease.[3,5] CLTI can also be caused by thromboembolism, Buerger's disease, trauma, dissection, vasculitis, fibromuscular dysplasia, entrapment syndromes, and cystic adventitial disease.[6] Patients with CLTI have a high risk of death and myocardial infarction; 20% die within 6 months and 50% within 5 years of their diagnosis. Mortality rates for patients with nonrevascularizable CLTI are even higher.[7]

CLTI is characterized by chronic ischemic rest pain or tissue loss. Given its poor prognosis with conservative management, intervention is

[a] Department of Medicine, Michigan State University, East Lansing, MI, USA; [b] Metro Health-University of Michigan Health, Grand Rapids, MI, USA
* Metro Health-University of Michigan Health Professional Building, 2122 Health Drive Southwest, Wyoming, MI 49519.
E-mail address: larry.diaz@metrogr.org

Intervent Cardiol Clin 9 (2020) 207–220
https://doi.org/10.1016/j.iccl.2019.12.006
2211-7458/20/© 2020 Elsevier Inc. All rights reserved.

typically required.[8] Anatomically, CLTI is typically characterized by multilevel (aortoiliac, femoropopliteal [FP], and infrapopliteal [IP]) disease, and more than 1 tibial artery is usually involved.[9–12] Infrainguinal PAD presents as isolated IP disease (approximately 33%) or combined FP and IP disease (approximately 67%).[13–17] Isolated IP disease is mainly seen in the elderly (>80 years old), diabetic patients, or patients with chronic kidney disease.[15] The diseased IP arteries are of relatively small caliber, often calcified, and associated with diffuse, multivessel stenoses and occlusions.[18] Isolated IP disease, is associated with a higher risk of amputation and a shorter amputation-free survival compared with combined FP and IP disease (median amputation-free survival, 17 months vs 37 months; $P = .001$).[16]

DIAGNOSTIC EVALUATION

The diagnosis of CLTI is routinely based on clinical symptoms, and traditionally confirmed by noninvasive limb hemodynamics such as the ankle–brachial index (ABI), toe–brachial index, and toe pressure.[19] ABI or toe–brachial index increases of more than 0.15 after mechanical therapy have been deemed as evidence of hemodynamic success in CLTI.[19] However, recent studies have shown that nearly one-third of patients with IP disease, rest pain, and tissue loss may present with a normal or mildly decreased ABI at baseline.[19,20] Another study of patients with CLTI with angiographically proven isolated IP disease showed that only 6% of patients had an ABI of less than 0.4, and 16% had an abnormal ankle pressure. Among patients with normal toe pressures, 29% had normal ABIs.[21] Emerging modalities such as skin perfusion pressure, transcutaneous oxygen pressure, fluorescent angiography, and subcutaneous oxygen microsensors may prove useful in the diagnosis and prognosis of patients with CLTI.[19]

Other noninvasive modalities include contrast-enhanced magnetic resonance angiography, and high-frequency duplex ultrasound (DUS) examination,[8,22] as well as digital subtraction angiography. The optimal preprocedural modality should be patient centered and largely depends on local expertise. The small caliber IP outflow vessels are best depicted by either time-resolved contrast-enhanced magnetic resonance angiography or super-selective digital subtraction angiography with the catheter positioned just above the IP trifurcation[22–24] (Fig. 1).

DUS results are operator dependent and, although the IP arterial evaluation is compromised by inflow occlusions, obesity, and calcifications, it can be useful in assessing pedal artery morphology, patency, and physiology.[25] In patients with advanced chronic kidney disease, intravenous administration of iodine contrast agents can cause contrast-induced nephropathy, and gadolinium may cause nephrogenic systemic fibrosis.[26] In an effort to decrease contrast-induced nephropathy and allergic reactions, carbon dioxide (CO_2) has been studied as a contrast agent during invasive procedures in the lower limbs. Minor complications from CO_2 angiography and interventions include leg pain, abdominal pain, diarrhea, and even rare lethal complications (nonobstructive mesenteric ischemia). A recent study compared the safety and efficacy of CO_2 and iodinated contrast in the angiographic evaluation of PAD patients using an automated CO_2 injector with selective and super-selective injections, showing that CO_2 was safe and efficacious for diagnostic purposes.[27] More recently, automated CO_2 angiography was used in patients with CLTI, showing that this modality was safe and efficacious in providing high-quality images of the IP and pedal circulation during diagnostic and therapeutic procedures[28] (Fig. 2).

PROCEDURAL PLANNING

Pretreatment imaging is intended to delineate the status of the inflow and IP vessels, pedal loops and arches, to plan access site and interventional approach. Newly described protocols to evaluate the pedal circulation, by measuring the pedal acceleration time with DUS,[29] have been introduced, and shown to be effective with even prognostic implications (Fig. 3). Most IP revascularization procedures should ideally be performed via antegrade ipsilateral access, because the ability to deliver coaxial force in a unilinear vector increases the likelihood of successful crossing of long, complex chronic total occlusions (CTOs). Antegrade access also provides the ability to perform distal injections to accurately assess the pedal vessels, and provides the ability to treat inframalleolar vessels in the event of embolization, dissection, or other distal complications. This access strategy should be combined with retrograde tibiopedal access when the CTO cap analysis indicates retrograde concavity of the distal cap. Optimal preprocedural imaging should identify the severity and length of the IP lesions, provide detailed information about collaterals (for transcollateral approaches), the distal pedal vasculature, the distal reconstitution of target vessels, and the status of the pedal arch.

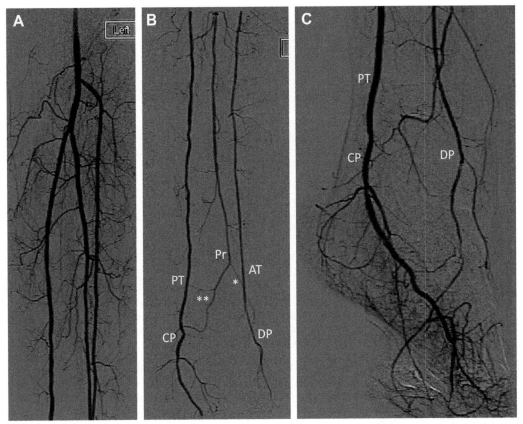

Fig. 1. Tibial- pedal DSA. (*A*) There is excellent opacification of the 3 major tibial arteries in their proximal and mid segments. (*B*) The AT and PT are seen in the mid and distal thirds of the leg, as well as their continuation as Dorsalis Pedis and Common Plantar branches beyond the ankle joint. The Peroneal (P) is seen tapering in the distal third of the leg and ends in a bifurcation that provides the ACA (*) and PCA (**) to the AT and PT respectively. (*C*) The PT provides the Common Plantar (CP) which in this example is the dominant pedal vessel. The DP is small. Further distally the tarsal and digital branches are seen.

THERAPEUTIC APPROACHES

Angiosome-directed therapy is the establishment of flow to the topographic area of the foot where the wound is located. To obtain procedural, technical, and clinical success, the IP vessel that feeds the ischemic angiosome should be the interventional target.

An angiosome is a 3-dimensional anatomic unit of tissue (consisting of skin, subcutaneous tissue, fascia, muscle, and bone) fed by a source artery and drained by specific veins. The foot and ankle angiosome is a topographic map conformed by 5 territories provided by 3 main arteries and their branches:

- The posterior tibial artery provides 3 angiosomes:
  The medial calcaneal (medial plantar aspect of the heel); the medial plantar and lateral plantar (supply the corresponding plantar surfaces).

- The peroneal artery provides 1 angiosome:
  The lateral calcaneal (lateral aspect of the heel and ankle)
- The anterior tibial artery provides 1 angiosome:
  The dorsalis pedis angiosome (supplying the dorsum of the foot) and anterior aspect of the ankle.

Angiosome-directed therapy can be achieved via direct flow (DF: in-line, pulsatile flow through the affected angiosome source artery), or indirect flow (IF: strategy whereby flow to the wound area is provided by collaterals fed by an arterial conduit that is revascularized in a neighboring angiosome), when DF is not considered technically feasible.

A prospective study compared the DF and IF strategies in 64 patients with CLTI with single-vessel runoff to the foot. Ulcer healing at 1, 3, and 6 months was superior with DF than with IF. However, there was no statistically significant

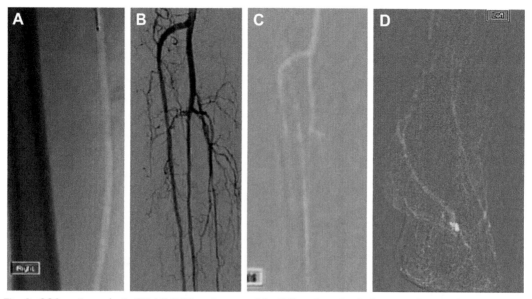

Fig. 2. CO2 angiography in CLI. (*A*) CO2 angiogram of the SFA and popliteal, showing adequate filling. (*B*) Iodinated contrast angiogram, showing well defined tibial anatomy. (*C*) CO2 angiogram of the same tibial arteries shown in Figure 4B. Note the significant difference in visualization. CO2 angiography is inferior. (*D*) CO2 pedal angiogram indicating flow in the pedal circulation.

difference in the limb salvage rate (LSR).[30] The latest prospective study in the subject enrolled 167 diabetic patients with CLTI and recorded interventions in 194 limbs. Wound healing in diabetic patients with CLTI seemed to be improved by intentional angiosome-oriented wound-targeted revascularization (DF), but no uniform benefit concerning major adverse limb events or limb preservation was observed. The

authors concluded that IF still represents an alternative for limb salvage in cases in which angiosome-guided revascularization (DF) fails.[31] One of the most significant hurdles in the real world is that DF to the ischemic angiosome may not be attainable in a large number of patients with CLTI. Berceli and colleagues[32] reported on the efficacy of dorsalis pedis bypass for ischemic forefoot and heel ulcerations.

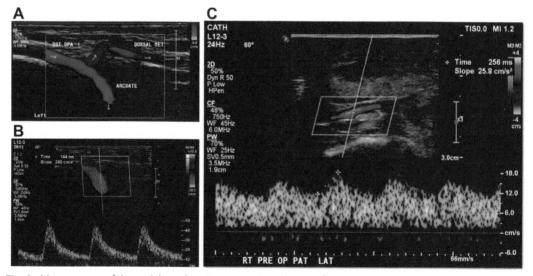

Fig. 3. Measurement of the pedal acceleration time. (*A*) Evaluation of the distal DP bifurcation, providing the dorsal metatarsal and the arcuate arteries. (*B*) Velocities in the Arcuate artery. (*C*) Evaluation of the Plantar Lateral. (*Images courtesy of* Jill Sommerset, RVT.)

According to the angiosome concept and this strategy, the forefoot would receive DF, whereas the heel would be perfused via IF. They achieved an LSR of 86%, indicating that heel ulcerations can heel with IF, even in the absence of an intact pedal arch, presumably through interangiosome connections for perfusion. As new techniques are being developed and carried into practice (US-guided tibial–pedal access and interventions, transcollateral tibial interventions, digital and transmetatarsal artery access and interventions), it seems that our ability to intervene in these complex patients[33,34] will continue to improve.

ANATOMIC CONSIDERATIONS

The updated 2015 Inter-Society Consensus for the Management of Peripheral Arterial Disease document[35] includes, for the first time, an anatomic classification for IP atherosclerotic disease, which attempts to address the multivessel component of the IP disease process typical of patients with CLTI. The occlusion of a single tibial artery rarely leads to clinical signs or symptoms. Thus, a clinically significant decrease in distal arterial perfusion, generally requires multilevel (aortoiliac and/or FP, in addition to the IP component) and multivessel involvement, which could result from the concurrence of multiple anatomic patterns of arterial lesions or occlusions. **Figs. 4** and **5** show tibial CTOs and common patterns of distal reconstitution.

CLINICAL CONSIDERATIONS

Asymptomatic patients with IP disease and those without clinical evidence of CLTI should not undergo revascularization to prevent CLTI, because the rate of progression to CLTI and/or amputation remains relatively low.[6,36–38] Patients with IP disease and claudication should ideally be treated with cilostazol, a supervised exercise program, and guideline-directed medical therapy before revascularization is considered. The most recent American College of Cardiology/American Heart Association guidelines emphasize that "the usefulness of endovascular procedures as a revascularization option for patients with claudication due to isolated IP artery disease is unknown."[6] Therefore, IP EVT is generally reserved for patients with CLTI. For patients with claudication and IP disease who are intolerant of medical therapy or continue to have symptoms despite maximal tolerated doses of guideline-recommended therapy, only those with greater than 50% diameter stenosis by angiography and multivessel tibial disease (≥2 tibial vessels) should be considered for revascularization.[13]

The primary goal of IP endovascular therapy (EVT) is to obtain relief from ischemic rest pain,

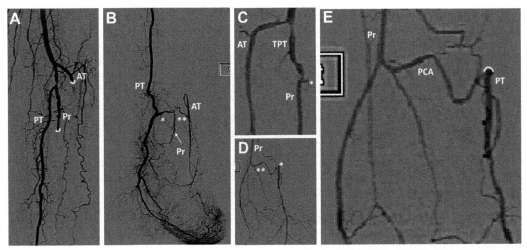

Fig. 4. Tibial CTOs. (*A*) AT and Peroneal (Pr) CTO, with high grade stenosis of the ostium of the PT. Notice the antegrade concavity of the occlusions in the AT and Pr. (*B*) Distal reconstitution of the AT via the Anterior communicating artery (**). The PT provides retrograde flow to the distal peroneal reconstitution via the Posterior Communicating Artery (*). (*C*) Severe disease of the TPT with ostial occlusion of the PT (*). (*D*) Distal reconstitution of the PT (*) via the Posterior communicating artery (PCA: **) from the Peroneal (Pr). (*E*) Zoomed image of the distal PT reconstitution via the Posterior Communicating Artery (PCA) from the Peroneal (Pfr). Notice the retrograde concave cap.

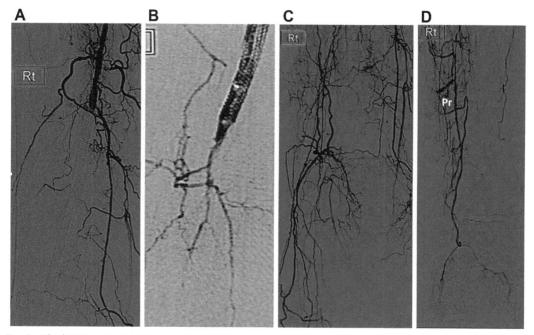

Fig. 5. Tibial CTOs. (*A*) Mid SFA occlusion. (*B*) P1 segment of the Popliteal is occluded after crossing the mid SFA occlusion. Angiography reveals no reconstitution. (*C*) Only collateral vessels are seen in the proximal and mid segments of the infrapopliteal segment. (*D*) Faint distal reconstitution of the Peroneal (Pr) via collaterals.

facilitate healing of ulcers or gangrene, prevent limb loss or limit the extent of amputation, and permit wound healing after any type of amputation. There has been an evolution in the treatment of IP disease. A vast body of literature exists pertaining to the surgical treatment of IP disease, primarily using the greater saphenous vein as a conduit, with various operative techniques. The use of spliced grafts, allograft material, or prosthetic material such as polytetrafluoroethylene, are considered less than ideal.[19] The PREVENT III trial[39] did provide outcomes for surgical bypass in the setting of a randomized multicenter clinical study of edifoligide, with 1404 patients with CLTI who underwent bypass: 65% had a distal anastomosis at the tibial or pedal arteries.[39] The 1-year primary patency rate was 61%, with 83.8% survival, and 88.5% LSR. Unfortunately, there is major mortality and morbidity associated with surgical bypass to treat IP disease in patients with CLTI, as shown in BASIL[17] and PREVENT III[39] (although these trials included patients with infrainguinal rather than isolated IP disease). Mortality occurred in 5.5% and 2.7% of patients, myocardial infarction in 7.0% and 4.7% of patients, stroke in 1.5% and 1.4% of patients, and surgical wound complications in 22.0% and 4.8% of patients in the BASIL and PREVENT III trials, respectively.

In comparison, a Japanese registry reported data describing risk adjusted 1-year outcomes for endovascular procedures in patients with CLTI.[40] This prospective multicenter study found that heart failure, wound infections, and underweight status (body mass index of <18.5 kg/m^2), increased the risk for a worse outcome, including a lower amputation-free survival rate.[40] At 3 years, the predictors of worse outcomes were body mass index of less than 18.5 kg/m^2, need for hemodialysis, and a Rutherford classification of 6 at baseline.[41]

Barshes and colleagues[42] determined that EVT and surgical bypass with endovascular revision as needed were more effective and less costly than wound care with or without amputation if the initial wound healing rates were approximately 50% and approximately 70%, respectively. BEST-CLTI should provide insight into the relative cost effectiveness of an endovascular versus surgery-first strategy.[43]

TECHNICAL CONSIDERATIONS

The endovascular-first proposal has gained traction since the publication of BASIL.[17] The adoption of this method has led to development of novel arterial access strategies, characterization of lesion morphology, and therapeutic approaches.

Ultrasound-Guided Versus Fluoroscopy-Guided Access

In a study to determine the safety and efficacy of using US guidance as the sole modality to obtain common femoral artery and tibial–pedal access among 86 patients with CLTI, US-guided access was successful in 95.3% of cases, including all in which tibial–pedal access was obtained (33.7%)[44] (Fig. 6).

These findings were validated in a cohort of 407 patients with CLTI in whom femoral and tibial–pedal access was obtained in 95% of cases.[45] In a large, multicenter, retrospective analysis of patients with CLTI, patients who exclusively underwent retrograde tibial–pedal access and intervention had a lower median fluoroscopy time, lower procedure time, shorter hospital stay, and lesser contrast volume than patients undergoing interventions via femoral or dual access (combined femoral and tibial–pedal),[46] suggesting that standalone retrograde arterial access or the use of tibial access as part of a preplanned dual access treatment strategy, is safe and efficacious for patients with advanced PAD and CLTI who have IP lesions[47] (Fig. 7).

Access Site Selection

Traditionally, IP endovascular interventions were approached via a contralateral femoral access. However, this strategy encounters failure rates of between 20% and 40% Consequently, operators have sought out alternative strategies, such as the use of a retrograde tibial–pedal access to approach CTOs from both above and below (dual access strategy).[48,49] The CTOP classification[50] has been developed to determine which access (accesses) is optimal and plan the treatment strategy. This classification was developed from a study of 114 patients with PAD and CLTI in whom morphology of CTO caps was analyzed by DUS examination and digital subtraction angiography. Lesions were then classified into 4 groups based on their respective morphology (Figs. 8 and 9).

In this study, CTO type I lesions were easiest and type IV were most difficult to cross in an antegrade fashion. The use of retrograde tibial–pedal access was beneficial for lesion lengths of greater than 10 cm, severe calcification, and CTO types II, III, and IV (80.3% of all lesions).[51]

Treatment Modalities
Balloon angioplasty

Percutaneous transluminal angioplasty (PTA) continues to represent the standard of care for IP EVT worldwide, even though outcomes remain suboptimal. Romiti and colleagues[52] reported the 3-year outcomes from a large meta-analysis where PTA was used as the primary treatment modality with an LSR of 82.4%. A

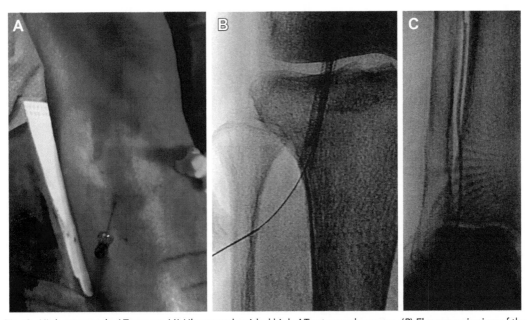

Fig. 6. High retrograde AT access. (*A*) Ultrasound-guided high AT retrograde access. (*B*) Fluoroscopic view of the retrograde access needle and a 0.018 wire to cross retrogradely into the P1 occlusion, and then into the antegrade catheter for "rendezvous" and access reversal. (*C*) Antegrade treatment of the AT into the foot.

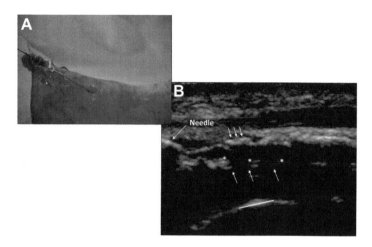

Fig. 7. Distal retrograde AT access. (A) Distal AT retrograde access. (B) US guided distal AT access: Arrows point to the arterial wall. The posterior wall of the artery is difficult to visualize due to drop out artifact (due to calcification). * * * shows the wire entering the vessel. The continuous line at the bottom of the picture is the bone landmark.

more recent meta-analysis of 3660 patients revealed that PTA in IP lesions results in inferior procedural and short-term outcomes relative to bare metal stents (BMS) and drug-eluting stents (DES).[46] The most recent of these meta-analyses included 6769 patients treated between 2005 and 2015 and concluded that PTA as primary treatment for IP disease leads to suboptimal procedural and 1-year outcomes.[53]

There has been an evolution of newer technologies, including drug-coated balloons (DCBs) and DES. In addition, several adjunctive endovascular devices, including atherectomy, cryoplasty, cutting balloons, laser, and most recently tack implants, bioabsorbable stents, and intravascular lithotripsy, which have demonstrated safety and efficiency when used in IP vessels. However, there are few comparative data demonstrating superior efficacy for these newer devices when compared with conventional, less expensive therapies. Given the associated cost of these newer devices, head-to-head studies comparing cost effectiveness are needed.[35]

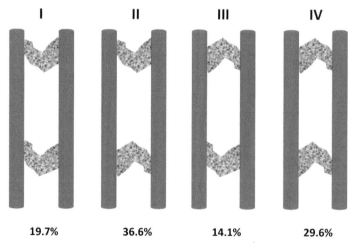

Fig. 8. CTOP classification. Type 1: Proximal and Distal caps have antegrade concavity: Proceed with traditional antegrade approach. Type 2: Proximal cap has antegrade concavity. Distal cap has retrograde concavity: Consider pre-planning dual access (antegrade ipsilateral CFA –or retrograde contralateral CFA if antegrade not feasible-) PLUS retrograde tibial-pedal access. Type 3: Proximal cap and distal cap are convex. This represents the most difficult subset of lesions. Consider pre-planning dual access (antegrade ipsilateral CFA –or retrograde contralateral CFA if antegrade not feasible-) PLUS retrograde tibial-pedal access. Type 4: Both the proximal and distal caps have a retrograde concavity. Consider performing retrograde tibial pedal access and TAMI technique. (From Saab F, Jaff MR, Diaz-Sandoval LJ, et al. Chronic Total Occlusion Crossing Approach BNased on Plaque Cap Morphology: The CTOP Classification. J Endovasc Ther 2018;25(3):284–291; with permission.)

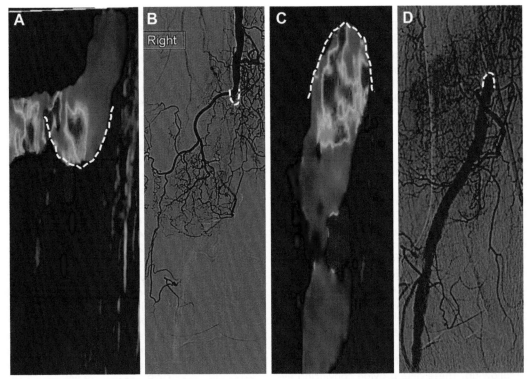

Fig. 9. CTOP type 2 CTO of the SFA. (*A*) Duplex ultrasound image of the proximal SFA cap with antegrade concavity. (*B*) Angiographic appearance of the proximal SFA cap with Critical Limb Ischemia CLI Diagnostics and Interventions HMP Communications

Bare metal stents

After BASIL,[17] the preferred endovascular approach for IP EVT was PTA with self-expanding nitinol BMS used as a bailout technique for dissections or suboptimal results. This strategy was then compared with primary stenting with a self-expanding BMS.[54] Ninety-two patients with IP PAD and severe claudication or CLTI were randomized 1:1 to either primary or provisional stenting with a self-expanding BMS. There was no difference in clinical improvement, freedom from TLR, mortality or amputation at 1 year between the groups.[54]

Drug-eluting stents

Data from 5 randomized, controlled rials[50,55–58] and several meta-analyses have provided robust evidence about the superiority of DES for IP disease, in comparison to PTA, BMS and DCBs.

The DESTINY[50] study randomized 140 patients with CLTI (Rutherford class 4 or 5 disease) with IP disease, comparing DES versus BMS (Xience V vs Multi-Link Vision; Abbott Laboratories, Abbott Park, IL). At the 1-year follow-up, there was no difference in functional outcomes and there were very few amputations. DES had superior patency (85% vs 54%;

$P = .0001$) and freedom from TLR (91% vs 66%; $P = .001$). The ACHILLES[55] trial randomized 200 patients with IP disease to DES (Cypher Select Sirolimus Eluting Stent, Cordis, Bridgewater, NJ) or PTA and found superior patency rates at 1 year for DES (75% vs 57.1%; $P = .025$). At 6 months, wound healing rates were superior with DES (95% vs 60%; $P = .048$), but at 1 year, the rates of complete wound closure were not statistically different. For patients with total lesion lengths of less than 120 mm, the 1-year restenosis rate for DES over PTA were 22.4% versus 41.9% ($P = .019$). This difference was more pronounced among diabetics (DES, 17.6% vs PTA, 53.2%; $P<.001$). There was no difference in mortality, amputation rates, or functional status. The YUKON-BTK[56] trial randomized 161 patients with severe claudication and CLTI to IP treatment with DES (Sirolimus eluting YUKON stent, Translumina, Hechingen, Germany) or BMS. Primary patency at 1 year was superior for DES (80.6% vs 55.6%; $P = .004$).

At 3 years of follow-up, event-free survival (65.8% vs 44.6%; $P = .02$), amputation (2.6% vs 12.2%; $P = .03$) and TLR rates (9.2% vs 20%; $P = .06$) were clearly superior for DES. The

IDEAS Randomized Controlled Trial[57] compared DES with a paclitaxel DCB (IN.PACT Amphirion, Medtronic, Brescia, Italy) in long (>70 mm) IP lesions in patients with Rutherford class 3 to 6 disease. Fifty patients were randomized to primary DES versus IP DCB PTA (DCB group). At 6 months, the angiographic restenosis rate was significantly lower in DES (28% vs 57.9%; $P = .046$). There were no significant differences in TLR (7.7% vs 13.6%; $P = .65$). In this comparison for longer IP lesions, DES were associated with significantly reduced restenosis rates at 6 months compared with DCB. The PADI trial[58] compared paclitaxel DES versus PTA-BMS in IP lesions of patients with CLTI. The 5-year follow-up data confirmed the long-term advantage of DES over PTA with provisional BMS (PTA-BMS) for patients with Rutherford classification 4 or higher disease with IP lesions. The 5-year clinical outcomes of amputation and event-free survival were superior for DES (amputation, 31.8% vs 20.4% [$P = .043$]; event-free survival, 26.2% vs 15.3% [$P = .041$]). Survival rates were comparable. The results showed higher patency rates after DES than after PTA-BMS at 1, 3, and 4 years of follow-up. These data provide convincing evidence (Class 1, LOE B) favoring IP DES over PTA and BMS for (1) improved patency, (2) reduced reinterventions, (3) reduced amputation, and (4) improved event-free survival.

Drug-coated balloons

The evidence supporting the use of DCB for IP lesions is less robust. The DEBATE-BTK[59] trial randomized 158 IP lesions in diabetic patients with CLTI from a single center to either DCB (In.Pact Amphirion, Medtronic, Minneapolis, MN) or PTA. The mean lesion length was significantly longer (approximately 100 mm) than those in the IP DES randomized trials. The primary end point (restenosis at 1 year) was significantly better for DCB (27% vs 74.3%; $P<.001$). The 12-month major adverse events occurred less frequently in the DCB group (31% vs 51%; $P = .02$). However, there was no difference in the rate of amputation, limb salvage, or mortality. The In.Pact Deep CLTI multicenter trial[60] prospectively enrolled 358 patients with CLTI with IP lesions and randomized them 2:1 to DCB versus PTA. The 12-month primary efficacy end points were not different between the groups. There was a nonsignificant trend toward higher amputation rates in the DCB group (8.8% vs 3.6%; $P = .08$). Novel devices and different platforms remain under investigation.

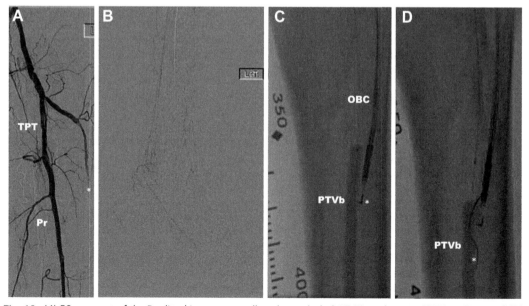

Fig. 10. (A) P3 segment of the Popliteal is seen, as well as the occluded AT (*), and patent TPT into Peroneal (Pr). The PT is occluded at the ostium, (B) "Desert Foot". (C) An antegrade Outback catheter has been advanced into the TPT and by US guidance, determined to be at the PT ostium. There is a balloon inflated in the Posterior Tibial Vein (accessed at the ankle) (PTVb). (D) The needle of the Outback is deployed into the balloon with contrast extravasation. The antegrade arterial wire is advanced into the retrograde balloon in the PT vein (which will act as a snare to retrieve the arterial wire out the venous sheath at the ankle).

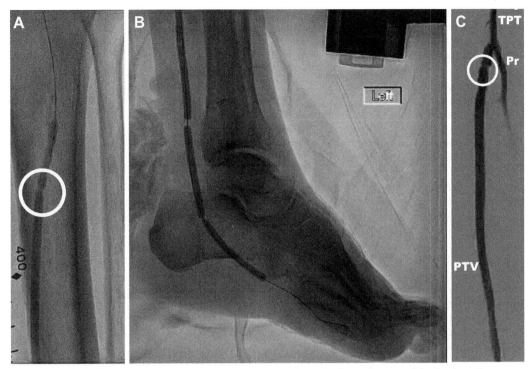

Fig. 11. (A) A balloon is inflated from the artery into the vein. The circle shows the area of the fistula with a "waist". (B) The Entire venous tract is dilated with a non-compliant balloon to perform "valvotomies". (C) Angiogram shows the TPT, Peroneal (Pr) and the PTV carrying arterial blood through the AV Fistula (Circle).

NEW FRONTIERS: INFRAMALLEOLAR ANGIOPLASTY AND DEEP VENOUS ARTERIALIZATION

The RENDEZVOUS registry studied 257 patients with IP and inframalleolar disease. All patients underwent IP EVT: 140 had adjunctive pedal artery angioplasty and 117 did not. The rate of wound healing was significantly higher (57.5% vs 37.3%; $P = .003$) and time to wound healing significantly shorter (211 days vs 365 days;

$P = .008$) in patients who received adjunctive inframalleolar PTA.[61]

Patients with CLTI who are considered to have no options typically present with a combination of small artery disease, diffuse arterial wall calcifications and the absence of patent pedal vessels (desert foot) leading to failure of revascularization attempts. For this unmet need, investigators have reported safety, feasibility, and promising results with the use of deep venous arterialization, a newly described

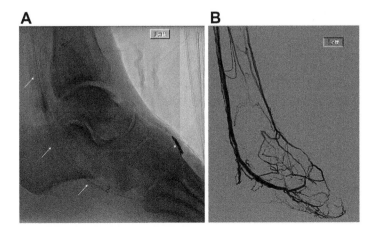

Fig. 12. (A) Viabhan stents are deployed in the venous conduit (Arrows) and Coils (*) deployed in venous branches to avoid "stealing". (B) Final angiogram.

endovascular and hybrid technique,[62,63] that creates an IP arteriovenous fistula with the purpose of bringing arterial blood through patent venous conduits to the foot (**Figs. 10–12**).

FUTURE DIRECTIONS

As the incidence of PAD and CLTI continue to increase, rapidly evolving revascularization techniques push the limits of meaningful outcomes analysis using the existing classification systems. Therefore, the Society for Vascular Surgery designed a new classification based on the evaluation of Wound, Ischemia, and foot Infection.[64] This system allows a more meaningful analysis of outcomes for endovascular and surgical therapies in this challenging and heterogeneous population and is likely to replace currently used classifications (ie, Rutherford-Becker), while providing more meaningful insights and predictive models. Better study design, more meaningful study end points, and multidisciplinary collaboration will provide higher quality research and care for this population.

DISCLOSURE

The author has nothing to disclose.

REFERENCES

1. Singh G, Brinza EK, Hildebrand J, et al. Midterm outcomes after infrapopliteal interventions in patients with critical limb ischemia based on the TASC II classification of below-the-knee arteries. J Endovasc Ther 2017;24(3):321–30.
2. Fowkes FGR, Rudan D, Rudan I, et al. Comparison of global estimates of prevalence and risk factors for peripheral artery disease in 2000 and 2010: a systematic review and analysis. Lancet 2013;382: 1329–40.
3. Nehler MR, Duval S, Diao L, et al. Epidemiology of peripheral arterial disease and critical limb ischemia in an insured national population. J Vasc Surg 2014;60(3):686–95.e2.
4. Farber A. Chronic limb-threatening ischemia. N Engl J Med 2018;379:171–80.
5. Howard DP, Banerjee A, Fairhead JF, et al. Population-based study of incidence, risk factors, outcome, and prognosis of ischemic peripheral arterial events: implications for prevention. Circulation 2015;132:1805–15.
6. Gerhard-Herman MD, Gornik HL, Barrett C, et al. AHA/ACC guideline on the management of patients with lower extremity peripheral artery disease: a report of the American College of Cardiology/American Heart Association Task Force

on Clinical Practice Guidelines. Circulation 2016; 135(12):e726–79.
7. Teraa M, Conte MS, Moll FL, et al. Critical limb ischemia. Current trends and future directions. J Am Heart Assoc 2016;5:e002938.
8. Norgren L, Hiatt WR, Dormandy JA, et al. Inter-society consensus for the management of peripheral arterial disease (TASC II). J Vasc Surg 2007; 45(suppl):S5–67.
9. Mustapha JA, Diaz-Sandoval LJ. Management of infrapopliteal arterial disease: critical limb ischemia. Interv Cardiol Clin 2014;3:573–92.
10. European Working Group on Critical Limb Ischemia. Second European consensus document on chronic critical leg ischaemia. Eur J Vasc Surg 1992;6(Suppl A):1–32.
11. Wolfe JH, Wyatt MG. Critical and subcritical ischaemia. Eur J Vasc Endovasc Surg 1997;13: 578–82.
12. Aboyans V, Desormais I, Lacroix P, et al. The general prognosis of patients with peripheral arterial disease differs according to the disease localization. J Am Coll Cardiol 2010;55(9):898–903.
13. Klein AJ, Jaff MR, Gray BH, et al. SCAI appropriate use criteria for peripheral arterial interventions: an update. Catheter Cardiovasc Interv 2017;90:E90–110.
14. Graziani L, Silvestro A, Bertone V, et al. Vascular involvement in diabetic subjects with ischemic foot ulcer: a new morphologic categorization of disease severity. Eur J Vasc Endovasc Surg 2007; 33:453–60.
15. Gray BH, Grant AA, Kalbaugh CA, et al. The impact of isolated tibial disease on outcomes in the critical limb ischemic population. Ann Vasc Surg 2010;24: 349–59.
16. Sadek M, Ellozy SH, Turnbull IC, et al. Improved outcomes are associated with multilevel endovascular intervention involving the tibial vessels compared with isolated tibial intervention. J Vasc Surg 2009;49:638–43.
17. Adam DJ, Beard JD, Cleveland T, et al. Bypass versus angioplasty in severe ischaemia of the leg (BASIL): multicentre, randomized controlled trial. Lancet 2005;366:1925–34.
18. Gray BH, Diaz-Sandoval LJ, Dieter RS, et al. SCAI expert consensus statement for infrapopliteal arterial intervention appropriate use. Catheter Cardiovasc Interv 2014;84:539–45.
19. Mustapha JA, Diaz-Sandoval LJ, Adams G, et al. Lack of association between limb hemodynamics and response to infrapopliteal endovascular therapy in patients with critical limb ischemia. J Invasive Cardiol 2017;29(5):175–80.
20. Bunte MC, Jacob J, Nudelman B, et al. Validation of the relationship between ankle–brachial and toe–brachial indices and infragenicular arterial

patency in critical limb ischemia. Vasc Med 2015; 20(1):23–9.

21. Shishehbor MH, Hammad TA, Zeller T, et al. An analysis of IN.PACT DEEP randomized trial on the limitations of the societal guidelines-recommended hemodynamic parameters to diagnose critical limb ischemia. J Vasc Surg 2016;63(5):1311–7.

22. Haider CR, Riederer SJ, Borisch EA, et al. High temporal and spatial resolution 3D time resolved contrast-enhanced magnetic resonance angiography of the hands and feet. J Magn Reson Imaging 2011;34:2–12.

23. Collins R, Burch J, Cranny G, et al. Duplex ultrasonography, magnetic resonance angiography, and computed tomography angiography for diagnosis and assessment of symptomatic, lower limb peripheral arterial disease: systematic review. BMJ 2007; 334(7606):1257.

24. Manzi M, Cester G, Palena LM, et al. Vascular imaging of the foot: the first step toward endovascular recanalization. Radiographics 2011;31:1623–36.

25. Hofmann WJ, Walter J, Ugurluoglu A, et al. Preoperative high-frequency duplex scanning of potential pedal target vessels. J Vasc Surg 2004;39: 169–75.

26. Stacul F, van der Molen AJ, Reimer P, et al. Contrast induced nephropathy: updated ESUR Contrast Media Committee guidelines. Eur Radiol 2011;21:2527–41.

27. Scalise F, Novelli E, Auguadro C, et al. Automated carbon dioxide digital angiography for lower-limb arterial disease evaluation: safety assessment and comparison with standard iodinated contrast media angiography. J Invasive Cardiol 2015;27:20–6.

28. Palena LM, Diaz-Sandoval LJ, Candeo A, et al. Automated carbon dioxide angiography for the evaluation and endovascular treatment of diabetic patients with critical limb ischemia. J Endovasc Ther 2016;23(1):40–8.

29. Sommerset J, Karmy-Jones R, Dally M, et al. Plantar acceleration time: a novel technique to evaluate arterial flow to the foot. Ann Vasc Surg 2019;60: 308–14.

30. Kabra A, Suresh KR, Vivekanand V, et al. Outcomes of angiosome and non-angiosome targeted revascularisation in critical lower limb ischemia. J Vasc Surg 2013;57:44–9.

31. Alexandrescu VA, Brochier S, Limbga A, et al. Healing of diabetic neuroischemic foot wounds with and without wound-targeted revascularization: preliminary observations from an 8-year prospective dual-center registry. J Endovasc Ther 2019;11. 1526602819885131.

32. Berceli SA, Chan AK, Pomposelli FB Jr, et al. Efficacy of dorsal pedal artery bypass in limb salvage for ischemic heel ulcers. J Vasc Surg 1999;30: 499–508.

33. Mustapha J, Saab F, McGoff T, et al. Tibio-pedal arterial minimally invasive retrograde revascularization in patients with advanced peripheral vascular disease: the TAMI TECHNIQUE, original case series. Catheter Cardiovasc Interv 2014;83:987–94.

34. Palena LM, Brocco E, Manzi M. The clinical utility of below-the ankle using "transmetatarsal artery access" in complex cases of CLI. Catheter Cardiovasc Interv 2014;83(1):123–9.

35. Jaff MR, White CJ, Hiatt WR, et al. An update on methods for revascularization and expansion of the TASC lesion classification to include below-the-knee arteries: a supplement to the Inter-Society Consensus for the Management of Peripheral Arterial Disease (TASC II). J Endovasc Ther 2015;22(5):663–77.

36. Leng G, Lee A, Fowkes F, et al. Incidence, natural history and cardiovascular events in symptomatic and asymptomatic peripheral arterial disease in the general population. Int J Epidemiol 1996;25: 1172–81.

37. Dormandy J, Mahir M, Ascady G, et al. Fate of the patient with chronic leg ischaemia. A review article. J Cardiovasc Surg 1989;30:50–7.

38. Jelnes R, Gaardsting O, Hougaard Jensen K, et al. Fate in intermittent claudication: outcome and risk factors. Br Med J 1986;293:1137–40.

39. Conte MS, Bandyk DF, Clowes AW, et al. Results of PREVENT III: a multicenter, randomized trial of edifoligide for the prevention of vein graft failure in lower extremity bypass surgery. J Vasc Surg 2006; 43:742–51.

40. Iida O, Nakamura M, Yamauchi Y, et al. Endovascular treatment for infrainguinal vessels in patients with critical limb ischemia. OLIVE Registry, a prospective, multicenter study in Japan with 12 month follow-up. Circ Cardiovasc Interv 2013;6:68–76.

41. Iida O, Nakamura M, Yamauchi Y, et al. 3-year outcomes of the OLIVE Registry, a prospective multicenter study of patients with critical limb ischemia: a prospective, multi-center, three-year follow-up study on endovascular treatment for infra-inguinal vessel in patients with critical limb ischemia. JACC Cardiovasc Interv 2015;8:1493–502.

42. Barshes NR, Chambers JD, Cohen J, et al. Cost-effectiveness in the contemporary management of critical limb ischemia with tissue loss. J Vasc Surg 2012;56:1015–24.

43. Menard MT, Farber A. The BEST-CLI trial: a multi-disciplinary effort to assess whether surgical or endovascular therapy is better for patients with critical limb ischemia. Semin Vasc Surg 2014;27: 82–4.

44. Mustapha JA, Saab F, Diaz L, et al. Utility and feasibility of ultrasound-guided access in patients with critical limb ischemia. Catheter Cardiovasc Interv 2013;81:1204–11.

45. Mustapha JA, Diaz-Sandoval LJ, Jaff MR, et al. Ultrasound-guided arterial access: outcomes among patients with peripheral artery disease and critical limb ischemia undergoing peripheral interventions. J Invasive Cardiol 2016;28(6):259–64.

46. Razavi MK, Mustapha JA, Miller LE. Contemporary systematic review and meta-analysis of early outcomes with percutaneous treatment for infrapopliteal atherosclerotic disease. J Vasc Interv Radiol 2014;25:1489–96, 1496.e1.

47. Mustapha JA, Saab F, McGoff TN, et al. Tibiopedal arterial minimally invasive retrograde revascularizatino (TAMI) in patients with peripheral arterial disease and critical limb ischemia. On behalf of the Peripheral Registry of Endovascular Clinical Outcomes (PRIME). Catheter Cardiovasc Interv 2019;1–8. https://doi.org/10.1002/ccd.28639.

48. Montero-Baker M, Schmidt A, Braunlich S, et al. Retrograde approach for complex popliteal and tibioperoneal occlusions. J Endovasc Ther 2008; 15:594–604.

49. Venkatachalam S, Bunte M, Monteleone P, et al. Combined antegrade-retrograde intervention to improve chronic total occlusion recanalization in high-risk critical limb ischemia. Ann Vasc Surg 2014;28(6):1439–48.

50. Bosiers M, Scheinert D, Peeters P, et al. Randomized comparison of everolimus-eluting versus bare-metal stents in patients with critical limb ischemia and infrapopliteal arterial occlusive disease. J Vasc Surg 2012;55:390–8.

51. Saab F, Jaff MR, Diaz-Sandoval LJ, et al. Chronic total occlusion crossing approach BNased on plaque cap morphology: the CTOP classification. J Endovasc Ther 2018;25(3):284–91.

52. Romiti M, Albers M, Brochado-Neto FC, et al. Meta-analysis of infrapopliteal angioplasty for chronic critical limb ischemia. J Vasc Surg 2008; 47:975–81.

53. Mustapha JA, Finton SM, Diaz-Sandoval LJ, et al. Percutaneous transluminal angioplasty in patients with infrapopliteal disease. Systematic review and meta-analysis. Circ Cardiovasc Interv 2016;9: e003468.

54. Schulte KL, Pilger E, Schellong S, et al. Primary Self-EXPANDing nitinol stenting vs balloon angioplasty with optional bailout stenting for the treatment of infrapopliteal artery disease in patients with severe intermittent claudication or critical limb ischemia (EXPAND Study). J Endovasc Ther 2015;22:690–7.

55. Scheinert D, Katsanos K, ACHILLES Investigators, et al. A prospective randomized multicenter comparison of balloon angioplasty and infrapopliteal stenting with the sirolimus-eluting stent in patients with ischemic peripheral arterial disease: 1-year results from the ACHILLES trial. J Am Coll Cardiol 2012;60:2290–5.

56. Rastan A, Brechtel K, Krankenberg H, et al. Sirolimus-eluting stents for treatment of infrapopliteal arteries reduce clinical event rate compared to bare-metal stents: long-term results from a randomized trial. J Am Coll Cardiol 2012;60: 587–91.

57. Siablis D, Kitrou PM, Spiliopoulos S, et al. Paclitaxel coated balloon angioplasty versus dug-eluting stenting for the treatment of infrapopliteal long-segment arterial occlusive disease: the IDEAS randomized controlled trial. JACC Cardiovasc Interv 2014;7:1048–56.

58. Spreen MI, Martens JM, Knippenberg B, et al. Long-term follow-up of the PADI trial: percutaneous transluminal angioplasty versus drug-eluting stents for infrapopliteal lesions in critical limb ischemia. J Am Heart Assoc 2017;6: e004877.

59. Liistro F, Porto I, Angioli P, et al. Drug-eluting balloon in peripheral intervention for below the knee angioplasty evaluation (DEBATE-BTK): a randomized trial in diabetic patients with critical limb ischemia. Circulation 2013;128(6):615–21.

60. Zeller T, Baumgartner I, Scheinert D, et al. Drug-eluting balloon versus standard balloon angioplasty for infrapopliteal arterial revascularization in critical limb ischemia: 12-month results from the IN.PACT DEEP randomized trial. J Am Coll Cardiol 2014;64:1568–76.

61. Nakama T, Watanabe N, Haraguchi T, et al. Clinical outcomes of pedal artery angioplasty for patients with ischemic wounds. Results from the multicenter Rendezvous Registry. JACC Cardiovasc Interv 2017; 10:79–90.

62. Kum S, Tan YK, Schreve MA, et al. Midterm outcomes from a pilot study of percutaneous deep vein arterialization for the treatment of no option critical limb ischemia. J Endovasc Ther 2017;24(5):619–26.

63. Ferraresi R, Casini A, Losurdo F, et al. Hybrid foot vein arterialization in no-option patients with critical limb ischemia: a preliminary report. J Endovasc Ther 2019;26(1):7–17.

64. Mills JL, Conte MS, Armstrong DG, et al. The society for vascular surgery lower extremity threatened limb classification system: risk stratification based on wound, ischemia, and foot infection (WIfI). J Vasc Surg 2014;59:220–34.

Acute Limb Ischemia Interventions

Saud Khan, MD, Beau M. Hawkins, MD*

KEYWORDS

- Acute limb ischemia • Peripheral artery disease • Peripheral vascular intervention

KEY POINTS

- Acute limb ischemia (ALI) is a sudden decrease in limb perfusion that threatens limb viability.
- ALI is a medical emergency carrying a high morbidity and mortality risk.
- Timely reperfusion is needed to salvage the limb and prevent amputation or death.
- ALI is categorized using the Rutherford classification, which guides clinicians on appropriate therapy and timing.
- Potential complications of ALI interventions include ischemia-reperfusion injury, compartment syndrome, and bleeding.

INTRODUCTION

Acute limb ischemia (ALI) is defined as a sudden decrease in limb perfusion that results in a threat to limb viability.[1] The estimated incidence of this condition is 140 per million per year,[1] occurring more frequently in the lower extremities than the upper. It is associated with a 1-year amputation rate of 11% and mortality rate of greater than 40%.[2] By definition, limb ischemia is considered acute if symptom onset is within 14 days of presentation, although it is important to acknowledge that advanced degrees of ALI may result in irreversible tissue damage within hours of symptom onset depending on baseline circulatory status, patient comorbidities, ALI etiology, and other factors. Clinical presentation includes the classic "6 P's": pain, paresthesia, pallor, poikilothermia, pulselessness, and paralysis. The constellation of symptoms that develop, and the rapidity with which it progresses, depends in part on the integrity of the preexisting arterial circulation. In patients with a prior history of symptomatic peripheral artery disease (PAD), the ALI presentation may be subtle and similar to a subacute worsening of preexisting claudication symptoms, particularly when a robust collateral circulation already exists. On the other hand, in those with no prior PAD, ALI often manifests as dramatic and severe symptoms developing very rapidly within the span of minutes to hours.

ACUTE LIMB ISCHEMIA ETIOLOGIES

The etiology of ALI is varied and includes multiple conditions that may acutely compromise the blood supply to the limb (Table 1). Embolic ALI occurs when debris from a primary source dislodges to situate in a more distal component of the arterial tree. Common sources for this embolic debris include left atrial appendage thrombus with atrial fibrillation, left ventricular thrombus in the setting of left ventricular aneurysm, or from preexisting arterial aneurysms, such as in the abdominal aorta. Paradoxic embolism also can occur in patients with deep vein thrombosis, where clot traverses a patent foramen ovale to lodge in a distal arterial bed. Thrombotic ALI occurs when an artery occludes due to in situ atherothrombosis involving an existing atherosclerotic plaque, or when an arterial aneurysm obstructs from mural thrombus. In addition, hypercoagulable states, such as antiphospholipid antibody syndrome and heparin-induced thrombocytopenia, may cause primary

Department of Medicine, Cardiovascular Section, University of Oklahoma Health Sciences Center, 800 Stanton L. Young Boulevard, AAT 5400, Oklahoma City, OK 73131, USA
* Corresponding author.
E-mail address: beau-hawkins@ouhsc.edu

Intervent Cardiol Clin 9 (2020) 221–228
https://doi.org/10.1016/j.iccl.2019.12.002
2211-7458/20/© 2019 Elsevier Inc. All rights reserved.

Table 1
Acute limb ischemia etiologies

Cause of Acute Limb Ischemia	Etiologies
Embolism	Atrial fibrillation Valvular heart disease Left ventricular thrombi Preexisting arterial aneurysms Paradoxic emboli from the venous circulation
Thrombosis	Atherosclerotic peripheral artery disease Thrombosis in an arterial aneurysm Hypercoagulable states (eg, antiphospholipid antibody syndrome, heparin-induced thrombocytopenia) Thrombosis of previous arterial bypass grafts Thrombosis of prior endovascular stents
Other	Trauma Arterial dissection Vasospasm Venous gangrene (eg, phlegmasia)

arterial thrombosis. Patients with preexisting bypass grafts of prior endovascular stents also may develop acute thrombosis. Other causes of ALI include trauma, arterial dissection, vasospasm, venous gangrene (eg, phlegmasia), and iatrogenic sources such as arterial instrumentation for diagnostic and interventional cardiovascular procedures.

REVASCULARIZATION STRATEGIES: SURGERY VERSUS ENDOVASCULAR TREATMENT

Both surgery and endovascular therapies can be successfully used in appropriate patients with ALI. The decision on the mode of revascularization used depends on several factors, including duration of ischemia, patient comorbidities, and available expertise and resources. In this light, these strategies are more fairly viewed as complementary rather than competitive. Regardless of the revascularization technique used, the goal is to achieve rapid inline flow to the distal limb to promote symptom relief and effective limb salvage. Selected studies comparing revascularization modalities are discussed as follows.

Ouriel and colleagues[3] compared primary catheter-directed thrombolysis (CDT) using urokinase with surgical intervention for ALI. A total of 114 patients were randomized to either CDT or surgical intervention. They reported similar limb salvage rates of 82%, although the CDT group had improved survival at 1 year (84% vs 58%, $P = .01$). Major bleeding events were more frequent in the CDT group (11% vs 2%, $P = .06$).

STILE (Results of a Prospective Randomized Trial Evaluating Surgery vs Thrombolysis for Ischemia of the Lower Extremity) also compared surgical intervention with CDT. In this study, 393 patients were randomized to surgical intervention or CDT. Of note, patients included had either ALI or chronic, critical limb ischemia. In the ALI cohort, CDT was associated with a reduction in major amputation (11% vs 30%, $P = .02$) and shorter hospital stay (9.7 days vs 14.3 days, $P = .04$). The CDT arm had higher rates of life-threatening hemorrhage (5.6% vs 0.7%, $P = .014$), as well as vascular complications (9.7% vs 3.5%, $P = .01$), but there was no significant difference in mortality (4.0% with CDT vs 4.9% with surgery, $P = .693$).[4]

Finally, TOPAS (A Comparison of Recombinant Urokinase with Vascular Surgery as Initial Treatment for Acute Arterial Occlusion of the Legs Trial) randomized 544 patients with ALI to either vascular surgery or CDT. The investigators observed no difference in the primary end point, amputation-free survival at 6 months (71.8% with CDT group vs 74.8% with surgery, $P = .43$). CDT was associated with fewer operative procedures at 6 months. Hemorrhagic complications were higher in the CDT group; however, mortality was not significantly different.[5]

In a Cochrane meta-analysis of randomized ALI studies comparing surgery with endovascular therapy, both strategies were associated with similar rates of death (odds ratio [OR] 0.67; 95% confidence interval [CI] 0.25–1.79; $P = .42$) and limb salvage (OR 0.88; 95% CI 0.62–1.23; $P = .44$) at 1 year. CDT was associated with increased risk of major hemorrhage at 30 days (OR 3.22; 95% CI 1.79–5.78; $P<.0001$). Given that the studies included in this meta-analysis were generally decades old, it remains unclear if the routine use of newer endovascular technologies or surgical techniques would differentially impact outcomes in the ALI population.[6]

In a propensity score–matched analysis using the National Inpatient Sample databases, Kolte and colleagues[7] compared endovascular with surgical revascularization in a propensity score–matched cohort of 7746, and found that endovascular revascularization was associated with lower in-hospital mortality (2.8% vs 4.0%, $P = .002$) and major bleeding (16.7% vs 21.0%, $P<.001$), but a higher vascular complication rate (1.4% vs 0.7%, $P = .002$). Rates of amputation did not differ significantly between the 2 groups (4.7% vs 5.1%, $P = .43$).

PATIENT SELECTION FOR TREATMENT

Selecting patients for ALI is a complex process that integrates severity of limb ischemia, estimated procedural risks, and decisions regarding best modality of revascularization. These factors are reviewed in detail in the discussion that follows.

ALI is categorized using the Rutherford classification scheme (Table 2). In Rutherford stage I, limb motor and sensory function are intact, and both arterial and venous Doppler signals are audible. In stage IIa, limbs have mild or no motor or sensory loss, and arterial Doppler signals are inaudible. In stage IIb, limbs have more advanced motor and sensory deficits, arterial signals are inaudible, and importantly, venous Doppler signals are present, signifying a limb that is viable with successful revascularization. Stage III limbs are not salvageable, even with revascularization, and are characterized by profound sensory loss, paralysis, and absent arterial and venous Doppler signals.[8]

After stratifying the ischemic limb using the Rutherford scheme, the patient must be rapidly assessed for any contraindications to anticoagulation, thrombolysis, and any major comorbidities that would influence decisions regarding revascularization modality (eg, surgery or endovascular approach). All patients should have basic laboratory tests performed, including a complete blood count, basic metabolic profile, and lactic acid and coagulation studies. Biochemical derangements should be aggressively corrected.

In patients with ALI in whom endovascular therapy is considered, it is paramount to screen for contraindications to thrombolysis, as most strategies will use this pharmacotherapy. Absolute contraindications include cerebrovascular event (excluding transient ischemic attack in the past 2 months), active bleeding diathesis, recent (<10 days) gastrointestinal bleed, neurosurgery within 3 months, and intracranial trauma within 3 months. Relative contraindications include cardiopulmonary resuscitation within 10 days, pregnancy, major nonvascular surgery or trauma within 10 days, uncontrolled hypertension (systolic blood pressure >180 mm Hg, diastolic blood pressure >110 mm Hg), puncture of a noncompressible vessel, intracranial tumor, and recent eye surgery.[1]

It should be noted, though, that these contraindications were established for patients undergoing systemic thrombolytic therapy. The risk of hemorrhagic complications with CDT may be less, given the typically lower doses of thrombolytics delivered.

All patients with salvageable limbs (categories I and II) should receive anticoagulation unless otherwise contraindicated.[9] Unfractionated heparin and low molecular weight heparin are the anticoagulants most commonly used. Anticoagulation serves to prevent further propagation of the clot. These patients may have other comorbidities for which they are taking antiplatelet and/or anticoagulant agents, which

Table 2					
Rutherford classification scheme					
Rutherford Class	**Prognosis**	**Sensory Findings**	**Motor Findings**	**Arterial Dopplers**	**Venous Dopplers**
I. Viable	Not immediately threatened	No sensory loss	No weakness	Audible	Audible
IIa. Marginally threatened	Salvageable with prompt revascularization	Minimal (eg, toes) or no sensory loss	No weakness	Inaudible	Audible
IIb. Immediately threatened	Salvageable with immediate revascularization	Sensory loss involving more than toes, rest pain	Mild-moderate weakness	Inaudible	Audible
III. Irreversible	Unsalvageable	Profound sensory loss, anesthesia	Profound weakness, paralysis	Inaudible	Inaudible

also may affect the patient's relative risk of bleeding.

Patients with Rutherford I and II ALI should receive revascularization in an attempt to facilitate limb salvage. The timing and modality used often is influenced by available expertise and resources, as well as patient characteristics. In general, the greater the severity of ischemia at presentation, the more rapidly revascularization should be accomplished. Current guidelines recommend CDT as an effective treatment for ALI. In addition, percutaneous mechanical thrombectomy (PMT) can be used as an adjunct to CDT in these patients. If CDT is not an option due to lack of local expertise or resources, surgical options should be considered for rapid restoration of blood flow.[9]

Patients with Rutherford III ALI should undergo primary amputation, as revascularization will not result in limb salvage. Although in certain situations revascularization may facilitate healing after amputation, care should be taken not to delay amputation, as doing so may increase the risk of limb loss.

PROCEDURAL CONSIDERATIONS

Access site selection is of paramount importance if proceeding with endovascular therapy. Bleeding is a common complication, given the frequent need for thrombolytics. Meticulous access technique, use of ultrasound and fluoroscopy, micropuncture needles, selection of sites with less bleeding (Fig. 1), and employment of the smallest-bore sheath size necessary can minimize bleeding risk.

Procedural technique to avoid distal embolization also should be used when treating patients with ALI. In the authors' opinion, distal embolic protection should be used routinely if performing thrombectomy, angioplasty, stenting, or other techniques in which fresh thrombus may dislodge and embolize downstream. Distal embolization can jeopardize the chances of

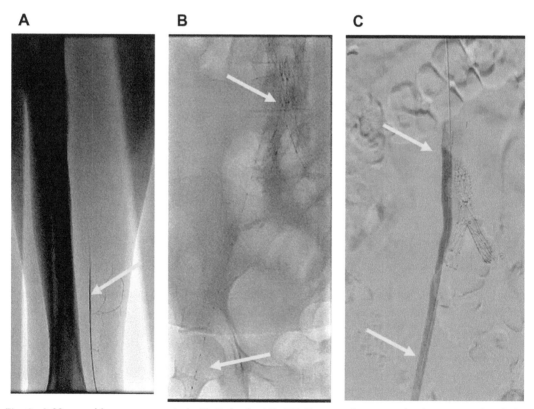

Fig. 1. A 38-year-old woman presented with Rutherford IIb ALI. Computed tomography demonstrated occlusion of the right bypass limb. She was declined for surgical therapy. (A) Ultrasound-guided access was obtained in the right posterior tibial artery (arrow). (B) An ultrasound-assisted thrombolysis catheter was placed across the occlusion from aorta to right common femoral artery (arrows), and CDT was initiated. (C) Relook angiography and angioplasty the following day resulted in restoration of flow through the graft limb (arrows). The patient was discharged the following day after an otherwise uneventful stay.

successful limb salvage even when more proximal inline flow has been established. Copious administration of intra-arterial vasodilators may lessen the risk of distal vessel occlusion if embolization occurs.

In addition, the manner in which thrombotic, occluded arteries are crossed merits attention. For example, traversing a thrombotic common iliac occlusion (Fig. 2) via a retrograde approach may "shovel" thrombus into the contralateral iliac potentially jeopardizing the good, asymptomatic limb. Crossing such lesions in antegrade fashion or protecting the contralateral side via balloon occlusion may be considered in such circumstances.

Multiple endovascular technologies are available for the treatment of ALI. CDT is a commonly used technique in which a thrombotic lesion is crossed, and an infusion catheter is left in the artery to continuously elute thrombolytic agent at low doses (0.5–2.0 mg/h) for 12 to 24 hours or longer (see Fig. 1). Relook angiography is then performed, often followed by definitive revascularization procedures (eg, angioplasty, stenting). The primary advantage of this technique is that thrombus resolution usually occurs before additional procedures are performed. On the other hand, this technique requires prolonged thrombolytic exposure time, which can increase bleeding risk, and such therapies are resource-intensive in that they require prolonged intensive care monitoring.

Several types of infusion catheters are available for use in CDT. Most, such as the Cragg-McNamara catheter (Medtronic, Dublin, Ireland), are end-hole catheters that are delivered across the lesion using standard workhorse wires. These catheters have additional side holes along the length of the catheter where low-dose thrombolytics elute over several hours. A unique catheter, the EKOS catheter (EKOS Corp., Bothell, WA), also has an additional filament housed in the infusion catheter that pulses ultrasonic energy during thrombolysis, which theoretically facilitates faster clot penetration and dissolution. Large, randomized trials comparing the efficacy of different CDT devices for ALI have not been conducted.

Thrombectomy is another technique used to treat ALI. Multiple devices are available, ranging from simple end-hole catheters (eg, suction thrombectomy) to dedicated mechanical devices that remove thrombus. One example is the Angiojet catheter (Boston Scientific, Marlborough, MA), which mechanically removes thrombus via rheolytic thrombectomy. It has an optional "power pulse" function that permits infusion of thrombolytic agents directly into the thrombus, during a short period of time (10–20 minutes), before the thrombolysed segment is evacuated. This technique is known as pharmaco-mechanical thrombolysis (Fig. 3). Another thrombectomy option is the Indigo device (Penumbra, Inc., Alameda, CA), which uses vacuum suction to mechanically extract clots. Advantages of thrombectomy primarily relate to the efficiency with which flow may be restored and the absence of second relook procedures when index results are satisfactory. In addition, thrombolytic use often can be avoided in patients deemed to be at high bleeding risk. Such a strategy is most effective when the thrombus burden is low, thrombotic material is relatively fresh, and anatomic characteristics (eg, vessel size and location) are favorable.

In reality, operators performing ALI work should be facile with and have access to multiple

A

B

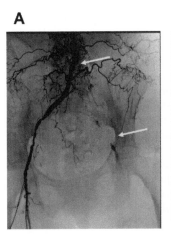 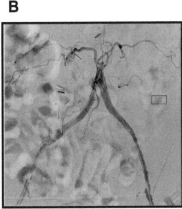

Fig. 2. A 60-year-old man presented with embolic ALI secondary to atrial fibrillation. (A) Angiography demonstrated a long, thrombotic left common iliac occlusion with faint reconstitution noted in the distal left external iliac artery (arrows). This lesion was crossed and thrombolysed via right common femoral access to avoid "pushing" thrombus into the right common iliac from a left retrograde approach. (B) Following CDT and covered stenting, brisk inflow was restored.

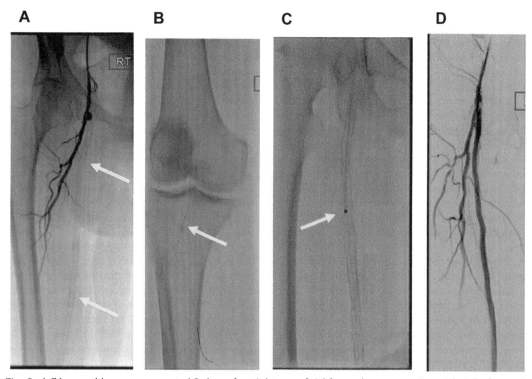

Fig. 3. A 74-year-old woman presented 3 days after right superficial femoral artery stenting with right foot pain and numbness. (A) Angiography showed acute stent thrombosis (arrows). (B) The lesion was crossed, and an embolic protection device was deployed in the popliteal artery (arrow). (C) Pharmaco-mechanical thrombectomy was performed using the power pulse function (arrow). (D) Following angioplasty, successful restoration of patency was achieved.

established tools. No 2 ALI cases are alike, and often multiple techniques are needed to achieve satisfactory outcomes.

COMPLICATIONS

As tissue ischemia persists, tissue damage may become irreversible. In addition, even when revascularization is achieved in a timely manner, further injury may occur from ischemia-reperfusion (IR) injury, sometimes resulting in compartment syndrome. Systemic complications also may occur, including the systemic inflammatory response syndrome and multiple organ dysfunction syndrome.

IR injury occurs after reestablishment of blood flow to a tissue after a period of malperfusion. Important mediators in the development of IR injury include cytokine release, formation of reactive oxygen species, and activation of the complement cascade. Cytokine release results in increased adhesion of leukocytes to the vascular endothelium and chemotaxis of leukocytes into the tissues. This leads to degranulation, development of reactive oxygen species,

and ultimately myocyte death. Cytokine release also can result in increased permeability of the vascular endothelium leading to profound interstitial edema.[10]

IR injury can increase extremity compartmental pressures, compromising perfusion to local tissues. Clinically, compartment syndrome presents as pain, paresthesia, diminished sensation, pallor, and muscle weakness, and in later stages, paralysis. These symptoms are similar to those of ALI, and thus a high index of suspicion is required to make the diagnosis. In addition, the compartment will feel tense on palpation, and invasive measurements will reveal elevated intracompartmental pressures. The diagnosis of compartment syndrome is clinical, and there is no single agreed on intracompartmental pressure threshold required. When suspected, urgent surgical evaluation is necessary, and it is reasonable for surgical evaluation at the time of revascularization in case symptoms of reperfusion injury or compartment syndrome subsequently develop. Although some propose the use of prophylactic fasciotomy after revascularization to improve the likelihood of limb salvage at 30 days, particularly in those with higher Rutherford class and more prolonged ischemia,[11] prophylactic fasciotomy is not without risk. Creatinine phosphokinase (CK), a marker of muscle necrosis, may be monitored in patients with ALI.

In cases of prolonged ALI or following compartment syndrome, rhabdomyolysis can occur following reperfusion. Rhabdomyolysis is marked by elevated levels of CK. Myoglobin can result in acute kidney injury (AKI) via acute tubular necrosis. Intravenous bicarbonate and mannitol are often used for prevention, although they have not shown consistent benefit in terms of reductions in AKI, need for dialysis, or mortality.[12] Intensive intravenous fluid resuscitation with saline is used for treatment.

The most common complication of endovascular therapy for ALI is bleeding. The rates of major hemorrhagic complications reported range from 6% to nearly 50%.[3–5,13–15] This wide variation is due in part to differences in the thrombolytic agent used, the dosing regimen used, and the criteria used to define major bleeding among various studies. The most frequent site of bleeding is at the vascular access site, although intracranial, gastrointestinal, retroperitoneal, and other sites of hemorrhage can occur. Patients who undergo CDT should be observed for symptoms and signs of hemorrhage, including frequent monitoring of vital signs, and periodic neurologic checks. Monitoring of hemoglobin and fibrinogen levels during CDT may identify and prevent clinically relevant bleeding, but it should be noted that there is not a standardized algorithm for checking these parameters during thrombolysis infusion. In addition, using the lowest effective doses possible of anticoagulants and thrombolytics is an important safeguard.

FOLLOW-UP

After revascularization for ALI, the nature of the outpatient follow-up will depend at least in part on the revascularization procedure performed, and the underlying etiology of the ALI.

Patients with underlying atherosclerotic PAD, those that underwent adjunctive angioplasty and stenting, and those who underwent bypass surgery for revascularization need assessment of cardiovascular risk factors, limb symptoms, and functional status. Patients with atherosclerotic vascular disease should be managed with lifestyle modifications, including exercise and smoking cessation, and treated with antiplatelet agents, statins, and angiotensin-converting enzyme inhibitors or angiotensin receptor blockers.

There are no consensus recommendations for imaging surveillance following endovascular treatment of ALI. Based on extrapolation from other forms of limb ischemia, it is reasonable to perform an ankle-brachial index (ABI) and duplex ultrasonography depending on patient anatomy and risk of restenosis.[9] A sufficient decrease in ABI may suggest a need for further investigation and possible intervention.[16] Ultrasound findings can help to indicate sites of stenosis,[16–18] and may also indicate impending graft failure[17,19,20] or stent failure.[21] Ultrasound surveillance following vein grafting has been shown to improve graft patency,[20,22] and to be effective in reducing major amputations.[23]

SUMMARY

ALI is a medical emergency with high morbidity and mortality requiring prompt recognition and treatment. Patients must be rapidly assessed and risk-stratified to facilitate decisions regarding optimal revascularization strategy. Interventions for patients with salvageable limbs include CDT, PMT devices, and surgical revascularization. Patients with ALI can develop multiple, potentially serious complications that can occur even in those receiving optimal treatment. Following initial acute management with revascularization, the underlying etiology for the ALI should be sought and treated to prevent recurrence.

DISCLOSURE

The authors have no relevant affiliations or financial involvement with any organization or entity with a financial interest in or financial conflict with the subject matter or materials discussed in the article. This includes employment, consultancies, honoraria, stock ownership or options, expert testimony, grants or patents received or pending, or royalties.

REFERENCES

1. Norgren L, Hiatt WR, Dormandy JA, et al. Inter-society consensus for the management of peripheral arterial disease (TASC II). Eur J Vasc Endovasc Surg 2007;33(Suppl 1):S1–75.

2. Baril DT, Ghosh K, Rosen AB. Trends in the incidence, treatment, and outcomes of acute lower extremity ischemia in the United States Medicare population. J Vasc Surg 2014;60(3):669–77.e2.

3. Ouriel K, Shortell CK, DeWeese JA, et al. A comparison of thrombolytic therapy with operative revascularization in the initial treatment of

acute peripheral arterial ischemia. J Vasc Surg 1994;19(6):1021–30.

4. Results of a prospective randomized trial evaluating surgery versus thrombolysis for ischemia of the lower extremity. The STILE trial. Ann Surg 1994;220(3):251–66 [discussion: 266–8].

5. Ouriel K, Veith FJ, Sasahara AA. A comparison of recombinant urokinase with vascular surgery as initial treatment for acute arterial occlusion of the legs. Thrombolysis or Peripheral Arterial Surgery (TOPAS) Investigators. N Engl J Med 1998; 338(16):1105–11.

6. Darwood R, Berridge DC, Kessel DO, et al. Surgery versus thrombolysis for initial management of acute limb ischaemia. Cochrane Database Syst Rev 2018;(8):CD002784.

7. Kolte D, Kennedy KF, Shishehbor MH, et al. Endovascular versus surgical revascularization for acute limb ischemia: a propensity-score matched analysis. Circ Cardiovasc Interv 2020;13:e008150.

8. Rutherford RB, Baker JD, Ernst C, et al. Recommended standards for reports dealing with lower extremity ischemia: revised version. J Vasc Surg 1997;26(3):517–38.

9. Gerhard-Herman MD, Gornik HL, Barrett C, et al. 2016 AHA/ACC guideline on the management of patients with lower extremity peripheral artery disease: executive summary: a report of the American College of Cardiology/American Heart Association Task Force on Clinical Practice Guidelines. J Am Coll Cardiol 2017;69(11):1465–508.

10. Eliason JL, Wakefield TW. Metabolic consequences of acute limb ischemia and their clinical implications. Semin Vasc Surg 2009;22(1):29–33.

11. Rothenberg KA, George EL, Trickey AW, et al. Delayed fasciotomy is associated with higher risk of major amputation in patients with acute limb ischemia. Ann Vasc Surg 2019;59:195–201.

12. Brown CV, Rhee P, Chan L, et al. Preventing renal failure in patients with rhabdomyolysis: do bicarbonate and mannitol make a difference? J Trauma 2004;56(6):1191–6.

13. Heymans S, Vanderschueren S, Verhaeghe R, et al. Outcome and one year follow-up of intra-arterial staphylokinase in 191 patients with peripheral arterial occlusion. Thromb Haemost 2000;83(5):666–71.

14. Swischuk JL, Fox PF, Young K, et al. Transcatheter intraarterial infusion of rt-PA for acute lower limb ischemia: results and complications. J Vasc Interv Radiol 2001;12(4):423–30.

15. Schrijver AM, de Vries JP, van den Heuvel DA, et al. Long-term outcomes of catheter-directed thrombolysis for acute lower extremity occlusions of native arteries and prosthetic bypass grafts. Ann Vasc Surg 2016;31:134–42.

16. Westerband A, Mills JL, Kistler S, et al. Prospective validation of threshold criteria for intervention in infrainguinal vein grafts undergoing duplex surveillance. Ann Vasc Surg 1997;11(1):44–8.

17. Mills JL, Harris EJ, Taylor LM Jr, et al. The importance of routine surveillance of distal bypass grafts with duplex scanning: a study of 379 reversed vein grafts. J Vasc Surg 1990;12(4):379–86 [discussion: 387–9].

18. Baril DT, Marone LK. Duplex evaluation following femoropopliteal angioplasty and stenting: criteria and utility of surveillance. Vasc Endovascular Surg 2012;46(5):353–7.

19. Bandyk DF, Cato RF, Towne JB. A low flow velocity predicts failure of femoropopliteal and femorotibial bypass grafts. Surgery 1985;98(4):799–809.

20. Stone PA, Armstrong PA, Bandyk DF, et al. Duplex ultrasound criteria for femorofemoral bypass revision. J Vasc Surg 2006;44(3):496–502.

21. Troutman DA, Madden NJ, Dougherty MJ, et al. Duplex ultrasound diagnosis of failing stent grafts placed for occlusive disease. J Vasc Surg 2014; 60(6):1580–4.

22. Lundell A, Lindblad B, Bergqvist D, et al. Femoropopliteal-crural graft patency is improved by an intensive surveillance program: a prospective randomized study. J Vasc Surg 1995;21(1):26–33 [discussion: 33–4].

23. Visser K, Idu MM, Buth J, et al. Duplex scan surveillance during the first year after infrainguinal autologous vein bypass grafting surgery: costs and clinical outcomes compared with other surveillance programs. J Vasc Surg 2001;33(1):123–30.

Interventional Therapies in Acute Pulmonary Embolism

Robert Zhang, MD, Taisei Kobayashi, MD, Steven Pugliese, MD,
Sameer Khandhar, MD, Jay Giri, MD*

KEYWORDS

- Pulmonary embolism • Catheter-directed thrombolysis • Catheter-directed embolectomy
- Cardiovascular mortality • Bleeding • Tissue plasminogen activator

---

KEY POINTS

- Catheter directed thrombolysis (CDL) and catheter-based embolectomy can be performed safely for patients presenting with intermediate or high-risk pulmonary embolism.
- CDL carries a 0.7% rate of intracranial hemorrhage and thus patient selection is paramount.
- While Catheter based embolectomy should carry a lower intracranial hemorrhage rate but is balanced by a higher risk of procedural respiratory or hemodynamic decompensation.
- Decisions regarding strategy of advanced therapies, timing, dosing of thrombolytics, patient selection can be facilitated by a multidisciplinary pulmonary embolism response team.

INTRODUCTION

Pulmonary embolism (PE) is the third leading cause of cardiovascular mortality among hospitalized patients.[1,2] It is estimated that 100,000 to 180,000 people die from PE annually in the United States.[3–5] Early risk stratification is critical to determine appropriate treatment and decrease morbidity and mortality. Patients with low-risk PE have excellent outcomes when treated with anticoagulation alone (<1% mortality at 1 month).[6] However, patients with intermediate-risk and high-risk PE have short-term mortality rates of 3% to 15% and greater than 30%, respectively.[7–10] The benefits of systemic thrombolysis in these populations are well-established, but accrue at the cost of life-threatening bleeding.[7,11] Concerns about the bleeding risks associated with systemic thrombolysis have prompted a growing interest in alternative options for management of this population, including catheter-directed thrombolysis (CDL) and catheter-directed embolectomy (CDE). This article discusses the current state of endovascular interventional therapy for acute PE, specific roles of CDL and CDE, and available technologies in this space.

PULMONARY EMBOLISM RISK STRATIFICATION

All major guidelines have used risk stratification to guide management. The American Heart Association classifies acute PE into 3 categories: massive, submassive, and low risk.[12] The European Society of Cardiology (ESC) has classified patients into analogous high-, intermediate-, and low-risk PE categories.[13] The main difference between these 2 PE classifications is within the intermediate or submassive category. The ESC acknowledges the complexity of the intermediate-risk category and further divides this into intermediate risk–high and intermediate risk–low.[13] In addition to using right heart strain to risk stratify the intermediate-risk group, the ESC guideline incorporates other clinical parameters such as the PE severity index and cardiac biomarkers in attempt to encompass a broader range of presentations. For the purposes of this review, risk categories will be described as high risk, intermediate risk, and low risk. Intermediate risk will encompass patients with PE and evidence of right heart strain without hypotension (ie, ESC criteria for intermediate risk/American Heart Association criteria for submassive).

Hospital of the University of Pennsylvania, 3400 Civic Center Boulevard, Philadelphia, PA 19104, USA
* Corresponding author.
E-mail address: jay.giri@uphs.upenn.edu

Intervent Cardiol Clin 9 (2020) 229–241
https://doi.org/10.1016/j.iccl.2019.12.003
2211-7458/20/© 2020 Elsevier Inc. All rights reserved.

Although the American Heart Association/ESC classifications serve as a means to risk stratify patients with acute PE, treatment decisions are not always straightforward. Anticoagulation remains the cornerstone of acute PE management for low-risk patients and they do very well with this therapy alone. Although anticoagulation does not actively lyse thrombus, it allows endogenous thrombolysis to work unopposed, preventing further clot propagation and reducing thromboembolic burden.[1] In patients with high-risk PE, more intensive interventions are generally warranted given the higher likelihood of mortality, but are accompanied by a higher bleeding risk. Among patients with intermediate-risk PE, there is no simple algorithm to guide whether a patient requires advanced therapy. Many factors influence treatment decisions, including but not limited to institutional expertise, bleeding risk, extent and location of thrombus, and various patient factors. The uncertainty around optimal therapy for the intermediate risk group is also related to the paucity of data supporting the efficacy and safety of available catheter-based therapies. Catheter-directed therapies have garnered interest on the one hand because of limitations with anticoagulation for intermediate-risk patients and on the other owing to the risks associated with systemic thrombolysis and surgical embolectomy. The following sections discuss the rationale, evidence, and safety for catheter-directed therapies in acute PE.

RATIONALE FOR CATHETER-DIRECTED THROMBOLYSIS

The goal of thrombolytic therapy in high-risk patients is to rapidly improve hemodynamic instability. In contrast, thrombolytic therapy in intermediate-risk patients is used to prevent possible hemodynamic collapse in those with right ventricular (RV) dysfunction and to expedite symptom resolution. Other potential but unproven benefits include prevention of recurrent PE, chronic thromboembolic pulmonary hypertension (CTEPH) and post-PE–related functional impairment. Enthusiasm for CDL is fueled by the hope of similar efficacy to systemic thrombolysis, but with a decreased risk of major or intracranial bleeding. Most studies with CDL use a fraction of the total thrombolytic dose recommended for systemic thrombolysis with similar efficacy in surrogate outcomes. Catheter-directed therapies may also avoid the theoretic issue of thrombolytic agents being shunted away from regions with thrombus and

toward unobstructed pulmonary arteries.[14] Theoretically, intrathrombus administration of thrombolytic therapy exposes a larger surface area of the clot to thrombolysis. This mechanism was described by Schmitz-Rode and colleagues,[14] who demonstrated that proximal vortex formation by obstructing emboli prevented a systemically administered drug from making effective contact with the thrombus. Given these theoretic benefits, a key clinical question is this: should catheter-directed lysis be used more often in high-risk patients and in selected patients with intermediate-risk PE?

SYSTEMIC THROMBOLYTIC THERAPY

Much of the evidence supporting CDL stems from studies of systemic thrombolysis. The Pulmonary Embolism International Thrombolysis (PEITHO) study was the largest randomized controlled trial (n = 1005) evaluating systemic thrombolysis in intermediate-risk PE. The study compared all-cause mortality and hemodynamic decompensation within 7 days of randomization between systemic thrombolysis and anticoagulation alone. Thrombolysis decreased the frequency of the primary endpoint (2.6% vs 5.6%; $P = .015$; number needed to treat, 33), but this was driven by a decrease in hemodynamic decompensation because the mortality rates were similar between the 2 arms.[11] These benefits were offset by increased rates of major extracranial bleeding (6.3% vs 1.5%; $P<.001$; number needed to harm [NNH], 20) and increased intracranial hemorrhage (ICH) in the tenecteplase group (2.0% vs 0.2%; $P = .003$; NNH, 45).[11]

In a meta-analyses of 16 randomized trials (n = 2115 patients) comparing thrombolysis with anticoagulation for acute PE (71% intermediate risk),[7] thrombolytic therapy was associated with decreased all-cause mortality (2.2% vs 3.9%; number needed to treat, 59) and recurrent PE (1.2% vs 3.0%; adjusted odds ratio [OR], 0.40; 95% confidence interval [CI], 0.22–0.74) at a mean follow-up of 82 days.[7] The decrease in all-cause mortality was observed even when the analysis was restricted to patients with intermediate risk PE (adjusted OR, 0.48; 95% CI, 0.25–0.92). However, this benefit was offset by an increase in ICH (1.5% vs 0.2%; adjusted OR, 4.78; 95% CI, 1.78–12.04; NNH, 79) and major bleeding (9.24% vs 3.42%; adjusted OR, 2.73; 95% CI, 1.91–3.91; NNH, 18).[7]

Current evidence does not support the routine use of thrombolytic therapy in unselected intermediate-risk patients with PE. However, studies evaluating CDL for intermediate-risk PE have emerged in recent years given concerns over treatment efficacy with anticoagulation alone.

Catheter-Directed Thrombolysis to Prevent Short-Term Complications of Acute Pulmonary Embolism

The data supporting CDL are limited to a small randomized trial and several single-arm prospective studies. Because of the difficulty in powering trials for clinically important outcomes, the majority of these studies have focused on short-term surrogate outcomes. In prior observational studies, an RV to left ventricular (LV) diameter ratio of greater than 0.9 was associated with mortality at 30 days and has become accepted as a reproducible and well-validated tool for assessing patients with PE at risk for adverse outcomes.[15–17]

Ultrasound-Assisted, Catheter-Directed Thrombolysis for Acute Intermediate-Risk Pulmonary Embolism (ULTIMA) was a randomized control trial that was able to demonstrate a greater reduction in RV/LV ratio in intermediate-risk patients when compared with anticoagulation alone without a difference in the complication rate.[18] The Pulmonary Embolism Response to Fragmentation, Embolectomy and Catheter Thrombolysis (PERFECT) and A prospective, Single arm, Multi-center Trial of EkoSonic Endovascular System and Activase for Treatment of Acute Pulmonary Embolism (SEATTLE II) trials were 2 single-arm prospective studies that also demonstrated a similar reduction in RV/LV ratio as well as a significant reduction of pulmonary artery (PA) systolic pressures.[19,20] Both the PERFECT and SEATLE II trial included a small number of patients with high-risk PE. In the PERFECT trial, both ultrasound-assisted thrombolysis (USAT) and CDL were used and the study showed no difference in outcomes between the 2 devices. Although the PERFECT and ULTIMA trials had no major bleeding events, the SEATLE II trial had an 11% major bleeding rate with no catastrophic bleeding and with most of the bleeding events related to access site complications. SEATTLE II raised concerns about CDL and prompted Tapson and colleagues[21] to study even lower doses of tissue plasminogen activator (tPA) in relation to efficacy and safety. The OPTALYSE PE trial studied 101 patients that were divided into 4 arms of varying doses and infusion times of alteplase (4–24 mg) with no control arm and demonstrated a similar reduction in RV/LV ratio at 48 hours across all 4 arms. It also demonstrated that higher doses of alteplase were associated with increased thrombus clearance (5.5% [95% CI, 1.7%–9.3%] in the lowest dose arm vs 25.7% [95% CI, 12.8%–38.6%] in the highest dose arm). Four major bleeding events occurred that did not correlate with alteplase dosing, 2 of which were ICH. One ICH was in the setting of receiving systemic thrombolysis as a bailout for an inadequate clinical response after CDL.

These prior studies demonstrated an improvement in the RV/LV ratio with CDL, and recently more detailed invasive hemodynamic data in intermediate-risk PE were published. In this cohort of patients, the authors demonstrated that 40% had a low cardiac index defined as less than 1.8 L/min/m during the initial right heart catheterization.[22] Although the mean PA pressures and cardiac index improved regardless of initial cardiac index, the improvement was more pronounced in those starting with a lower cardiac index. After CDL treatment, the mean PA pressure and cardiac index improved significantly with CDL. This finding raises the possibility of using invasive and noninvasive functional hemodynamic assessments to select intermediate risk patients for CDL.

Although there are many methodologic limitations inherent in available studies, there are several key takeaways. Indirect comparisons demonstrate that CDL is significantly more effective in reducing the RV/LV ratio (Table 1) than anticoagulation alone. Given that several studies have shown CDL improves short-term surrogate outcomes in patients with intermediate-risk acute PE, CDL likely benefits carefully selected patients in this population, although larger randomized, controlled trials are needed to identify these patients.

Based on current limited evidence, there continues to be significant uncertainty regarding the safety of CDL; however, the key benefit of CDL is the profound decrease in amount of thrombolytic used. Based on the OPTALYSE-PE trial as well as prior studies such as Moderate Pulmonary Embolism Treated with Thrombolysis (MOPETT) and a study by Wang and colleagues,[23,24] the current optimal dose of tPA is unknown and remains an area of active investigation. The OPTALYSE-PE trial suggests that higher doses of tPA are associated with faster thrombus resolution. The significance of this finding is unknown, but may be important given that many PE survivors have decreased exercise tolerance months and years after the event. These studies were also not designed to assess the long-term outcomes of CDL such as functional impairment, recurrent PE, CTEPH, and

Table 1
Comparison of studies assessing RV/LV ratio with use of advanced therapies versus anticoagulation

Study	N	Study Design	Mean Age (y)	Treatment	tPA Dose (mg)	Intermediate-Risk PE, n (%)	High-Risk PE, n (%)	Reduction in RV/LV Ratio
ULTIMA 2013[18]	30	RCT	63	USAT	20	30 (100%)	0 (0)	0.29 (22%) at 24 h
SEATTLE II 2015[19]	150	Single arm	59	USAT	24	119 (79.3)	31 (20.7)	0.42 (24%)
PERFECT 2015[20]	101	Single arm	60.3	USAT/CDL	28 (mean) variable	73 (72.3)	28 (27.7)	89.1% (95% CI, 76.8–94.4) had ↓ RV strain on echo
OPTALYSE PE 2018[21]	101	RCT	60	USAT	4–28	101 (100)	0 (0)	0.35–0.48 (22.6%–26.3%)
FLARE 2018[54]	106	Single arm	55.6	FlowTriever	0	106 (100)	0 (0)	0.39 (25%)
Fasullo et al,[57] 2011	37	RCT	72.1	Systemic tPA	50	37 (100)	0 (0)	0.38 (27%)
Becattini et al,[58] 2010	23	RCT	62.9	Systemic tPA	30–50	23 (100)	0 (0)	0.31 (24%) at 24 h
ULTIMA 2013[18]	29	RCT	63	AC	0	29 (100)	0 (0)	0.03 (2.5%)
Fasullo et al,[57] 2011	35	RCT	57	AC	0	35 (100)	0 (0)	0.2 (14%)
Becattini et al,[58] 2010	28	RCT	64.5	AC	0	28 (100)	0 (0)	0.1 (8%) at 24 h

Abbreviations: AC, anticoagulation; RCT, randomized control trial.

mortality. Last, there have been no data directly comparing the outcomes of systemic thrombolytic therapy to CDL and, thus, the differences in efficacy and safety between the 2 treatment modalities remain unknown.

Thrombolytic Therapy to Prevent Long-Term Complications of Acute Pulmonary Embolism

Post-PE syndrome and CTEPH are recognized long-term complications of acute PE. The pathophysiology of post-PE syndrome and CTEPH is thought to be multifactorial, including incomplete thrombus resolution, elevated PA pressures, and persistent RV dysfunction, as well as residual perfusion defects.[25–27] Some observational studies have demonstrated elevated PA pressures in patients with acute PE treated with anticoagulation alone at 6 to 28 months of follow-up.[25,26] A prospective observational analysis demonstrated 29% of patients who survive an acute PE will have persistent perfusion defects on V/Q scan at 12 months.[28] Patients with persistent perfusion defects were more likely to have dyspnea, higher PA pressures, and shorter distances on the 6-minute walk test. Additionally, the OPTALYSE PE study was able to demonstrate that higher doses of thrombolytic therapy was associated with faster clot resolution.[21] The clinical significance of this finding is unknown, but may be important given that incomplete clot resolution occurs in one-fourth to one-third of patients after acute PE.[29] Most thrombus resolution seems to plateau after 3 months owing to clot remodeling into a permanent fibrous scar.[29] This finding suggests that there may be a benefit to early clot resolution, although long-term follow-up in selected patients from the PEITHOs trial did not demonstrate a benefit in systemic thrombolytics over anticoagulation in the incidence of CTEPH or persistent functional limitation.[30] With currently available information, it is unclear whether upfront advanced therapy with CDL reduces long-term symptom burden. This topic remains an active area of investigation.

Devices for Catheter-Directed Lysis

The 2 most commonly used non–ultrasound-assisted catheters are the Uni-Fuse (Angiodynamics Inc, Latham, NY) and Cragg-McNamara (Covidien, Plymouth, MN) catheters. Both carry an indication from the US Food and Drug Administration for infusion of thrombolytics into the peripheral vasculature, without a specific indication for PE. Both are 4F to 5F multisidehole catheters. The most common ultrasound-assisted catheter is the EkoSonic Endovascular System (EKOS Corporation, Bothell, WA). The EKOS device (https://btgplc.com/en-US/EKOS/Home) uses multiple small ultrasound transducers inserted into the catheter to help facilitate thrombolytic delivery into the thrombus. The ultrasound energy is theorized to alter the local architecture of the fibrin clot by dissociating fibrin strands and increasing available receptor sites for tPA.[31] This technique may increase the efficacy of USAT and allows for shorter infusion times compared with standard CDL. There have been no randomized trials in acute PE comparing USAT versus traditional CDL in acute PE. In the PERFECT registry, there was no difference in technical or clinical success between the two.[20] Two retrospective studies also found no statistical differences in clinical and hemodynamic outcomes or complication rates between the 2 methods.[32,33] In a nonrandomized trial of 33 patients, USAT led to improved treatment outcome based on thrombus removal, decrease the duration of thrombolytic infusion time, and fewer treatment-related hemorrhagic complications.[34] A randomized trial comparing conventional CDL versus USAT in iliofemoral DVT found no difference between the modalities in clinical or ultrasound outcomes at 12 months.[35] Current available data do not suggest that USAT (which is associated with increased cost) improves thrombolytic efficacy when added to conventional CDL, but a current ongoing randomized head-to-head trial (SUNSET sPE NCT02758574) aims to address this question.[36] In this study, patients who have radiographic or biochemical evidence of submassive PE are randomized 1:1 to USAT or standard CDL. The primary outcome of this study is clearance of pulmonary thrombus burden assessed by postprocedure computed tomography angiography. Secondary outcomes include resolution of RV strain, improvement in PA pressures, and 3- and 12-month echocardiographic, functional, and quality-of-life measures.[36]

The Bashir Endovascular Catheter (Thrombolex Inc, Doylestown, PA) is an expandable nitinol basket with multiple sideholes that allow for thrombolytic agents to be infused directly into clot while also facilitating mechanical thrombus disruption. This device is currently being evaluated in a prospective single-arm study for PE. Technical considerations of CDL and a summary of devices can be found in **Table 2**.

Safety of Catheter-Directed Lysis

As expected, the most commonly reported complications with CDL involve bleeding. The

Table 2
Devices used in catheter directed therapies

Device	Mechanism	Technical Considerations	Associated Prospective Studies
EkoSonic	USAT	5F catheter. Remain on full dose anticoagulation during the procedure with goal ACT of >200 s. Subtherapeutic heparin dose after thrombolytic infusion is initiated. Fibrinogen/PTT levels checked every 4–6 h, consider reducing or stopping infusion if fibrinogen <100–150. May need cardiac anesthesiologist if anesthesia is required. Caution in patients with LBBB to avoid iatrogenic CHB.	ULTIMA, SEATTLE II, OPTALYSE PE
Cragg-McNamara	CDL		
Unifuse	CDL		
AngioVac	Venoveno bypass with large filter in between to catch/remove thrombus	Two access sites. 26F access for inflow, 22F for outflow. Requires a perfusionist.	
FlowTreiver	Mechanical aspiration with 3 nitinol self-expanding disks to help to remove the thrombus	20F catheter. Continuous aspiration may lead to blood loss.	FLARE
Penumbra Indigo	Mechanical aspiration	8F catheter. Continuous aspiration may result in blood loss.	EXTRACT-PE (under investigation)
AngioJet	High flow saline jet producing negative pressure allowing aspiration of thrombus	8F catheter. Bradycardia, hypotension.	

Abbreviations: ACT, activated clotting time; CHB, complete heart block; LBBB, left bundle branch block; PTT, partial thromboplastin time.

definition of major and minor bleeding often varies between trials, which makes it difficult to directly compare studies or combine bleeding rates. Given that the optimal dose of tPA remains under active investigation, the thrombolytic dosage and duration used in previous studies is also highly variable. In the 6 largest and most recent prospective trials consisting of 556 patients that underwent USAT (PERFECT, OPTALYSE, ULTIMA, SEATTLE II, Bloomer and colleagues,[37] and Ozcinar and colleagues[38]), the pooled estimate for major bleeding was 4.3% (95% CI, 1.1%–7.5%) and the estimated ICH rate was 0.7% (95% CI, 0.0%–1.3%).[39] These rates seem to be lower than those observed in a meta-analysis of systemic thrombolytic therapy (n = 1061), where major bleeding and ICH

occurred in 9.2% and 1.5% of patients, respectively.[7] It is important to note that the average age of patients the 6 largest prospective studies evaluating CDL was 62 years old, whereas the majority of major bleeding in the meta-analysis of systemic thrombolysis occurred in patients aged more than 65 years. The younger age in the catheter-based studies may exaggerate the safety profile of CDL and this technology needs to be studied more extensively in the older population. Additionally, early studies in a controlled environment often underestimate true complication rates and higher rates of major bleeding should be expected in general use. Although indirect evidence may suggest lower rates of bleeding complications with CDL compared with systemic therapy, additional prospective comparative studies are needed to confirm this finding.

Other potential complications of CDL include cardiac tamponade from cardiac perforation, ventricular arrhythmias with catheter advancement through the RV, papillary muscle/tricuspid valve trauma with the use of stiff wires, worsening hemodynamics owing to distal embolization of proximal nonocclusive thrombi, and transient complete heart block in those with a baseline left bundle branch block.[40] These complications are rare given the low profile of these catheters in comparison with larger embolectomy devices and, to our knowledge, have not been reported in the literature. Pulmonary hemorrhage from PA rupture is also a potential complication but it has been rarely reported. The largest retrospective analysis of pulmonary hemorrhage associated with PA catheter placement (n = 32,422) identified an incidence of 0.03%.[41] A summary of bleeding events in recent trials involving CDL are listed in **Table 3**.

Patient Selection for Catheter-Directed Lysis

All patients with acute PE should receive prompt anticoagulation unless contraindicated.[12] Patients with low-risk PE should be treated with anticoagulation alone with many eligible for outpatient therapy.[42–44] The use of thrombolysis is not recommended in low-risk patients because their short-term mortality rates are 1% with anticoagulation.[12] At the other extreme, patients with hemodynamic instability warrant strong consideration of advanced treatment options, including systemic or catheter-based therapy because they have a high incidence of adverse outcomes.[12] There is a paucity of data supporting the best interventional approach in these patients and head-to-head randomized, controlled trials in this patient population are difficult for a number of reasons. Only 5% of PEs are high risk, which makes recruiting a study powered to detect clinically meaningful outcomes challenging. Many patients have relative or absolute contraindications (**Table 4**) to systemic thrombolysis (47% in 1 study), limiting the ability to randomize patients.[9] Based on available evidence, it is reasonable for patients with high-risk PE with contraindications to systemic thrombolytics or failed thrombolysis to undergo CDL or be considered for surgical or catheter-based thrombectomy, assuming clinical expertise is available. Therapeutic options in the high-risk category should be individualized with the help of a multidisciplinary team.

Management of intermediate-risk patients is controversial. Traditionally, anticoagulation alone has been sufficient to prevent further morbidity in these patients, but some studies suggest that a subset of these patients with RV dysfunction may be at risk for early decompensation despite initial stability.[12] Recognizing that clinical progression from intermediate-risk to high-risk PE can occur rapidly, patients with intermediate-risk PE should be monitored closely for deterioration with escalation of therapy if needed.

In view of the equivocal data presented, it is prudent to rigorously examine the risks and benefits of thrombolytic therapy in each patient in the intermediate-risk category. PE-related functional impairment and objective signs of impaired end organ perfusion (such as elevated lactate), elevated heart rates, relative hypotension, and severity of hypoxia should also be taken into consideration when deciding on thrombolysis. Owing to the equivocal data of advanced therapies in acute PE in the intermediate-risk group along with rapidly evolving therapeutic options, multidisciplinary PE response teams have been created to help with immediate risk stratification and rapid triaging.[45,46] At present, the available literature is insufficient to support the routine use of CDL for intermediate risk patients. However, it is important to recognize that there may be a subset of intermediate-risk PE patients that may benefit from CDL and ongoing research efforts should work to better identify this group.

CATHETER-BASED EMBOLECTOMY

Catheter-based embolectomy refers to nonlytic, nonsurgical, catheter-based therapies for acute PE that seek to remove thrombus and relieve obstruction of the pulmonary arteries. The data behind catheter-based embolectomy are relatively sparse, but growing. Furthermore, the variety of devices in catheter-based embolectomy make it more difficulty to study. We next focus on the general indications and considerations of catheter-based embolectomy, the risks and benefits of these therapies, and then review specific devices.

Rationale and Indications for Catheter-Based Embolectomy

At least one-third of patients with acute PE have some contraindications to systemic thrombolytics and up to 10% of patients who receive thrombolytic therapy remain in shock.[47,48] For these patients, surgical embolectomy may be considered, but surgical expertise is often limited to selected centers and surgical

Table 3
Complication rates with catheter-directed lysis

Study[REF]	N	Mean Age (y)	Study Design	tPA Dose (mg)	No. of High-Risk PE Patients	No. of Intermediate-Risk PE Patients	Major Bleeding Rate, n (%)	ICH, n (%)
ULTIMA 2013[18]	59	63	Randomized controlled trial	20	0	30[a]	0 (0) CDL vs 0 (0) AC	0 (0)
SEATTLE II 2015[19]	150	59	Prospective single arm	24	31	119	15 (10)	0 (0)
PERFECT 2015[20]	101	60.3	Prospective single arm	28 (mean), variable	28	73	0 (0)	0 (0)
Bloomer et al,[37] 2017	137	59	Prospective single arm	17 (median), 2–48	16	121	13 (9.4)	2 (1.4)
OPTALYSE PE 2018[21]	101	60	Randomized controlled trial	4–24	0	101	4 (4)	2 (2)
Total	519 treated with CDL				75	444 treated with CDL	31 (6.0)	4 (0.77)

[a] Twenty-nine patients were treated with anticoagulation.

Table 4	
Contraindications to systemic thrombolysis	
Absolute Contraindications	**Relative Contraindications**
Prior intracranial hemorrhage	Systolic blood pressure >180 or diastolic >110
Known structural cerebral lesion	History of ischemic stroke >3 mo
Known malignant neoplasm	Major surgery within the last 3 wk, recent invasive procedure
Ischemic stroke within 3 mo	Trauma or prolonged cardiopulmonary resuscitation >10 min
Suspected aortic dissection	Recent extracranial bleeding (2–4 wk)
Active bleeding (excluding menses)	Age >75
Recent head trauma or brain injury	Pregnancy, active peptic ulcer, pericarditis, diabetic retinopathy

embolectomy can have high morbidity and mortality, especially in patients who have failed thrombolytic therapy. Percutaneous pulmonary embolectomy may be an attractive option for these patients and should be considered in those with persistent hemodynamic instability despite thrombolytic therapy or in those who have contraindications to thrombolytics.[12,13] An important adjunctive therapy in these cases is mechanical circulatory support, either extracorporeal membrane oxygenation or isolated percutaneous RV support.[49,50] Mechanical circulatory support can be used to buy time for a patient's RV to recover while on anticoagulation, serving as a bridge to more definitive treatment (CDL, CDE, surgical embolectomy), or as a bailout in the case of intraprocedural hemodynamic decompensation.

As with CDL, catheter-based embolectomy in patients with intermediate-risk acute PE remains controversial. Patients that should be considered are those with a higher risk of developing hemodynamic instability and those with significant symptoms, persistent

desaturation, or significant functional limitation despite adequate anticoagulation. In general, patients also must meet anatomic criteria when considering percutaneous pulmonary embolectomy. Thrombus in the central, lobar, or interlobar arteries should be the targets of emboli, and anything more distal is unlikely to benefit owing to anatomic restrictions of the catheter navigating into smaller vessels.[51] Given the paucity of data and lack of standard approach regarding catheter-based embolectomy, patient selection should involve a multidisciplinary discussion among specialists with expertise in each therapeutic option.

Specific Catheters and Techniques
Catheter-based thrombus maceration
Clot maceration can be performed using a modified pigtail catheter with a guidewire that exits from a side hole of the pigtail loop. Manual rotation attempts to break down fresh thrombus into smaller fragments that can embolize downstream and allow forward flow. Peripheral balloons can also be used for this purpose. These techniques may be helpful in hypotensive patients with totally occluded proximal branches to allow forward flow and partially decompress the right ventricle until further treatment, such as local thrombolysis takes effect.[52] It is not clear if maceration is helpful by itself because the majority of reported cases have been performed in conjunction with thrombolytic therapy.[52] In the current era with dedicated embolectomy devices available, this technique has been rendered largely obsolete (see Table 2).

Rheolytic thrombectomy
This technology uses high-speed saline jets that travel backward from the tip of the catheter creating a vacuum and thrombus fragmentation effects. While embedded in the thrombus, it can also provide pulse delivery of thrombolytic agents. This device has been associated with profound bradycardia and a high incidence of procedure-related complications (hemoptysis from presumed pulmonary hemorrhage, major hemorrhage at access and non-access site locations) when used in PE patients.[53] The US Food and Drug Administration has issued a Black Box warning regarding its use in PE treatment.

FlowTriever
Currently there is only 1 prospective, multicenter, single arm study (FLARE) that evaluated the FlowTriever system (Inari Medical, Irvine, CA) in 106 patients with acute PE.[54] Patients with proximal PE and RV/LV ratio of 0.9 or higher

were eligible for enrollment and, notably, the study excluded patients who had recent thrombolytic use. The primary endpoint was change in RV/LV ratio at 48 hours, which was significantly reduced by 0.39 (25%) (95% CI, 1.53–1.15; $P<.0001$) from baseline. To put these results into context, the change in RV/LV ratio with FlowTriever embolectomy was similar to trials evaluating CDL and significantly better than anticoagulation alone at the 24- to 48-hour timepoint (see Table 1). Notably, there was no ICH or access site major bleeding. Four patients had clinical deterioration, which included 1 intraprocedural pulmonary hemorrhage requiring lower lobectomy. Two patients had minimal thrombus removal during thrombectomy and experienced respiratory deterioration during or immediately after the procedure, requiring intubation. One patient arrested in the setting of periprocedural agitation, requiring increasing sedation. These major adverse events emphasize the tradeoff between CDL and CDE, bleeding on one side and risk of decompensation in the other.

The FlowTriever (Inari Medical) is the only CDE device cleared by the US Food and Drug Administration and features a 20F aspiration guide catheter (termed AGC or Triever 20) and a restoration catheter that is advanced inside the catheter over a wire and placed near the thrombus (https://www.inarimedical.com/flow-triever/). The device has undergone several iterations over the past few years and the latest version has significantly more suction power (104 mL/s) than the first version. The AGC is typically placed near the clot and owing to the large suction force created will often remove large pieces of thrombus. There is now a 16F device for more distal clots in subsegmental vessels and also a larger 24F device to extract larger proximal clots en bloc. The second component of this system consists of 3 self-expanding nitonol mesh disks that are advanced through the larger AGC or Triever catheter to engage, disrupt, and retract the clot back into the AGC. This technique is typically used when the clot is adherent to the vessel wall or more distal. The discs come in different sizes to target varying sizes and locations of the pulmonary arterial circulation. Once the clot is loosened, it can be aspirated through the AGC. Given the need for continuous aspiration through a large-bore device, careful attention should be paid to blood loss during the procedure. At the conclusion of the case, the 20F to 26F venous sheath is removed and a mattress suture is applied. Patients remain on heparin throughout the procedure and can remain on heparin immediately afterward as well. The initial FLARE Trial was in intermediate-risk patients, but there are growing data for use even in massive pulmonary emboli.

AngioVac

The AngioVac catheter (AngioDynamics) is a 22F catheter with a funnel shaped, balloon-expandable layered tip that can remove thrombus through a centrifugal pump (https://www.angio-dynamics.com/products/3/AngioVac/). It also has an 18F reinfusion canula that creates a venovenous bypass circuit with a large filter in between to remove aspirated thrombus. This procedure requires 2 access points and usually requires a perfusionist to be present to set up and operate the system. The major benefit of this system is that it can suction large amounts of blood and thrombus without significant blood loss. The major limitation of this device in treatment of acute PE are its large size, inflexibility, and the need for procedural support from a perfusion team. This makes it difficult to steer through the tortuous anatomy to get to the PA. The data on the use of AngioVac for pulmonary emboli are sparse. There are no randomized controlled trials or large retrospective analyses on the use of this device in acute PE. Much of the data have been extrapolated from use for iliocaval vein thrombosis. Published experiences in acute PE are limited to case reports and small case series.[55] The largest systematic review of AngioVac providing safety data included 57 patients in whom the device as used for various indications (iliocaval thrombus, right atrial thrombus, and PE); there were 6 access site hematomas, 1 fatal retroperitoneal bleed, and 1 ICH.[56]

Penumbra Indigo

The Indigo system (Penumbra Inc, Alameda, CA) device is a smaller bore suction aspiration device that has been used in the peripheral arterial and venous circulations as well as in neurovascular cases. The Indigo embolectomy system (Penumbra, Inc) is a flexible 8F small-bore aspiration catheter that is connected to a continuous suction vacuum system (https://www.penumbrainc.com/peripheral-device/indigo-system/). A wire separator is moved back and forth at the tip of the catheter to clear clot and improve aspiration of thrombus. The major benefit of the Indigo system is the small size and ease of delivery to the pulmonary arteries. The major drawbacks of the system are that it requires aspiration, which can result in substantial blood loss, and that the catheter caliber may not be large enough to effectively perform embolectomy on larger, central thrombi. To minimize blood loss, the catheter is usually placed more distally closer to the clot and aspiration is performed by slowing pulling back while visualizing the amount of blood flowing into the cannister. If a significant amount of blood is returning into the cannister, the catheter likely disengaged the thrombus and then the operator should reposition the catheter to reengage the thrombus. The device was studied in a prospective, single-arm, multicenter trial in patients with PE and an RV/LV ratio of greater than 0.9 (EXTRACT-PE; NCT03218566). Preliminary results from EXTRACT-PE showed that the use of the Indigo aspiration system in acute PE resulted in an RV/LV reduction of 0.43 and a major adverse event rate (pulmonary hemorrhage) of 1.7% at 48 hours.

Safety of Catheter-Based Embolectomy

Many of the same procedural-related complications that occur with CDL also exist with catheter-based embolectomy. However, non-access site bleeding risk with catheter-based embolectomy is typically lower than CDL as no thrombolytic therapy must be concomitantly administered. This was consistent with the 0.9% (1/104) rate of major bleeding events in the FLARE trial. However, thrombectomy devices may carry an increased risk of intraprocedural complications compared with CDL given that the catheters and devices are much larger and stiffer wires used to guide advancement of larger devices into the pulmonary vasculature may result in structural damage to the heart or pulmonary vessels.

SUMMARY

Historically, there have been 2 main treatment modalities for acute PE: systemic thrombolysis and anticoagulation. Although anticoagulation remains the cornerstone of acute PE therapy, the role of catheter-based therapies is rapidly evolving to fill an unmet clinical need in PE treatment. Although systemic thrombolysis is effective in acute PE, the benefits are often offset by the high risk of bleeding. CDL may offer a potentially lower bleeding profile despite similar efficacy, although there are no available head-to-head randomized, controlled trials. Optimal tPA dosing remains an area of active investigation. Patients with absolute contraindications to thrombolytic therapy or those who require rapid thrombus removal may be candidates for catheter-based embolectomy.

The current evidence does not support the routine use of catheter-directed therapy in preference to anticoagulation alone in intermediate-risk patients. A select subgroup of these patients may benefit from catheter-based therapies and decision making in this setting may be facilitated by the use of a multidisciplinary PE response teams.

DISCLOSURE

Dr S. Khandhar has served as a primary investigator for Inari Medical. Dr J. Giri reports Board of Directors of PERT Consortium, advisory board of Astra Zeneca, consulting fees from Phillips Medical. Drs R. Zhang, T. Kobayashi, and S. Pugliese have nothing to report.

REFERENCES

1. Centers for Disease Control and Prevention (CDC). Venous thromboembolism in adult hospitalizations - United States, 2007-2009. MMWR Morb Mortal Wkly Rep 2012;61(22):401–4.
2. Tapson VF. Acute pulmonary embolism. N Engl J Med 2008;358(10):1037–52.
3. Park B, Messina L, Dargon P, et al. Recent trends in clinical outcomes and resource utilization for pulmonary embolism in the United States: findings from the nationwide inpatient sample. Chest 2009;136(4):983–90.
4. Horlander KT, Mannino DM, Leeper KV. Pulmonary embolism mortality in the United States, 1979-1998: an analysis using multiple-cause mortality data. Arch Intern Med 2003;163(14):1711–7.
5. Rathbun S. Cardiology patient pages. The Surgeon General's call to action to prevent deep vein thrombosis and pulmonary embolism. Circulation 2009;119(15):e480–2.
6. Jimenez D, Kopecna D, Tapson V, et al. Derivation and validation of multimarker prognostication for normotensive patients with acute symptomatic pulmonary embolism. Am J Respir Crit Care Med 2014;189(6):718–26.
7. Chatterjee S, Chakraborty A, Weinberg I, et al. Thrombolysis for pulmonary embolism and risk of all-cause mortality, major bleeding, and intracranial hemorrhage: a meta-analysis. JAMA 2014;311(23): 2414–21.
8. Becattini C, Agnelli G, Lankeit M, et al. Acute pulmonary embolism: mortality prediction by the 2014 European Society of Cardiology risk stratification model. Eur Respir J 2016;48(3):780–6.
9. Kasper W, Konstantinides S, Geibel A, et al. Management strategies and determinants of outcome in acute major pulmonary embolism: results of a multicenter registry. J Am Coll Cardiol 1997;30(5): 1165–71.

10. Goldhaber SZ, Visani L, De Rosa M. Acute pulmonary embolism: clinical outcomes in the International Cooperative Pulmonary Embolism Registry (ICOPER). Lancet 1999;353(9162):1386–9.

11. Meyer G, Vicaut E, Danays T, et al. Fibrinolysis for patients with intermediate-risk pulmonary embolism. N Engl J Med 2014;370(15):1402–11.

12. Jaff MR, McMurtry MS, Archer SL, et al. Management of massive and submassive pulmonary embolism, iliofemoral deep vein thrombosis, and chronic thromboembolic pulmonary hypertension: a scientific statement from the American Heart Association. Circulation 2011;123(16):1788–830.

13. Konstantinides SV, Torbicki A, Agnelli G, et al. 2014 ESC guidelines on the diagnosis and management of acute pulmonary embolism. Eur Heart J 2014; 35(43):3033–69, 3069a-3069k.

14. Schmitz-Rode T, Kilbinger M, Gunther RW. Simulated flow pattern in massive pulmonary embolism: significance for selective intrapulmonary thrombolysis. Cardiovasc Intervent Radiol 1998;21(3): 199–204.

15. Schoepf UJ, Kucher N, Kipfmueller F, et al. Right ventricular enlargement on chest computed tomography: a predictor of early death in acute pulmonary embolism. Circulation 2004;110(20): 3276–80.

16. van der Meer RW, Pattynama PM, van Strijen MJ, et al. Right ventricular dysfunction and pulmonary obstruction index at helical CT: prediction of clinical outcome during 3-month follow-up in patients with acute pulmonary embolism. Radiology 2005; 235(3):798–803.

17. Trujillo-Santos J, den Exter PL, Gomez V, et al. Computed tomography-assessed right ventricular dysfunction and risk stratification of patients with acute non-massive pulmonary embolism: systematic review and meta-analysis. J Thromb Haemost 2013;11(10):1823–32.

18. Kucher N, Boekstegers P, Muller OJ, et al. Randomized, controlled trial of ultrasound-assisted catheter-directed thrombolysis for acute intermediate-risk pulmonary embolism. Circulation 2014;129(4): 479–86.

19. Piazza G, Hohlfelder B, Jaff MR, et al. A prospective, single-arm, multicenter trial of ultrasound-facilitated, catheter-directed, low-dose fibrinolysis for acute massive and submassive pulmonary embolism: the SEATTLE II study. JACC Cardiovasc Interv 2015;8(10):1382–92.

20. Kuo WT, Banerjee A, Kim PS, et al. Pulmonary embolism response to fragmentation, embolectomy, and catheter thrombolysis (PERFECT): initial results from a prospective multicenter registry. Chest 2015;148(3):667–73.

21. Tapson VF, Sterling K, Jones N, et al. A randomized trial of the optimum duration of acoustic pulse thrombolysis procedure in acute intermediate-risk pulmonary embolism: the OPTALYSE PE trial. JACC Cardiovasc Interv 2018;11(14):1401–10.

22. Khandhar SJ, Mehta M, Cilia L, et al. Invasive hemodynamic assessment of patients with submassive pulmonary embolism. Catheter Cardiovasc Interv 2019. https://doi.org/10.1002/ccd.28491.

23. Sharifi M, Bay C, Skrocki L, et al. Moderate pulmonary embolism treated with thrombolysis (from the "MOPETT" Trial). Am J Cardiol 2013;111(2):273–7.

24. Wang C, Zhai Z, Yang Y, et al. Efficacy and safety of low dose recombinant tissue-type plasminogen activator for the treatment of acute pulmonary thromboembolism: a randomized, multicenter, controlled trial. Chest 2010;137(2):254–62.

25. Stevinson BG, Hernandez-Nino J, Rose G, et al. Echocardiographic and functional cardiopulmonary problems 6 months after first-time pulmonary embolism in previously healthy patients. Eur Heart J 2007;28(20):2517–24.

26. Kline JA, Steuerwald MT, Marchick MR, et al. Prospective evaluation of right ventricular function and functional status 6 months after acute submassive pulmonary embolism: frequency of persistent or subsequent elevation in estimated pulmonary artery pressure. Chest 2009;136(5):1202–10.

27. Sista AK, Miller LE, Kahn SR, et al. Persistent right ventricular dysfunction, functional capacity limitation, exercise intolerance, and quality of life impairment following pulmonary embolism: systematic review with meta-analysis. Vasc Med 2017;22(1): 37–43.

28. Sanchez O, Helley D, Couchon S, et al. Perfusion defects after pulmonary embolism: risk factors and clinical significance. J Thromb Haemost 2010; 8(6):1248–55.

29. Klok FA, van der Hulle T, den Exter PL, et al. The post-PE syndrome: a new concept for chronic complications of pulmonary embolism. Blood Rev 2014; 28(6):221–6.

30. Konstantinides SV, Vicaut E, Danays T, et al. Impact of thrombolytic therapy on the long-term outcome of intermediate-risk pulmonary embolism. J Am Coll Cardiol 2017;69(12):1536–44.

31. Braaten JV, Goss RA, Francis CW. Ultrasound reversibly disaggregates fibrin fibers. Thromb Haemost 1997;78(3):1063–8.

32. Liang NL, Avgerinos ED, Marone LK, et al. Comparative outcomes of ultrasound-assisted thrombolysis and standard catheter-directed thrombolysis in the treatment of acute pulmonary embolism. Vasc Endovascular Surg 2016;50(6):405–10.

33. Rao G, Xu H, Wang JJ, et al. Ultrasound-assisted versus conventional catheter-directed thrombolysis for acute pulmonary embolism: a multicenter comparison of patient-centered outcomes. Vasc Med 2019;24(3):241–7.

34. Lin PH, Annambhotla S, Bechara CF, et al. Comparison of percutaneous ultrasound-accelerated thrombolysis versus catheter-directed thrombolysis in patients with acute massive pulmonary embolism. Vascular 2009;17(Suppl 3):S137–47.

35. Engelberger RP, Stuck A, Spirk D, et al. Ultrasound-assisted versus conventional catheter-directed thrombolysis for acute iliofemoral deep vein thrombosis: 1-year follow-up data of a randomized-controlled trial. J Thromb Haemost 2017;15(7):1351–60.

36. Avgerinos ED, Mohapatra A, Rivera-Lebron B, et al. Design and rationale of a randomized trial comparing standard versus ultrasound-assisted thrombolysis for submassive pulmonary embolism. J Vasc Surg Venous Lymphat Disord 2018;6(1):126–32.

37. Bloomer TL, El-Hayek GE, McDaniel MC, et al. Safety of catheter-directed thrombolysis for massive and submassive pulmonary embolism: results of a multicenter registry and meta-analysis. Catheter Cardiovasc Interv 2017;89(4):754–60.

38. Ozcinar E, Cakici M, Dikmen Yaman N, et al. Thrombus resolution and right ventricular functional recovery using ultrasound-accelerated thrombolysis in acute massive and submassive pulmonary embolism. Int Angiol 2017;36(5):428–37.

39. Kannel WB, Dannenberg AL, Levy D. Population implications of electrocardiographic left ventricular hypertrophy. Am J Cardiol 1987;60(17):85i–93i.

40. Taslakian B, Sista AK. Catheter-directed therapy for pulmonary embolism: patient selection and technical considerations. Interv Cardiol Clin 2018;7(1):81–90.

41. Kearney TJ, Shabot MM. Pulmonary artery rupture associated with the Swan-Ganz catheter. Chest 1995;108(5):1349–52.

42. Piran S, Le Gal G, Wells PS, et al. Outpatient treatment of symptomatic pulmonary embolism: a systematic review and meta-analysis. Thromb Res 2013;132(5):515–9.

43. Zondag W, den Exter PL, Crobach MJ, et al. Comparison of two methods for selection of out of hospital treatment in patients with acute pulmonary embolism. Thromb Haemost 2013;109(1):47–52.

44. Kearon C, Akl EA, Ornelas J, et al. Antithrombotic therapy for VTE disease: CHEST guideline and expert panel report. Chest 2016;149(2):315–52.

45. Barnes GD, Kabrhel C, Courtney DM, et al. Diversity in the pulmonary embolism response team model: an organizational survey of the national PERT consortium members. Chest 2016;150(6):1414–7.

46. Barnes G, Giri J, Courtney DM, et al. Nuts and bolts of running a pulmonary embolism response team: results from an organizational survey of the National PERT Consortium members. Hosp Pract (1995) 2017;45(3):76–80.

47. Stein PD, Matta F. Thrombolytic therapy in unstable patients with acute pulmonary embolism: saves lives but underused. Am J Med 2012;125(5):465–70.

48. Wan S, Quinlan DJ, Agnelli G, et al. Thrombolysis compared with heparin for the initial treatment of pulmonary embolism: a meta-analysis of the randomized controlled trials. Circulation 2004;110(6):744–9.

49. Elder M, Blank N, Kaki A, et al. Mechanical circulatory support for acute right ventricular failure in the setting of pulmonary embolism. J Interv Cardiol 2018;31(4):518–24.

50. Ain DL, Albaghdadi M, Giri J, et al. Extra-corporeal membrane oxygenation and outcomes in massive pulmonary embolism: two eras at an urban tertiary care hospital. Vasc Med 2018;23(1):60–4.

51. Jaber WA, McDaniel MC. Catheter-based embolectomy for acute pulmonary embolism: devices, technical considerations, risks, and benefits. Interv Cardiol Clin 2018;7(1):91–101.

52. Schmitz-Rode T, Janssens U, Duda SH, et al. Massive pulmonary embolism: percutaneous emergency treatment by pigtail rotation catheter. J Am Coll Cardiol 2000;36(2):375–80.

53. Kuo WT, Gould MK, Louie JD, et al. Catheter-directed therapy for the treatment of massive pulmonary embolism: systematic review and meta-analysis of modern techniques. J Vasc Interv Radiol 2009;20(11):1431–40.

54. Tu T, Toma C, Tapson VF, et al. A prospective, single-arm, multicenter trial of catheter-directed mechanical thrombectomy for intermediate-risk acute pulmonary embolism: the FLARE study. JACC Cardiovasc Interv 2019;12(9):859–69.

55. Donaldson CW, Baker JN, Narayan RL, et al. Thrombectomy using suction filtration and venovenous bypass: single center experience with a novel device. Catheter Cardiovasc Interv 2015;86(2):E81–7.

56. Worku B, Salemi A, D'Ayala MD, et al. The AngioVac device: understanding the Failures on the Road to Success. Innovations (Phila) 2016;11(6):430–3.

57. Fasullo S, Scalzo S, Maringhini G, et al. Six-month echocardiographic study in patients with submassive pulmonary embolism and right ventricle dysfunction: comparison of thrombolysis with heparin. Am J Med Sci 2011;341(1):33–9.

58. Becattini C, Agnelli G, Salvi A, et al. Bolus tenecteplase for right ventricle dysfunction in hemodynamically stable patients with pulmonary embolism. Thromb Res 2010;125(3):e82–6.

Intervention for Iliofemoral Deep Vein Thrombosis and May-Thurner Syndrome

Taufiq Salahuddin, MD[a],
Ehrin J. Armstrong, MD, MSc, MAS[a,b],*

KEYWORDS

- Iliofemoral deep vein thrombosis (DVT) • Proximal deep vein thrombosis
- May-Thurner syndrome • Iliac vein compression syndrome
- Catheter-directed thrombolysis (CDT) • Venous stenting

KEY POINTS

- Patients with iliac vein compression (May-Thurner syndrome [MTS]) are more likely to develop iliofemoral DVT, and patients with iliofemoral DVT may have an increased prevalence of MTS.
- Postthrombotic syndrome (PTS) presents with signs and symptoms of venous hypertension and is more likely to occur after iliofemoral DVT than more distal DVT.
- Iliac vein compression from MTS (with or without thrombosis) is an important cause of unilateral venous symptoms, including pain, edema, venous claudication, and skin ulcers.
- Whereas clot removal via catheter-directed thrombolysis (CDT) remains controversial for iliofemoral DVT, reduced clot burden via CDT may help prevent PTS or reduce its severity.
- Stenting for symptomatic MTS improves symptoms and quality of life, has low morbidity, and has good patency rates in follow-up.

INTRODUCTION

Iliofemoral deep venous thrombosis (IFDVT) and May-Thurner syndrome (MTS) are 2 distinct clinical entities that are closely intertwined. In this *Clinics* article, we discuss the relation of IFDVT with MTS as well as procedural intervention for both.

May-Thurner Syndrome

MTS is defined by extrinsic compression of the iliocaval veins (also known as iliac vein compression syndrome or iliocaval compression syndrome), most commonly between the arterial system and bony structures. Compression of the iliac vein may predispose patients to IFDVT, and conversely, patients with IFDVT have a relatively high prevalence of MTS.

The most common variant of MTS, first described by May and Thurner in 1957, is compression of the left iliac vein between the overlying right common iliac artery and fifth lumbar vertebrae.[1] Cockett and colleagues recognized iliac compression syndrome in the next decade, and also described its relation to postthrombotic syndrome (PTS).[2] Causes, in addition to compression by the arterial system, may include extrinsic tumor compression, uterine enlargement, aortoiliac aneurysm, retroperitoneal fibrosis, and osteophytes.

The true prevalence of MTS is unknown, as patients may not have symptoms or require treatment for iliac vein compression.[3] MTS is identified as an etiology in 2% to 5% of patients presenting with a symptomatic lower-extremity venous disorders.

---

[a] Cardiology Section, Rocky Mountain Regional VA Medical Center, 1700 North Wheeling Street, Aurora, CO 80045, USA; [b] Interventional Cardiology, Vascular Laboratory, Rocky Mountain Regional VA, Division of Cardiology, University of Colorado, University of Colorado School of Medicine, Aurora, CO, USA
* Corresponding author. Cardiology Section, Rocky Mountain Regional VA Medical Center, 1700 North Wheeling Street, Aurora, CO 80045, USA.
E-mail address: ehrin.armstrong@gmail.com

Intervent Cardiol Clin 9 (2020) 243–254
https://doi.org/10.1016/j.iccl.2019.11.003

The prevalence of MTS in patients presenting with IFDVT may approximate 50% to 60%.[4,5] Some studies report even higher rates.[6]

Even in the absence of IFDVT, anatomic compression from MTS can itself be symptomatic.[7] Venous obstruction may result in unilateral extremity pain and swelling, lower-extremity edema, skin discoloration, or ulceration from venous hypertension, and/or venous claudication. MTS has also been associated with pelvic congestion syndrome in female patients.[8]

Iliofemoral Deep Vein Thrombosis

IFDVT accounts for approximately 25% of all lower-extremity DVTs and is associated with increased risk of pulmonary embolism, limb malperfusion, DVT recurrence, and PTS compared with below the knee DVT.[9–13]

When PTS occurs, it adversely affects quality of life (QOL).[14] The pathophysiology of PTS is incompletely understood but thought to be partially related to venous reflux and obstruction due to destruction of venous valves after DVT. Symptoms of PTS are similar to those present in other forms of venous hypertension.[15]

Because MTS predisposes to IFDVT and IFDVT may lead to PTS, MTS should be considered during the evaluation and treatment of IFDVT and PTS. It is worth noting that iliac compression and venous outflow obstruction can lead to signs and symptoms similar to PTS even in the absence of venous thrombosis. The goal of procedural intervention for any of these entities is to relieve the signs and symptoms of venous hypertension.

Herein, we review endovascular procedural interventions for symptomatic IFDVT and MTS: CDT, with or without stenting, for IFDVT, and stenting for MTS.

EVIDENCE BASE FOR ENDOVASCULAR INTERVENTION

Iliofemoral Deep Vein Thrombosis

There have been several trials comparing catheter-directed therapy (CDT) plus anticoagulation versus anticoagulation alone in IFDVT. The main goals of therapy have been to minimize venous congestion symptoms and the incidence and severity of PTS. Previous trials of CDT[16–18] and 1 trial of surgical thrombectomy[19] reported favorable outcomes with intervention for IFDVT, but these were collectively limited by nonrandomized design, small sample size, and single-center enrollment. One such trial, Thrombus Obliteration by Rapid Percutaneous Intervention in Deep Venous Occlusion, was a randomized single-center study that included proximal iliofemoral

and popliteal DVT and showed reduction in recurrent venous thromboembolism and development of PTS at 6 months, comparing endovascular therapy with thrombectomy, balloon venoplasty, stenting, and/or local low-dose thrombolytic therapy (37% received thrombolytic therapy). These benefits persisted to at least 2.5 years.[20,21]

The highest-quality evidence relating to CDT for IFDVT comes from 2 multicenter randomized controlled trials, Catheter-Directed Thrombolysis versus Standard Treatment for Acute Iliofemoral Deep Vein Thrombosis (CaVenT) and Pharmacomechanical Catheter-Directed Thrombolysis for Deep Vein Thrombosis (ATTRACT). CaVenT, an open-label, multicenter, randomized controlled trial that enrolled 209 patients,[22] demonstrated improved iliofemoral patency (65.9% vs 47.4%, $P = .012$) and a lower rate of PTS (41.1% vs 55.6%, $P = .047$) for CDT compared with anticoagulation alone at 24-month follow-up with similar results demonstrated at 5 years.[22] However, CDT did not improve long-term QOL.[23] ATTRACT was of design similar to CaVenT and randomized 692 patients with acute proximal (femoral, common femoral, or iliac veins) DVT to CDT versus anticoagulation alone.[24] ATTRACT found no difference in the incidence of its primary endpoint, development of PTS between 6 and 24 months (47% vs 48%; $P = .56$). However, the secondary endpoint moderate-to-severe PTS occurred less often with CDT (18% vs 28%, $P = .04$) and Villalta scores (a metric reflecting PTS severity, Table 1) were lower at all time points during follow-up ($P<.01$ for comparison) in the CDT group when compared with anticoagulation alone.

A prespecified substudy of ATTRACT, which included only those with IFDVT (n = 391 patients; 57% of the overall trial population),[25] found no difference between incidence of PTS between 6 and 24 months in anticoagulation alone versus CDT groups. Secondary endpoint analyses, similar to the overall trial, did indicate a benefit of CDT, with the CDT group having less moderate-to-severe PTS and severe PTS (18% vs 28%, $P = .021$; and 8.7% vs 15%, $P = .048$, respectively). The stronger results in the iliofemoral group suggest that (1) the secondary endpoint benefit observed in the full trial cohort may have been driven primarily by the subset with IFDVT and (2) the patients who may benefit most in prevention of CDT are those with greater extent of iliofemoral thrombus. CDT also resulted in greater reduction of leg pain and swelling through 30 days, reduced PTS severity by Villalta scores, and greater improvement in venous disease-specific QOL from baseline to 24 months.[25]

Table 1
Villalta scale for assessment of postthrombotic syndrome severity

Villalta Score components

Symptoms	Clinical signs
Pain	Edema
Cramps	Skin induration
Heaviness	Hyperpigmentation
Pruritus	Redness
Paresthesia	Pain during calf compression
	Venous ectasia
	Venous ulcers (present or absent)

Scoring: Each sign or symptom is rated as 0 (absent), 1 (mild), 2 (moderate), or 3 (severe), except for venous ulcers, which are either present or absent

Grading scale	
0–4 points	No PTS
5–14 points	Mild-to-moderate PTS
>15 points *or* presence of venous ulcers	Severe PTS

Some observational studies suggest that there is a lower rate of reocclusion after thrombectomy followed by stenting than thrombectomy without stenting.[4,6] In addition, if MTS is present, retrospective observational data suggest that stenting may help maintain patency.[26] CaVenT and ATTRACT have been criticized for their low rates of stent implantation, which were not mandated as part of the trial protocol. In CaVenT and ATTRACT, 16.7% and 28% (39% among those with IFDVT) of the CDT groups were treated with stenting, respectively.

Iliac Compression (May-Thurner) without Acute Deep Vein Thrombosis
Chronic venous occlusions
Recent data suggest that patients with symptomatic chronic venous occlusions benefit from procedural intervention with clot removal and stenting. The Accelerated thrombolysis for PTS using EKOS (ACCESS PTS) study (Mark Garcia, unpublished, presented in 2018), included 78 treated patients with chronic IFDVT of at least 6 months duration and persistent symptoms despite conservative treatment for at least 3 months. Intervention with ultrasound-accelerated CDT improved symptom-based outcomes by Villalta and Venous Insufficiency

Epidemiologic and Economic Study–QOL scores with low complication rates.[27]

Compression without thrombosis
There have been several studies of stenting for venous outflow obstruction in patients with symptomatic iliac vein compression (MTS). These studies, mostly single-center observational studies, generally indicate relief of symptoms, such as improved pain, reduced edema, and improved venous stasis ulcer healing, with good long-term patency and little morbidity.[28–30] The largest assessment consisted of 982 chronic nonmalignant femoroiliocaval vein obstructive lesions that were stented and showed favorable outcomes after assessment by Comprehensive Classification System for Chronic Venous Disorders scores, QOL by CIVIQ, and hemodynamics.[28]

Stenting for nonthrombotic iliac vein lesions seems to be safe and to improve symptoms and QOL without requiring correction of venous reflux. A double-blinded randomized controlled trial comparing 58 patients with medical treatment alone versus medical treatment plus iliac vein stenting in a population with venous symptoms demonstrated a significant decline in pain and venous clinical severity score (VCSS) scores with medical therapy plus stenting and reported excellent patency rates.[31] In a trial of nonthrombotic iliac vein lesions (319 patients and 332 limbs), patients undergoing stenting experienced complete relief of swelling in approximately half of patients, complete relief of pain in approximately 70%, and complete stasis ulcer healing in approximately 70% of limbs. The rates of these events were not dependent on correction of venous reflux.[7]

INDICATIONS
Iliofemoral Deep Vein Thrombosis
In patients with IFDVT, treatment should start with full therapeutic anticoagulation at the time of diagnosis, unless contraindicated. Unfractionated heparin (UFH) is preferred as the initial choice if patients are being considered for thrombus reduction strategies, although current guidelines recommend initial use of low-molecular-weight heparin (LMWH) rather than UFH in patients with proximal DVT being initiated on warfarin because LMWH has been associated with less recurrent venous thromboembolism and fewer major bleeding events.[32] Factor Xa inhibitors have similar efficacy to LMWH.[33] Because LMWH and Factor Xa inhibitors are renally cleared, their use should

be avoided if the estimated glomerular filtration rate is less than 30 mL/min/m^2.

Indications for procedural intervention are mainly related to symptoms and clot burden with goals of preserving normal circulation and valve function as well as minimizing the occurrence of PTS. Systemic thrombolysis for IFDVT is not recommended because of its risk of major bleeding and inferior efficacy compared with endovascular techniques.[34] Patient considerations for endovascular intervention have been discussed previously[35] and are summarized in Table 2.

Surgical intervention may also be considered for limb preservation in the case of phlegmasia. However, although there have been no head-to-head trials, lack of evidence for superiority and increased risk with surgery favor endovascular options for IFDVT if they are available (hospital transfer may be considered if it is not).[34]

Catheter-Directed Thrombolysis for Iliofemoral Deep Vein Thrombosis

CDT for IFDVT remains controversial. The highest-quality evidence from randomized controlled trials suggests that, although there may not be a difference in the subsequent rates of PTS, CDT may decrease PTS severity and improve QOL. Consequently, the decision for CDT should be based on clinical judgment. Patient factors, extent of thrombus, risk of developing PTS, and shared decision making with the patient should be considered (see Table 2).

In the case of IFDVT with concurrent MTS, clot removal with stenting is likely to be of greater benefit. Presence of acute DVT can be considered a manifestation of symptomatic MTS, which is itself an indication for stenting.

May-Thurner Syndrome

Because stenting for MTS has been shown to have low morbidity and good patency with relief of symptoms, any patient with symptoms and identifiable iliac vein compression should be considered for stenting. The decision for intervention should be driven primarily by symptoms of venous outflow obstruction and guidance by history and physical examination. History of DVT may also increase the clinical indication for stenting.

CONTRAINDICATIONS

Contraindications to CDT and stent placement are mostly related to bleeding risk. Absolute contraindications are active internal bleeding or disseminated intravascular coagulation, recent cerebrovascular event, including transient ischemic attacks, neurosurgery, or intracranial trauma.

In addition to standard bleeding risk assessment, relative contraindications advised in previous trials have included life expectancy less than 2 years, chronic nonambulatory status, hemoglobin less than 9 mg/dl, or international normalized ratio greater than 1.6 before warfarin use.[36]

Patients with acute IFDVT who have contraindications to anticoagulation should be considered for inferior vena cava (IVC) filter implantation to minimize the likelihood of a massive pulmonary embolism.

PROCEDURAL TECHNIQUE

Imaging

Diagnosis of MTS has been described by various modalities, including noninvasive venous imaging with duplex ultrasonography, computed tomography (CT), or magnetic resonance (MR) venography, catheter-based venography, and intravascular ultrasonography. Although sensitivity is lowest for duplex ultrasonoraphy, it is often the initial test because of its noninvasive and low-cost nature. MR is rarely used. CT is useful in identifying iliac vein compression, especially with techniques, such as use of minimal luminal area for ipsilateral reference areas,[37] but intravascular ultrasonography (IVUS) remains the gold standard.

Venography is significantly limited when compared with IVUS. A comparison of IVUS and venography in 155 limbs of 152 patients found that venography missed stenotic lesions, misidentified their severity and location, and also misidentified the location of the iliac-caval confluence and distal landing zone in most limbs.[38] Additional venography techniques, such as anteroposterior venography may help by identifying collaterals and pancaking, but IVUS should still be performed.[39]

Oblique imaging during venography can also be helpful. Fig. 1 demonstrates a case of bilateral iliac vein compression that was minimally apparent on anteroposterior imaging, but obvious with oblique imaging. IVUS confirmed severe iliac vein stenosis that was treated with stent implantation.

Catheter-Directed Thrombolysis for Iliofemoral Deep Vein Thrombosis

Specific methods for CDT have been described in guidelines and in supplements of CDT trials.[22,24] In brief, catheter access with ultrasound guidance is recommended to help

Table 2
Patient selection for catheter-directed thrombolysis in iliofemoral deep venous thrombosis and stenting in May-Thurner syndrome

CDT for IFDVT

Extent of thrombus	Greater extent of thrombus increases risk for developing subsequent PTS and clinical indication for clot removal, although there are no agreed on criteria to guide this assessment.
Severity of symptoms	Mild symptoms may be treated conservatively with anticoagulation and clinical follow-up; CDT helps provide symptomatic relief when symptoms are severe.
Thrombus duration	Thrombus retraction and solidification after 21 d may limit efficacy of lysis.[23,34]
Baseline activity level of patient	Younger, more active patients are more likely to experience short- and long-term limitations from acute symptoms and/or subsequent development of PTS than patients who are wheelchair-bound or have low levels of activity.
Failure of conservative therapy	Patients with worsening symptoms despite conservative treatment (anticoagulation, compression) may benefit from CDT.
Presence of underlying conditions	Presence and treatment plan of underlying conditions, such as MTS or neoplasia should be considered in the decision for CDT.
Bleeding risk or contraindications	The decision for intervention should be carefully weighed against likelihood of bleeding complications, especially in high-risk patients.

Stenting for MTS

Presence of acute thrombosis	Acute thrombosis is considered a manifestation of symptomatic MTS, which is an indication for stent implantation. CDT should be considered.
Symptom severity	Venous symptoms should be considered. Stenting is generally indicated for MTS with symptoms, such as edema, paresthesia, pain, venous claudication, skin erythema, or ulceration.

Abbreviations: CDT, catheter-directed thrombolysis; DVT, deep vein thrombosis; IFDVT, iliofemoral deep vein thrombosis; MTS, May-Thurner syndrome.

Evidence is not strong enough to make CDT routine for IFDVT. Randomized, controlled clinical trials suggest that clot reduction and removal with CDT may reduce the incidence of postthrombotic syndrome (PTS), especially moderate-to-severe PTS. Factors to consider when considering CDT for IFDVT are summarized.

Stent implantation is generally indicated for cases of symptomatic iliac vein compression (MTS).

minimize bleeding complications and can be through any lower-extremity vein or the internal jugular vein. Venography should be performed to examine the extent of thrombus; however, IVUS should also be used in essentially all cases.

Initial CDT involves intrathrombus delivery of a recombinant tissue plasminogen activator, most commonly alteplase. If the popliteal vein is occluded or the IVC is involved, ATTRACT investigators were required to use "infusion-first CDT" in which recombinant tissue plasminogen activator (rt-PA) infusion was first attempted for a duration less than 30 hours. For all other patients, physicians attempted single-session thrombus removal with rapid rt-PA with the AngioJet Rheolytic Thrombectomy System (Boston Scientific) or the Trellis Peripheral Infusion System (Medtronic). If complete thrombus resolution is not achieved in a single session, rt-PA can be infused afterward for up to 24 hours through a multi-sidehole catheter.

Dosing of rt-PA as described in ATTRACT is as follows: (1) for infusions, 0.01 mg/kg/h, maximum 1.0 mg/h; (2) for AngioJet/Trellis delivery during single-session therapy, initial dose range 0.25 to 0.33 mg/cm thrombus length (estimated from the initial venogram), minimum 4 mg; (3) ≤25 mg during first session; (4) ≤5 mg during each follow-up session; and (5) ≤35 mg for all sessions and infusions combined.[24]

Cleanup of residual thrombus can include balloon maceration, catheter aspiration, Angiojet or Trellis thrombectomy, and/or additional rt-PA infusion. Stenting was encouraged in lesions in iliac and/or common femoral veins with

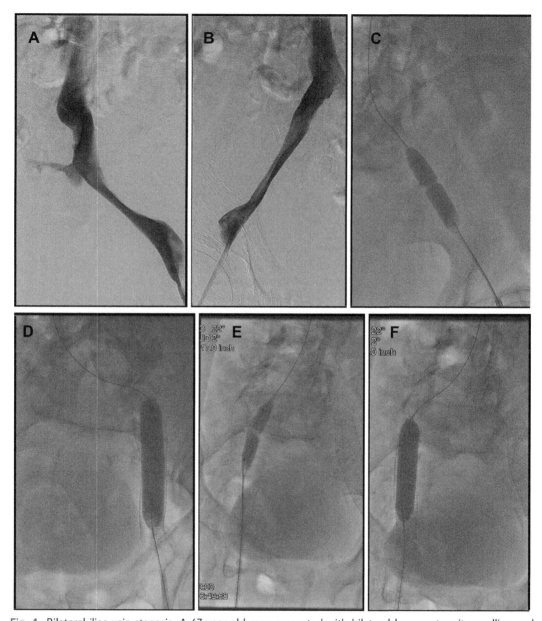

Fig. 1. Bilateral iliac vein stenosis. A 67-year-old man presented with bilateral lower-extremity swelling and chronic venous stasis changes. Anteroposterior venography did not demonstrate any significant disease. (A) Left iliofemoral venography demonstrated a significant stenosis with oblique imaging. (B) Similarly, oblique imaging demonstrated significant right iliac vein stenosis. (C) Balloon angioplasty of the left iliac vein demonstrated a waist during balloon inflation, consistent with scarring/intravascular webbing. (D) A stent was placed in the left iliac vein. (E) A similar stenosis was demonstrated in the right iliac vein. (F) A stent was also placed in the right iliac vein. The patient developed complete resolution of his symptoms at 1 month of follow-up.

greater than 50% stenosis, robust collateral filling, and/or mean pressure gradient greater than 2 mm Hg after percutaneous transluminal balloon angioplasty for obstructive lesions.

Treatment is discontinued after 90% thrombus removal or if there is a serious complication. Sheath removal should occur at least 1 hour after the last rt-PA or heparin bolus dose. Bed rest is recommended with leg immobilization for 6 hours, with ambulation as tolerated afterward.

Therapeutic anticoagulation during CDT should be with twice daily LMWH or UFH infusion (6–12 units/kg/h, maximum 1000 units/h).

Additional heparin boluses can be given at physician discretion. Anticoagulation should be resumed 2 hours after hemostasis is obtained following sheath removal, with resumption of UFH with no bolus or continuation of twice daily LMWH dosing. Warfarin can be initiated on the same day of sheath removal if this is the chosen long-term anticoagulation strategy.

Endovascular Therapy for May-Thurner Syndrome

Stent implantation for MTS should follow standard procedural technique for percutaneous endovascular angioplasty and stenting. IVUS should be used in virtually all cases, as discussed above. Predilation should be used to assess the size of the vessel as well as other anatomic factors, such as intravascular webs. Stent size should mirror normal anatomic size of the vessel undergoing stent implantation.

Device (Stent) Selection

It should be noted that most devices used for CDT, including in the CaVenT and ATTRACT trials, were used off-label. Most stents used for treatment of iliofemoral obstruction have been Wallstents, which are not specifically designed for venous stenting. Dedicated venous stents have only recently been developed and include the VICI stent (Veniti, Inc/Boston Scientific), the Venovo stent (Bard), the Zilver Vena (Cook), the Sinus Venous (Optimized), and the ABRE stent (Medtronic).[40] Of these, only the VICI and Venovo are Food and Drug Administration approved for iliofemoral vein stenting.[41] Dedicated venous (nitinol) stents provide more accurate positioning due to the lack of foreshortening on deployment compared with Wallstents, adequate outward and compression radial force, crush resistance, and flexibility that allows the stents to take the shape of the iliac vein. These dedicated venous stents are also available in multiple lengths better suited for iliac vein stenting. Characteristics of various stents used to treat iliac vein compression as outlined by Radaideh and colleagues[40] and are summarized in **Table 3**. **Fig. 2** demonstrates use of a VICI stent for the treatment of left common iliac vein compression.

Initial clinical trial results for these newer stents suggest excellent patency. In a multicenter, international, single-arm feasibility trial of the VICI stent (n = 30), 1-year outcomes have been excellent, with high patency rates, safety, and no stent fractures.[42] The VIRTUS study, which evaluated the VICI stent in an expanded group (presented in January 2019, unpublished) included 170 patients with chronic disease, 75% of whom had thrombotic lesions and 25% of whom had a nonthrombotic lesions (MTS). The primary patency rate was 84% at 12 months, and 98.8% of patients were free from major adverse events at 30 days, both of which exceeded predefined performance goals. Similarly, initial results from the VERNACULAR study for iliac vein compression were also presented in early 2019 but have not yet been published. This study demonstrated a primary patency benefit for Venovo venous stent (Bard) compared with historical controls at 12 months with low rates of 30-day major adverse events and significant benefit in pain and QOL scores by VCSS and CIVIQ.[43]

COMPLICATIONS AND THEIR MANAGEMENT

Some trials have demonstrated higher bleeding risk with CDT than anticoagulation alone,[24] but the bleeding was not life-threatening. Access site complications are usually minor and should be managed in the standard fashion.

Back pain is common after iliofemoral stent placement and should resolve within 2 to 3 weeks in most patients. In severe cases of back pain, which may result from stent compression of nerves in the lower lumbar and upper sacral region, stent explantation may be rarely required.[44]

Stent fracture and stent migration are also possible. To avoid stent fracture, overlap of stents should be avoided on 1 cm on each side of the inguinal ligament.[44] In many cases, fractures may be asymptomatic. On the other hand, stent migration can be life-threatening and include complications, such as entrapment in the tricuspid valve. Placement of stents with adequate diameter and length helps avoid stent migration.[44]

PERIPROCEDURAL ISSUES

The Society of Interventional Radiology recommends monitoring with complete bed rest and immobility during the thrombolysis period.[45] One prospective nonrandomized trial of 24 patients suggests that intermittent pneumatic compression results in better CDT success.[46] Early ambulation is not associated with progression of DVT or development of pulmonary embolism and should be encouraged after the bed rest period after sheath removal.[47]

Table 3
Characteristics of stents used to treat iliac venous disease

Stent (Manufacturer)	VICI (Boston Scientific)	Venovo (Bard)	Sinus Venous (Optimed)	Zilver Vena (Cook)	ABRE (Medtronic)	Wallstent (Boston Scientific)
Material	Nitinol	Nitinol	Nitinol	Nitinol	Nitinol	Elgiloy
Expansion	Self-expanding	Self-expanding	Self-expanding; balloon expandable at kissing portion	Self-expanding	Self-expanding	Self-expanding
Sheath size	9 F	8–10 F	10 F	6 F	9 F	6–10 F
Foreshortening	10%–15%	None	None	None	None	30%–40%
Radial force	++++	++++	+++	++	++	+
Diameter, mm	Up to 16	Up to 20	Up to 18	Up to 16	Up to 20	Up to 24
Length, mm	60–120	40–160	60–150	60, 100, 140	40–150	20–94
FDA approved for venous indication?	Yes	Yes	No	No	No	Pending

LONG-TERM FOLLOW-UP: CLINICAL, IMAGING, AND SO FORTH

Anticoagulation for Iliofemoral Deep Vein Thrombosis

The choice of agent and duration of long-term anticoagulation for IFDVT is discussed in current guidelines[34] and should take into account whether or not the patient has cancer and whether a DVT was provoked or unprovoked. Long-term anticoagulation traditionally used warfarin, although oral direct Factor Xa inhibitors have been shown to be noninferior to warfarin for the treatment of DVT. Specifically, rivaroxaban and apixaban were associated with less bleeding than warfarin. In general, anticoagulation should be continued for 3 months at

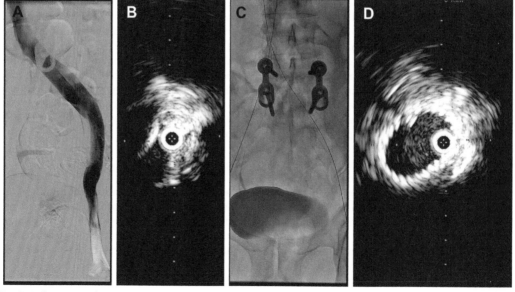

Fig. 2. Left common iliac vein compression. A 62-year-old man presented with unilateral left chronic venous stasis symptoms. (A) Iliac venography did not show any obvious stenosis. (B) Intravascular ultrasonography demonstrated scarring of the vein and a focal, severe stenosis at the origin of the left common iliac artery. (C) A VICI venous stent was implanted. (D) Intravascular ultrasonography demonstrated excellent expansion.

Table 4
Long-term anticoagulation considerations for iliofemoral deep vein thrombosis or after stent implantation for May-Thurner syndrome

Agent	Advantages	Disadvantages
Choice of agent		
Warfarin	Low cost	INR monitoring
Factor Xa inhibitors	Similar efficacy with less bleeding (rivaroxaban and apixaban) compared with warfarin	Contraindicated for eGFR <30 mL/min/m^2, must consider hepatic function, higher cost, shorter duration of action, fewer options for reversal

Scenario	Low-Moderate Bleeding Risk	High Bleeding Risk
Duration of anticoagulation		
First unprovoked IFDVT	Indefinite therapy	3 mo
Second unprovoked IFDVT	Indefinite therapy	3 mo
IFDVT with active malignancy	Extended therapy with period reassessment of risk (eg, annually)	
IFDVT provoked by surgery	3 mo	
IFDVT with nonsurgical transient risk factor	3 mo	
Stent implantation for MTS without acute thrombosis	At least 1 mo	1 mo

Abbreviations: eGFR, estimated glomerular filtration rate; F, French.

minimum, with longer duration of anticoagulation being preferred for patients at low bleeding risk (**Table 4**). Renal and hepatic clearance should also be considered before starting Factor Xa inhibitors.

Anticoagulation After Stent Placement for May-Thurner Syndrome

In the case of stenting for iliac compression without thrombosis, full anticoagulation is recommended for at least a month for compression as antiplatelet agents are less effective in the venous system. These recommendations are based primarily on expert opinion.

Considerations for long-term anticoagulation are summarized in **Table 4**.

Postthrombotic Syndrome

Despite optimal therapy and anticoagulation, recognition and treatment of PTS after IFDVT is of high importance. PTS occurs in 20% to 50% of patients after IFDVT and negatively affects QOL.[14] Providers must monitor periodically for PTS, because its late onset at 12 to 24 months may cause it to be underrecognized. In addition, residual thrombus is a strong risk factor for recurrent DVT and subsequent PTS.[12]

PTS has been reviewed previously,[48] and its symptoms may vary significantly in severity. The Villalta scoring system for PTS severity has been validated and is proposed to standardize PTS scoring in current guidelines.[49] Scoring criteria are summarized in **Table 1**.

Prevention and treatment of PTS are controversial. Following the randomized, multicenter, placebo-controlled SOX trial,[50] and the smaller, single-center studies without placebo control that preceded it,[34] it is unclear whether compression therapy can prevent PTS. Treatment may include conservative treatment with compression or pharmacologic therapy or invasive therapy with surgery or venous stenting.[48] However, given its low risk, compression therapy should be considered for all patients (except those with symptomatic peripheral artery disease, in whom compression is contraindicated[51]) after IFDVT, especially if patients have symptoms of venous congestion. Similarly, exercise has been postulated to prevent PTS but has not had confirmed benefit.[52]

Monitoring

Venous stents are vulnerable to stent compression, especially after MTS.[53] Stent compression is almost impossible to detect with contrast venography but can be identified using ultrasonography. Monthly surveillance may be appropriate if there are residual PTS symptoms. In patients with MTS, surveillance every 6 months may be appropriate if resolution of symptoms is maintained.[53]

SUMMARY

IFDVT and compression of the iliac veins MTS are separate entities that are closely intertwined. All patients with IFDVT should be promptly initiated on anticoagulation unless contraindicated. Routine intervention for IFDVT with CTD remains controversial. The current evidence base does not support CDT as first-line therapy for all patients with IFDVT, but CDT helps prevent complications of moderate-to-severe PTS with comparable safety to anticoagulation alone.[25] Future studies with higher rates of stenting after CDT in IFDVT patients may help clarify the benefit of routine endovascular intervention for IFDVT.

In general, stenting of iliac veins for symptomatic MTS is successful with good patency rates in follow-up and low complication rates. New advances in stent technology with dedicated venous nitinol stents have improved patency as well as symptoms and QOL compared with previous stents.

DISCLOSURE

No relevant disclosures.

REFERENCES

1. May R, Thurner J. The cause of the predominantly sinistral occurrence of thrombosis of the pelvic veins. Angiology 1957;8(5):419–27.
2. Cockett FB, Thomas ML, Negus D. Iliac vein compression—its relation to iliofemoral thrombosis and the post-thrombotic syndrome. BMJ 1967; 2(5543):14–9.
3. Kibbe MR, Ujiki M, Goodwin AL, et al. Iliac vein compression in an asymptomatic patient population. J Vasc Surg 2004;39(5):937–43.
4. Mickley V, Schwagierek R, Rilinger N, et al. Left iliac venous thrombosis caused by venous spur: treatment with thrombectomy and stent implantation. J Vasc Surg 1998;28(3):492–7.
5. Kasirajan K, Gray B, Ouriel K. Percutaneous Angio-Jet thrombectomy in the management of extensive deep venous thrombosis. J Vasc Interv Radiol 2001; 12(2):179–85. Avaialble at: http://www.ncbi.nlm.nih.gov/pubmed/11265881. Accessed September 4, 2019.
6. Hartung O, Benmiloud F, Barthelemy P, et al. Late results of surgical venous thrombectomy with iliocaval stenting. J Vasc Surg 2008;47(2):381–7.
7. Raju S, Neglen P. High prevalence of nonthrombotic iliac vein lesions in chronic venous disease: a permissive role in pathogenicity. J Vasc Surg 2006;44(1):136–44.
8. Khan TA, Rudolph KP, Huber TS, et al. May-Thurner syndrome presenting as pelvic congestion syndrome and vulvar varicosities in a nonpregnant adolescent. J Vasc Surg Cases Innov Tech 2019; 5(3):252–4.
9. Nyamekye I, Merker L. Management of proximal deep vein thrombosis. Phlebology 2012;27(SUPPL. 2):61–72.
10. Plate G, Ohlin P, Eklof B, et al. Pulmonary embolism in acute iliofemoral venous thrombosis. Br J Surg 1985;72:912–5.
11. Young T, Tang H, Hughes R. Vena caval filters for the prevention of pulmonary embolism. Cochrane Database Syst Rev 2010;(2):CD006212.
12. Douketis JD, Crowther MA, Foster GA, et al. Does the location of thrombosis determine the risk of disease recurrence in patients with proximal deep vein thrombosis? Am J Med 2001;110(7):515–9.
13. Kahn SR, Shrier I, Julian JA, et al. Determinants and time course of the postthrombotic syndrome after acute deep venous thrombosis. Ann Intern Med 2008;149(10):698–707.
14. Kahn SR, Hirsch A, Shrier I. Effect of postthrombotic syndrome on health-related quality of life after deep venous thrombosis. Arch Intern Med 2002; 162(10):1144.
15. Rabinovich A, Kahn SR. How I treat the postthrombotic syndrome. Blood 2018;131(20):2215–22.
16. Comerota AJ, Throm RC, Mathias SD, et al. Catheter-directed thrombolysis for iliofemoral deep venous thrombosis improves health-related quality of life. J Vasc Surg 2000;32(1):130–7.
17. AbuRahma AF, Perkins SE, Wulu JT, et al. Iliofemoral deep vein thrombosis: conventional therapy versus lysis and percutaneous transluminal angioplasty and stenting. Ann Surg 2001;233(6):752–60.
18. Elsharawy M, Elzayat E. Early results of thrombolysis vs anticoagulation in iliofemoral venous thrombosis. A randomised clinical trial. Eur J Vasc Endovasc Surg 2002;24(3):209–14. Avaialble at: http://www.ncbi.nlm.nih.gov/pubmed/12217281. Accessed September 3, 2019.
19. Plate G, Akesson H, Einarsson E, et al. Long-term results of venous thrombectomy combined with a temporary arterio-venous fistula. Eur J Vasc Surg 1990;4(5):483–9. Avaialble at: http://www.ncbi.nlm.nih.gov/pubmed/2226879. Accessed September 3, 2019.
20. Sharifi M, Mehdipour M, Bay C, et al. Endovenous therapy for deep venous thrombosis: the

TORPEDO trial. Catheter Cardiovasc Interv 2010; 76(3):316–25.

21. Sharifi M, Bay C, Mehdipour M, et al. Thrombus obliteration by rapid percutaneous endovenous intervention in deep venous occlusion (TORPEDO) trial: midterm results. J Endovasc Ther 2012;19(2): 273–80.

22. Enden T, Haig Y, Kløw NE, et al, CaVenT Study Group. Long-term outcome after additional catheter-directed thrombolysis versus standard treatment for acute iliofemoral deep vein thrombosis (the CaVenT study): a randomised controlled trial. Lancet 2012;379:31–8. Available at: www.the-lancet.com.

23. Haig Y, Enden T, Grøtta O, et al. Post-thrombotic syndrome after catheter-directed thrombolysis for deep vein thrombosis (CaVenT): 5-year follow-up results of an open-label, randomised controlled trial. Lancet Haematol 2016;3(2):e64–71.

24. Vedantham S, Goldhaber SZ, Julian JA, et al. Pharmacomechanical catheter-directed thrombolysis for deep-vein thrombosis. N Engl J Med 2017; 377(23):2240–52.

25. Comerota AJ, Kearon C, Gu C-S, et al. Endovascular thrombus removal for acute iliofemoral deep vein thrombosis. Circulation 2019;139(9):1162–73.

26. Husmann MJ, Heller G, Kalka C, et al. Stenting of common iliac vein obstructions combined with regional thrombolysis and thrombectomy in acute deep vein thrombosis. Eur J Vasc Endovasc Surg 2007;34(1):87–91.

27. Garcia M, Sterling K, Jaff M, et al. 3:00 PM abstract no. 351 Distinguished Abstract Access PTS Study: ACCElerated thrombolySiS for post-thrombotic syndrome using the acoustic pulse thrombolysis EkoSonic® endovascular system: midterm results of a multicenter study. J Vasc Interv Radiol 2018;29(4):S151.

28. Neglén P, Hollis KC, Olivier J, et al. Stenting of the venous outflow in chronic venous disease: long-term stent-related outcome, clinical, and hemodynamic result. J Vasc Surg 2007;46(5). https://doi.org/10.1016/j.jvs.2007.06.046.

29. Kölbel T, Lindh M, Åkesson M, et al. Chronic iliac vein occlusion: midterm results of endovascular recanalization. J Endovasc Ther 2009;16(4):483–91.

30. Lamont JP, Pearl GJ, Patetsios P, et al. Prospective evaluation of endoluminal venous stents in the treatment of the May-Thurner syndrome. Ann Vasc Surg 2002;16(1):61–4.

31. Rossi FH, Kambara AM, Izukawa NM, et al. Randomized double-blinded study comparing medical treatment versus iliac vein stenting in chronic venous disease. J Vasc Surg Venous Lymphat Disord 2018;6(2):183–91.

32. Erkens PM, Prins MH. Fixed dose subcutaneous low molecular weight heparins versus adjusted dose unfractionated heparin for venous thromboembolism. In: Prins MH, editor. Cochrane Database of Systematic Reviews. Chichester (United Kingdom): John Wiley & Sons, Ltd; 2010:CD001100.

33. Büller HR, Davidson BL, Decousus H, et al. Fondaparinux or enoxaparin for the initial treatment of symptomatic deep venous thrombosis. Ann Intern Med 2004;140(11):867.

34. Liu D, Peterson E, Dooner J, et al. Diagnosis and management of iliofemoral deep vein thrombosis: clinical practice guideline. CMAJ 2015;187(17): 1288–96.

35. Endovascular today—the ABCs of iliofemoral DVT. 2017. Avaialble at: https://evtoday.com/2017/07/supplement/the-abcs-of-iliofemoral-dvt/. Accessed September 12, 2019.

36. Elbasty A, Metcalf J. Safety and efficacy of catheter direct thrombolysis in management of acute iliofemoral deep vein thrombosis: a systematic review. Vasc Specialist Int 2017;33(4):121–34.

37. Shammas NW, Shammas GA, Jones-Miller S, et al. Predicting iliac vein compression with computed tomography angiography and venography: correlation with intravascular ultrasound. J Invasive Cardiol 2018; 30(12):452–5. Avaialble at: http://www.ncbi.nlm.nih.gov/pubmed/30504513. Accessed September 9, 2019.

38. Raju S, Montminy ML, Thomasson JD, et al. A comparison between intravascular ultrasound and venography in identifying key parameters essential for iliac vein stenting. J Vasc Surg Venous Lymphat Disord 2019. https://doi.org/10.1016/j.jvsv.2019.03.015.

39. Lau I, Png CYM, Eswarappa M, et al. Defining the utility of anteroposterior venography in the diagnosis of venous iliofemoral obstruction. J Vasc Surg Venous Lymphat Disord 2019;7(4):514–21.e4.

40. Radaideh Q, Patel NM, Shammas NW. Iliac vein compression: epidemiology, diagnosis and treatment. Vasc Health Risk Manag 2019;15:115–22.

41. Murphy EH. Endovascular Today—surveying the 2019 venous stent landscape. Endovasc Today 2019. Avaialble at: https://evtoday.com/2019/07/surveying-the-2019-venous-stent-landscape/. Accessed September 16, 2019.

42. Razavi M, Marston W, Black S, et al. The initial report on 1-year outcomes of the feasibility study of the VENITI VICI VENOUS STENT in symptomatic iliofemoral venous obstruction. J Vasc Surg Venous Lymphat Disord 2018;6(2):192–200.

43. Liu D, Homayoon B, Chung J. Endovascular Today—twelve-Month VERNACULAR data for venovo venous stent presented at SIR 2019. Endovasc Today 2017. Avaialble at: https://evtoday.com/2019/03/28/twelve-month-vernacular-data-for-venovo-venous-stent-presented-at-sir-2019. Accessed September 7, 2019.

44. Black S, Morris R. Endovascular Today—the un-knowns of venous stenting: why do good cases go bad?. 2019. Avaialble at: https://evtoday.com/2019/07/the-unknowns-of-venous-stenting-why-do-good-cases-go-bad/?utm_source=iContact&utm_medium=email&utm_campaign=evt-enews&utm_content=EVT+Most+Read+US. Accessed September 7, 2019.

45. Vedantham S, Thorpe PE, Cardella JF, et al. Quality improvement guidelines for the treatment of lower extremity deep vein thrombosis with use of endo-vascular thrombus removal. J Vasc Interv Radiol 2006;17(3):435–48.

46. Ogawa T, Hoshino S, Midorikawa H, et al. Intermit-tent pneumatic compression of the foot and calf improves the outcome of catheter-directed throm-bolysis using low-dose urokinase in patients with acute proximal venous thrombosis of the leg. J Vasc Surg 2005;42(5):940–4.

47. Aissaoui N, Martins E, Mouly S, et al. A meta-anal-ysis of bed rest versus early ambulation in the man-agement of pulmonary embolism, deep vein thrombosis, or both. Int J Cardiol 2009;137(1): 37–41.

48. Baldwin MJ, Moore HM, Rudarakanchana N, et al. Post-thrombotic syndrome: a clinical review. J Thromb Haemost 2013;11(5):795–805.

49. Kahn SR, Partsch H, Vedantham S, et al. Definition of post-thrombotic syndrome of the leg for use in clinical investigations: a recommendation for stan-dardization. J Thromb Haemost 2009;7(5):879–83.

50. Kahn SR, Shapiro S, Wells PS, et al. Compression stockings to prevent post-thrombotic syndrome: a randomised placebo-controlled trial. Lancet 2014; 383(9920):880–8.

51. Aschwanden M, Jeanneret C, Koller MT, et al. Ef-fect of prolonged treatment with compression stockings to prevent post-thrombotic sequelae: a randomized controlled trial. J Vasc Surg 2008; 47(5):1015–21.

52. Shrier I, Kahn SR, Steele RJ. Effect of early physical activity on long-term outcome after venous throm-bosis. Clin J Sport Med 2009;19(6):487–93.

53. Raju S. Ten lessons learned in iliac venous stenting. Endovasc Today 2016;15(7):40–4. Avaialble at: https://evtoday.com/2016/07/ten-lessons-learned-in-iliac-venous-stenting/. Accessed September 7, 2019.

Venous Ablation

Sahil Agrawal, MD[a], Walid Saber, MD, RPVI[b,c,d,*]

KEYWORDS

• Venous insufficiency • Varicose veins • Venous ablations

KEY POINTS

• Chronic venous insufficiency is a common vascular disorder.
• The symptom burden can be significant and disabling.
• Available therapeutic strategies are safe and effective, including conservative and minimally invasive catheter-directed endovenous ablations.

EPIDEMIOLOGY

Chronic venous insufficiency (CVI) resulting from venous reflux afflicts 15% to 20% of the population yet remains under-recognized and under-treated.[1] Venous reflux occurs when the unidirectional valves in the veins of the lower extremities are rendered incompetent, resulting in venous hypertension over time. Such valvular incompetence can be the primary pathology or can occur secondary to impaired calf pump function or follow previous injury from deep venous thrombosis (DVT).[2] Although the exact mechanism of primary valvular incompetence remains debated, it is clear that in CVI blood flows in a retrograde manner each time an erect posture is attained.[3] Hydrostatic pressure from the resultant column of blood can reach near arterial levels in the lower legs and the resultant venous hypertension can lead to venous engorgement, dilation, prominence and tortuosity. Venous reflux can affect the superficial great saphenous veins (GSV) or short saphenous veins, especially at their junction with the femoral and popliteal veins, respectively, the deep intramuscular veins or the perforator veins that connect the 2 systems, either in isolation or in combination.

RISK FACTORS

Given the strong familial clustering, a genetic predisposition to primary valvular incompetence has been proposed whereby patients are predisposed to poor elasticity and saphenofemoral junction incompetence.[4] A hormonal influence is possible; venous reflux disease is significantly more prevalent in females and the risk increases even further with pregnancy. An increased incidence is also noted with older age.[5] Other risk factors include elevated intra-abdominal pressures related to obesity and pregnancy, as well as occupations that require prolonged standing or sitting.[6]

SYMPTOMS

A large number of patients with CVI may be asymptomatic and present with cosmetic concerns related to varicose veins and skin hyperpigmentation. Often times, the only symptom is leg edema, which is worse at the end of day, with prolonged standing, and in warmer weather. Some patients may report pain or pruritus at the site of varicose veins, or leg discomfort described as achiness, heaviness, cramping, throbbing, or restlessness.[7] Extravasation of erythrocytes and fluid, and deposition of hemosiderin in the dermis from venous hypertension leads to skin hyperpigmentation typical of CVI. Stasis dermatitis characterized by erythema and, scaly, sometimes pruritic lesions on the distal legs results from the chronic edema and can be mistaken for cellulitis.[8] Continued progression of CVI and chronic dermatitis leads to lipodermatosclerosis, which is characterized by

---

[a] Warren Clinic Cardiology of Tulsa, Saint Francis Hospital, 6161 South Yale Avenue, Tulsa, OK 74136, USA;
[b] Interventional Vascular Services, Non-invasive Vascular Lab, Landmark Medical Center, Woonsocket, RI, USA;
[c] Brown University, Providence, RI, USA; [d] Oceanstate Cardiovascular & Vein Center, 191 Social Street, Suite 100, Woonsocket, RI 02895, USA
* Corresponding author. Oceanstate Cardiovascular & Vein Center, 191 Social Street, Suite 100, Woonsocket, RI 02895.
E-mail address: wsaber@oscvc.com

Intervent Cardiol Clin 9 (2020) 255–263
https://doi.org/10.1016/j.iccl.2019.12.007

erythema and induration.[9] Superficial thrombophlebitis may sometimes develop, presenting as a tender, erythematous, and indurated cord or nodule in the distribution of a superficial vein. Varicose veins may rupture and bleed after a trauma, especially when located over bony prominences. The most dreaded complication of CVI is tissue loss with development of a venous ulcer, classically over the medial malleolus and affects approximately 1% of patients with CVI.[10] Complete healing of leg ulcers is frequently difficult and requires prolonged wound treatment. Last, varicose veins are associated with an increase in risk of DVT.[11] These symptoms can negatively impact quality of life (QOL), with QOL scores in the most severe cases worse than individuals suffering from chronic lung disease, back pain, and arthritis.[2,12]

DIAGNOSIS

In patients with suspected venous insufficiency related to reflux, color flow duplex venous ultrasound examination is indicated for morphologic and functional assessment of the venous system. According to the most commonly used criterion, reflux is defined as reversed flow lasting more than 0.5 seconds after distal manual augmentation.[13]

Several additional observations should be made on the duplex examination:

1. What venous systems are involved—superficial, deep, perforators?
2. What is the extent and location of incompetence?
3. What is the reflux time and volume?
4. Is there concomitant iliac venous obstruction or compression?
5. Is there evidence of previous DVT?

Use of the clinical, etiologic, anatomic, pathophysiologic (CEAP) classification is recommended to standardize description of clinical severity of venous disease and describe contributing pathology. This schema takes into account severity (C1–6), etiology (E), anatomy (A), and pathophysiology (P) (Fig. 1).[14] The most common tool used to assess symptom burden is the venous clinical severity score (VCSS), a 10-item clinician-administered evaluation, with each item assigned a value 1 to 3, for a total score of up to 30.[15]

TREATMENT

Selection of treatment modalities is governed by cause and location of pathology, as well as symptom severity and patient preference. The goals of treatment are symptom improvement, prevention of complications related to CVI, and promotion of ulcer healing in patients with tissue loss. Treatment options include conservative measures with lifestyle modification, compression therapy, and the use of oral and topical phlebotonics as first-line therapy[16–20] an surgical interventions, as well as local and endovenous ablative therapies, with a multimodality approach needed in the majority of patients.

Cosmetic concerns, symptoms refractory to noninvasive measures, recurrent hemorrhage, and superficial thrombophlebitis are indications for invasive therapy. Most payers require a trial of compression stockings (often 3 months) before providing coverage for more invasive therapies.[21] Historically, treatment of CVI was primarily surgical, consisting of ligation and stripping of the GSV and short saphenous vein at the saphenofemoral junction and saphenopopliteal junction, respectively, with concurrent distal phlebectomy of bulging symptomatic varicosities as needed.[22,23] However, in addition to incurring patient anxiety, these procedures required a relatively prolonged recovery period of up to 2 weeks and were associated with typical surgical complications, including hematoma, cellulitis, and abscess formation in up to 3% of patients.[24] Recurrence rates were often high as well, with up to 30% of patients requiring additional procedures at extended follow-up.[25]

Endovenous Ablation

Endovenous ablation therapy uses either radiofrequency ablation (RFA) or laser energy (endovenous laser therapy [EVLT]) to induce thermal injury to the endothelium with the intention to promote thrombotic closure of the saphenous veins. Commercially available devices include the VNUSClosureFast RFA system (Fig. 2) and the Angiodynamics, Inc, VenaCure EVLT system (Fig. 3). Laser catheters are available in an array of different wavelengths and tip constructions. RFA and EVLT are primarily used for trunk incompetence; however, nontruncal veins and perforators may be treated with these catheters as long as their course is straight enough to allow endoluminal advancement of the catheter.

Sclerotherapy and phlebectomy are primarily used for isolated tributary or perforator incompetence or recurrent varicose veins, as well as in combination with other procedures. Patients with visible varicose veins or telangiectasias should undergo saphenous vein ablation before local management of varicosities, because this strategy may decrease the need for treatment.

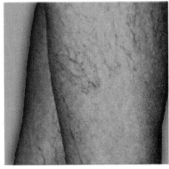

C1–Telangiectasia or reticular veins
(i.e., spider veins)

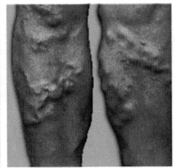

C2–Varicose veins, larger than 3 mm

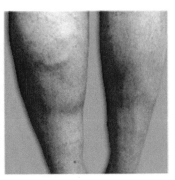

C3–Edema
(fluid in the skin)

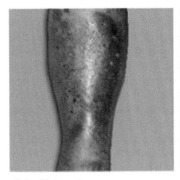

C4–Skin changes
(i.e., pigmentation, eczema, lipodermatosclerosis)

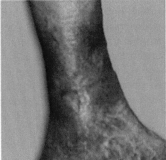

C5–Healed venous ulcer

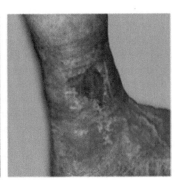

C6–Active venous ulcer

Fig. 1. CEAP clinical classification for staging CVI severity. (*Courtesy of* Angiodynamics, Inc., Latyham, NY; with permission.)

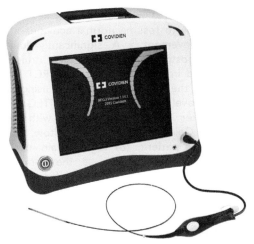

Fig. 2. VNUSClosureFast RFA system. (Reproduced with permission of Medtronic, Inc.)

Saphenous vein ablation should also be performed first in those patients who are found to have a combination of saphenous and perforator reflux, because perforator reflux often resolves after saphenous ablation. Endovenous ablation may be performed under local anesthesia or conscious sedation in an outpatient suite. A warm room and blankets help to prevent venous spasm. The saphenous vein of interest is punctured with a micropuncture needle under ultrasound guidance, as distal in the limb as technically feasible. A compatible working sheath (typically 7F) is then inserted to allow passage of the RFA or EVLT catheter in a distal to proximal direction. If GSV ablation is being attempted, the catheter tip should be placed and ablation begun at least 2.5 cm distal to the saphenofemoral junction. This positioning is essential to decrease the risk of endovenous heat-induced thrombosis of the deep venous system, which occurs in about 0.2% to 1.3% of

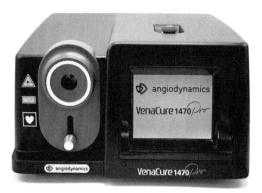

Fig. 3. VenaCure EVLT system. (*Courtesy of* Angiodynamics, Inc., Latyham, NY; with permission.)

patients.[26] Before ablation is commenced, local tumescent anesthesia is administered by injecting a cocktail of saline mixed with sodium bicarbonate and lidocaine in the perivenous fascia along the entire length of the vein segment being ablated to improve patient comfort and protect the overlying skin from thermal injury. A 21-G needle and a pedal-operated peristaltic pump are usually used for this purpose.

The procedure is generally safe and well-tolerated by patients. Potential complications include thrombophlebitis (7%), dermal pigmentation (5%), paresthesia (1%–2%), hematoma (0%–7%), postoperative pain, skin burns, and cutaneous nerve injury.[27] As discussed elsewhere in this article, endovenous heat-induced thrombosis with thrombus extension in to the deep venous system is reported to occur with an incidence of approximately 1%. Pulmonary embolism is rare after endovenous ablation.[13,27]

Postprocedure discomfort is easily managed with nonsteroidal anti-inflammatory drugs. Patients should be instructed to elevate the treated leg as much as feasible and to wear compression stockings continuously for the first 2 days. A repeat duplex ultrasound examination is typically performed in 2 days to assess for treatment success and to rule out a DVT. Anticoagulation should be initiated if thrombus extension into the deep venous system is noted. If the thrombus extends up to but not into the saphenofemoral or saphenopopliteal junction, a repeat ultrasound examination should be performed in 1 week.

Early endovenous ablation of superficial venous reflux, in addition to compression therapy and wound dressings, decreases the time to healing of venous leg ulcers, increases ulcer-free time, and is highly likely to be cost-effective based on results of the Early Venous Reflux Ablation (EVRA) randomized controlled trial (RCT).[28] In patients with spider telangiectasias or reticular veins in addition to larger varicose veins, treatment of saphenous venous varicosities should be performed first, because relieving venous reflux may resolve or improve these superficial varicosities, thereby decreasing the need for subsequent local therapies. Endovenous ablation of saphenous veins should be avoided in patients with deep venous obstruction or reflux because of an increased risk of venous ulceration.

The treatment efficacy and recurrence rates of endoluminal procedures—both RFA and EVLT—are comparable to the postoperative outcomes following saphenofemoral ligation and stripping.[29,30] The 3-year pooled success rates were 84% for RFA, 94% for EVLT, and 78% for surgical stripping when treating saphenous varicosities.[31] In another study, 98% of randomized patients with greater saphenous vein reflux were symptom free at 1 year whether treated with EVLT or with surgical stripping.[32] The durability of endovenous ablation therapies seems to be sustained, with 5-year follow-up of an RCT showing failure rates of 6.3% for surgery, 5.8% for RFA, and 6.8% for EVLT ($P<.001$).[33]

RFA was compared with EVLT (using an 810-nm wavelength catheter) in a prospective, double-blind RCT. In the 159 patients enrolled, complete occlusion on duplex ultrasound examination was noted in all patients in both groups at 1 week with comparable venous occlusion rates (97% for RFA and 96% for EVLT) at the 3-month follow-up. RFA was associated with less postoperative pain and bruising, with similar QOL scores and times to return to normal activities.[34] Similar results were reported in another RCT that compared RFA using the VNUSClosureFast system with EVLT; pain scores were lower with RFA with similar times to resume normal activities and QOL improvement.[35] A significantly lower level of postprocedure pain and bruising were noted in the RFA arm of an RCT that compared the outcomes of EVLT using an 810-nm wavelength catheter (BioLITEC system, Biolitec AG, Jena, Germany) with RFA (Olympus Celon RFiTT system, Teltow, Germany) in 66 patients (87 legs). Again, occlusions rates were similar at the 9-month follow-up (78% vs 74%) with no differences in degree of improvement and in time to return to normal activity.[36]

The advantages of endovenous ablation are several. In the multicenter endovenous radiofrequency obliteration (closure) versus ligation and vein stripping (EVOLVeS) RCT, which compared

RFA with high ligation and stripping; recovery times were faster and QOL scores were higher with less postoperative pain and fewer adverse events in the RFA group at 2 years of follow-up. Occlusion and recurrence rates were similar in both groups.[37] Faster return to work with shorter length of disability were also reported by Darwood and colleagues[38] after endovenous ablation compared with surgery. In addition, endovenous ablation obviated the needs for general anesthesia,[39] as well as the higher risk of hematoma, infection, and nerve injury seen with surgery.[40,41] Further, the estimated direct cost of performing endovenous radiofrequency was found to be significantly lower that for surgical stripping, because the former can be performed in an outpatient setting and uses fewer personnel.[42]

Nonthermal Nontumescent Techniques

RFA and EVLT are classified as thermal tumescent techniques, and have the inherent disadvantage of a low but potential risk of thermal injury to surrounding tissues causing pain, pigmentation and occasionally skin burns,[43,44] hence the need for tumescence anesthesia. Novel ablative techniques, which include non-compounded foam, endovenous chemical adhesive, and combined mechanical/chemical sclerosant (mechanochemical ablation [MOCA]) do not require tumescent anesthesia of the tissue adjacent to the treated vein and are referred to as nonthermal nontumescent techniques. Sclerosing agents when used as a foam displace venous blood and increase endothelial contact, thereby augmenting their sclerosing ability.[45]

Foam Sclerosant

Varithena (Fig. 4) (previously Varisolve and polidocanol endovenous microfoam) is the only commercially approved, ready-made injectable sclerosing foam in the United States. It was developed and produced by Provensis Ltd, a BTG International group pharmaceutical company (London, UK). The final product was refined to a gas combination of 65% oxygen, 35% carbon dioxide, and a trace of nitrogen (<0.8%).

Varithena was approved after the 2 phase III placebo controlled RCTs, VANISH I (n = 275) and VANISH II (n = 232).[46,47] The efficacy and safety of Varithena in treating the symptoms and appearance of visible varicosities in patients with saphenofemoral junction incompetence owing to GSV or major accessory vein reflux was assessed. Three concentrations, 0.5%, 1.0%, and 2.0% of Varithena were compared

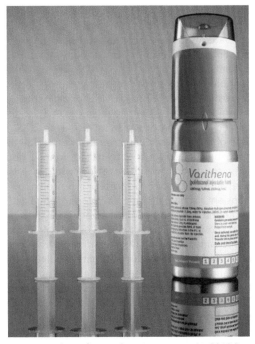

Fig. 4. Varithena foam sclerosing system. (© 2019 Boston Scientific Corporation or its affiliates. All rights reserved.)

with placebo (agitated saline solution) and control (Varithena 0.125%). Primary, secondary, and tertiary outcome measures were assessed at baseline and/or 8 weeks after treatment. Of note, the outcomes in both trials were pooled (VANISH I [0.5%, 1.0%, 2.0%] and VANISH II [0.5% and 1.0%] versus placebo) because the studies were not adequately powered to analyze differences between separate concentrations of Varithena and placebo.

The primary end point was symptom improvement as measured in an electronic diary using a VVSymQ instrument, which was a tool developed and validated by the BTG group, and involved recording symptoms such as leg heaviness and aching.[48] A mean improvement of 6.3 points in the VVSymQ score, equivalent to a reported change of moderately to much improved, was considered a meaningful change.[48] Pooled data from VANISH I and II demonstrated that 77.7% of patients treated with Varithena (0.5%, 1.0%, and 2.0%) reported moderate to much improved symptom relief, compared with 13.3% of placebo-treated patients, from baseline to 8 weeks.

Safety data from Varithena focused on venous thrombosis, neurologic complications and anaphylactic reactions. In the VANISH I and II trials, 27 of 275 (9.8%) and 24 of 232 (10.3%) patients, respectively, were diagnosed with a venous thrombus with all thrombi detected on protocol duplex ultrasound scans and none of the patients in the Varithena trials spontaneously presenting with a symptomatic thrombus. Of patients with proximal DVT, 70% received anticoagulants with a median time to stabilization or resolution of 87 days.[49] The incidence of neurologic and visual adverse events in the pooled Varithena group (n = 437) was 2.7%.[49] One of the 1333 patients treated with Varithena, described an episode of twinkling lights 1 hour after treatment, which resolved without issue and another patient reported symptoms of a transient ischemic attack with no sequelae.[49] Varithena has also been tested on those patients with known right to left shunt, usually via a patent foramen ovale.[50] Despite demonstration of cerebral MCA bubbles in 60 patients (including 54 patients with a patent foramen ovale), no patient developed any serious neurologic events. The biggest limitation of using this modality is cost of the product, which can be substantial.

Mechanochemical Ablation

The ClariVein (Fig. 5) MOCA device (Merit Medical, South Jordan, UT), is a nonthermal nontumescent ablation device that combines an endovenous mechanical method using a rotating wire at 3500 rotations per minute, which then injures the venous intima with simultaneous injection of liquid sclerosant.[51]

In a study of 29 patients with primary GSV reflux with average VCSS of 4.5 and with a clinical CEAP score between 2 and 4, the primary closure rate was 96.7% at 260 days with no reported pain during the procedure, skin injury or DVT. The authors concluded that the ClariVein device was safe and effective in the treatment of venous reflux.[51]

The MARADONA trial was designed to directly compare the anatomic and clinical success rate of MOCA compared with RFA with the goal to recruit 230 patients in each group (460 patients in total).[52] Patients will be followed up for 5 years. The 2-year results[53] and data for a total of 213 patients (46.3% of intended number of patients) randomized, of whom 209 were treated (105 in the MOCA group and 104 in the RFA group), showed that the overall median pain scores during the first 14 days were lower after MOCA (0.2 vs 0.5 after RFA; P = .01). At 30 days, there was no difference in complications or health-related QOL scores (Aberdeen Varicose Vein Questionnaire [AVVQ]: MOCA, 8.9; RFA, 7.6; P = .23). Hyperpigmentation was reported in 7 patients in the MOCA group and 2 patients in the RFA group (P = .038). The 1- and 2-year anatomic success rates were lower after MOCA (83.5% and 80.0%) compared with RFA (94.2% and 88.3%; P = .025 and .066), mainly driven by partial recanalizations. After 2 years of follow-up, no differences were observed in the number of complete failures. Similar clinical success rates at 1 year (MOCA, 88.7%; RFA, 93.2%; P = .32) and 2 years (MOCA, 93.0%; RFA, 90.4%; P = .70) and no differences in HRQOL scores on the AVVQ at 1 year (MOCA, 7.5; RFA, 7.0; P = .753) and 2 years (MOCA, 5.0%; RFA, 4.8%; P = .573) were observed. Possible complications after MOCA include superficial thrombophlebitis, hematoma, and mild hyperpigmentation at the puncture site, as well as the possibility of the rotating wire tip causing patient discomfort.[51]

Cyanoacrylate Glue

Cyanoacrylate (CA) glue (VenaSeal, Medtronic, Minneapolis, MN) (Fig. 6), which was initially developed by Sapheon Inc., and later acquired by Covidien and then Medtronic, makes use of n-butyl CA, an adhesive liquid monomeric agent that quickly polymerizes and becomes solid when it comes into contact with blood producing an inflammatory endothelial response and, ultimately, fibrosis.[54] It was introduced in medical practice more than 40 years ago to treat gastric bleeding from varicosities, intracranial bleeding owing to arteriovenous malformations, and in a variety of other indications with high safety profiles reported in patients followed for 10 years after administration.[54–56]

The first human trial for CVI recruited was a prospective nonrandomized study of 38 patients with GSV incompetence.[57] The mean GSV diameter at the saphenofemoral junction was 8.0 ± 2.2 mm and the mean length of vein treated was 33.8 ± 9.1 cm. The mean volume of CA glue used was 1.3 mL (range, 0.6–2.3 mL). At 1 year, the complete occlusion rate was 92.1%.[57]

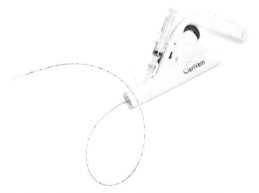

Fig. 5. ClariVein. (*Courtesy of* Merit Medical Systems, Inc., South Jordan, UT; with permission.)

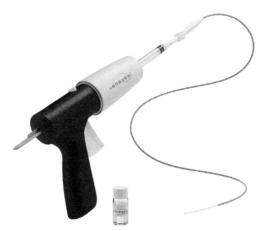

Fig. 6. The VenaSeal Closure System. (*Courtesy of Medtronic, Minneapolis, MN; with permission.*)

A prospective 7-center study of 70 patients was conducted in 4 European countries to abolish GSV reflux by endovenous CA embolization without tumescent anesthesia or postprocedure compression stockings.[58] Clinical examination, QOL assessment, and duplex ultrasound evaluation were performed at 2 days and after 1, 3, 6, and 12 months. The complete occlusion rate was 92.9% at 12 months.[58] The VCSS and AVVQ both demonstrated significant improvement at 12 months[58] Side effects were generally mild; a phlebitic reaction occurred in 8 cases (11.4%) with a median duration of 6.5 days (range, 2–12 days). Pain without a phlebitic reaction was observed in 5 patients (8.6%) for a median duration of 1 day (range, 0–12 days).[58]

VeClose was a trial involving 10 US centers and 222 patients with GSV reflux in veins up to 12 mm diameter who were randomized to treatment with CA or RFA.[59] The primary study end point, complete closure of the GSV at 3 months, occurred in 99% and 96% of those randomized to CA and RFA, respectively. The investigators concluded that CA was noninferior to RFA; however, the results were obtained using predictive statistical models to compensate for missing data (31/222). At 3 months, the VCSS, AVVQ, and generic QOL all showed significant improvement compared with baseline (3.5 [$P<.01$]; 8 [$P<.01$]; and 0.03 [$P = .01$], respectively). There was a nonsignificant increased incidence of phlebitis in the CA group (20 events vs 15 events; $P = .36$). Most cases were mild and successfully treated with over-the-counter nonsteroidal anti-inflammatory drugs. Venous access and mean intraprocedural pain scores for both methods were similar.[59] Long-term follow-up at 24 and 36 months continued to show clinical success with so significant complications.[60,61]

SUMMARY

CVI resulting from venous reflux is a very common peripheral vascular disorder for which multiple effective and safe catheter-based therapies are available. These should be tailored to the clinical situation at hand.

DISCLOSURE

Dr W. Saber has a consulting relation with Medtronic, INC.

REFERENCES

1. Bootun R, Davies AH. Long-term follow-up for different varicose vein therapies: is surgery still the best? Phlebology 2016;31(1 Suppl):125–9.
2. Abenhaim L, Kurz X. The VEINES study (VEnous Insufficiency Epidemiologic and Economic Study): an international cohort study on chronic venous disorders of the leg. VEINES Group. Angiology 1997;48(1):59–66.
3. Raffetto JD, Mannello F. Pathophysiology of chronic venous disease. Int Angiol 2014;33(3): 212–21.
4. Cornu-Thenard A, Boivin P, Baud JM, et al. Importance of the familial factor in varicose disease. Clinical study of 134 families. J Dermatol Surg Oncol 1994;20(5):318–26.
5. Fan CM. Epidemiology and pathophysiology of varicose veins. Tech Vasc Interv Radiol 2003;6(3): 108–10.
6. Laurikka JO, Sisto T, Tarkka MR, et al. Risk indicators for varicose veins in forty- to sixty-year-olds in the Tampere varicose vein study. World J Surg 2002;26(6):648–51.
7. Eberhardt RT, Raffetto JD. Chronic venous insufficiency. Circulation 2014;130(4):333–46.
8. Partsch H. Varicose veins and chronic venous insufficiency. Vasa 2009;38(4):293–301.
9. Choonhakarn C, Chaowattanapanit S, Julanon N. Lipodermatosclerosis: a clinicopathologic correlation. Int J Dermatol 2016;55(3):303–8.
10. Bonner ER. Venenstudie der Deutschen Gesellschaft für Phlebologie. Phlebology 2003;1–14.
11. Decousus H, Quere I, Presles E, et al. Superficial venous thrombosis and venous thromboembolism: a large, prospective epidemiologic study. Ann Intern Med 2010;152(4):218–24.
12. Kurz X, Lamping DL, Kahn SR, et al. Do varicose veins affect quality of life? Results of an international population-based study. J Vasc Surg 2001; 34(4):641–8.
13. Labropoulos N, Tiongson J, Pryor L, et al. Definition of venous reflux in lower-extremity veins. J Vasc Surg 2003;38(4):793–8.
14. Eklof B, Rutherford RB, Bergan JJ, et al. Revision of the CEAP classification for chronic venous

disorders: consensus statement. J Vasc Surg 2004; 40(6):1248–52.

15. Rutherford RB, Padberg FT Jr, Comerota AJ, et al. Venous severity scoring: an adjunct to venous outcome assessment. J Vasc Surg 2000;31(6): 1307–12.

16. Ey I. Venous and lymphatic disease. In: Dries DJ, editor. Schwartz's principles of surgery. 8th edition. New York: McGraw-Hill; 2005. p. 823–5.

17. Gohel MS, Barwell JR, Taylor M, et al. Long term results of compression therapy alone versus compression plus surgery in chronic venous ulceration (ESCHAR): randomised controlled trial. BMJ 2007;335(7610):83.

18. Piazza G. Varicose veins. Circulation 2014;130(7): 582–7.

19. Raju S, Hollis K, Neglen P. Use of compression stockings in chronic venous disease: patient compliance and efficacy. Ann Vasc Surg 2007; 21(6):790–5.

20. Bush R, Comerota A, Meissner M, et al. Recommendations for the medical management of chronic venous disease: the role of Micronized Purified Flavanoid Fraction (MPFF). Phlebology 2017; 32(1_suppl):3–19.

21. Gloviczki P, Comerota AJ, Dalsing MC, et al. The care of patients with varicose veins and associated chronic venous diseases: clinical practice guidelines of the Society for Vascular Surgery and the American Venous Forum. J Vasc Surg 2011;53(5 Suppl):2S–48S.

22. Böhler K. Surgery of varicose vein insufficiency. Wien Med Wochenschr 2016;166:293–6.

23. Hach W. Medizingeschichte der Krossektomie. Phlebologie 2012;41:142–9.

24. Critchley G, Handa A, Maw A, et al. Complications of varicose vein surgery. Ann R Coll Surg Engl 1997; 79(2):105–10.

25. Fischer R, Chandler JG, De Maeseneer MG, et al. The unresolved problem of recurrent saphenofemoral reflux. J Am Coll Surg 2002;195(1):80–94.

26. Brar R, Nordon IM, Hinchliffe RJ, et al. Surgical management of varicose veins: meta-analysis. Vascular 2010;18(4):205–20.

27. Wittens C, Davies AH, Baekgaard N, et al. Editor's choice - management of chronic venous disease: clinical practice guidelines of the European Society for Vascular Surgery (ESVS). Eur J Vasc Endovasc Surg 2015;49(6):678–737.

28. Gohel MS, Heatley F, Liu X, et al. A randomized trial of early endovenous ablation in venous ulceration. N Engl J Med 2018;378(22):2105–14.

29. Merchant RF, Pichot O, Closure Study Group. Long-term outcomes of endovenous radiofrequency obliteration of saphenous reflux as a treatment for superficial venous insufficiency. J Vasc Surg 2005;42(3):502–9 [discussion: 509].

30. Rasmussen L, Lawaetz M, Bjoern L, et al. Randomized clinical trial comparing endovenous laser ablation and stripping of the great saphenous vein with clinical and duplex outcome after 5 years. J Vasc Surg 2013;58(2):421–6.

31. van den Bos R, Arends L, Kockaert M, et al. Endovenous therapies of lower extremity varicosities: a meta-analysis. J Vasc Surg 2009;49(1):230–9.

32. Christenson JT, Gueddi S, Gemayel G, et al. Prospective randomized trial comparing endovenous laser ablation and surgery for treatment of primary great saphenous varicose veins with a 2-year follow-up. J Vasc Surg 2010;52(5):1234–41.

33. Lawaetz M, Serup J, Lawaetz B, et al. Comparison of endovenous ablation techniques, foam sclerotherapy and surgical stripping for great saphenous varicose veins. Extended 5-year follow-up of a RCT. Int Angiol 2017;36(3):281–8.

34. Nordon IM, Hinchliffe RJ, Brar R, et al. A prospective double-blind randomized controlled trial of radiofrequency versus laser treatment of the great saphenous vein in patients with varicose veins. Ann Surg 2011;254(6):876–81.

35. Shepherd AC, Gohel MS, Brown LC, et al. Randomized clinical trial of VNUS ClosureFAST radiofrequency ablation versus laser for varicose veins. Br J Surg 2010;97(6):810–8.

36. Goode SD, Chowdhury A, Crockett M, et al. Laser and radiofrequency ablation study (LARA study): a randomised study comparing radiofrequency ablation and endovenous laser ablation (810 nm). Eur J Vasc Endovasc Surg 2010;40(2):246–53.

37. Lurie F, Creton D, Eklof B, et al. Prospective randomised study of endovenous radiofrequency obliteration (closure) versus ligation and vein stripping (EVOLVeS): two-year follow-up. Eur J Vasc Endovasc Surg 2005;29(1):67–73.

38. Darwood RJ, Theivacumar N, Dellagrammaticas D, et al. Randomized clinical trial comparing endovenous laser ablation with surgery for the treatment of primary great saphenous varicose veins. Br J Surg 2008;95(3):294–301.

39. Gibson KD, Ferris BL, Pepper D. Endovenous laser treatment of varicose veins. Surg Clin North Am 2007;87(5):1253–65.

40. Braithwaite B, Hnatek L, Zierau U, et al. Radiofrequency-induced thermal therapy: results of a European multicentre study of resistive ablation of incompetent truncal varicose veins. Phlebology 2013;28(1):38–46.

41. Kugler NW, Brown KR. An update on the currently available nonthermal ablative options in the management of superficial venous disease. J Vasc Surg Venous Lymphat Disord 2017;5(3):422–9.

42. Eidson JL 3rd, Atkins MD, Bohannon WT, et al. Economic and outcomes-based analysis of the

care of symptomatic varicose veins. J Surg Res 2011;168(1):5–8.

43. Anwar MA, Lane TR, Davies AH, et al. Complications of radiofrequency ablation of varicose veins. Phlebology 2012;27(Suppl 1):34–9.

44. Dexter D, Kabnick L, Berland T, et al. Complications of endovenous lasers. Phlebology 2012; 27(Suppl 1):40–5.

45. Tessari L, Cavezzi A, Frullini A. Preliminary experience with a new sclerosing foam in the treatment of varicose veins. Dermatol Surg 2001;27(1):58–60.

46. King JT, O'Byrne M, Vasquez M, et al. Treatment of truncal incompetence and varicose veins with a single administration of a new polidocanol endovenous microfoam preparation improves symptoms and appearance. Eur J Vasc Endovasc Surg 2015; 50(6):784–93.

47. Todd KL 3rd, Wright DI, Group V-I. Durability of treatment effect with polidocanol endovenous microfoam on varicose vein symptoms and appearance (VANISH-2). J Vasc Surg Venous Lymphat Disord 2015;3(3):258–64.e1.

48. Paty J, Turner-Bowker DM, Elash CA, et al. The VVSymQ(R) instrument: use of a new patient-reported outcome measure for assessment of varicose vein symptoms. Phlebology 2016;31(7):481–8.

49. Star P, Connor DE, Parsi K. Novel developments in foam sclerotherapy: focus on varithena(R) (polidocanol endovenous microfoam) in the management of varicose veins. Phlebology 2018;33(3):150–62.

50. Regan JD, Gibson KD, Rush JE, et al. Clinical significance of cerebrovascular gas emboli during polidocanol endovenous ultra-low nitrogen microfoam ablation and correlation with magnetic resonance imaging in patients with right-to-left shunt. J Vasc Surg 2011;53(1):131–7.

51. Elias S, Raines JK. Mechanochemical tumescentless endovenous ablation: final results of the initial clinical trial. Phlebology 2012;27(2):67–72.

52. van Eekeren RR, Boersma D, Holewijn S, et al. Mechanochemical endovenous ablation versus RADiOfrequeNcy ablation in the treatment of primary great saphenous vein incompetence (MARA-DONA): study protocol for a randomized controlled trial. Trials 2014;15:121.

53. Holewijn S, van Eekeren R, Vahl A, et al. Two-year results of a multicenter randomized controlled trial comparing mechanochemical endovenous ablation to RADiOfrequeNcy ablation in the treatment of primary great saphenous vein incompetence (MARADONA trial). J Vasc Surg Venous Lymphat Disord 2019;7(3):364–74.

54. Idle MR, Monaghan AM, Lamin SM, et al. N-butyl-2-cyanoacrylate (NBCA) tissue adhesive as a haemostatic agent in a venous malformation of the mandible. Br J Oral Maxillofac Surg 2013;51(6): 565–7.

55. Linfante I, Wakhloo AK. Brain aneurysms and arteriovenous malformations: advancements and emerging treatments in endovascular embolization. Stroke 2007;38(4):1411–7.

56. Min RJ, Almeida JI, McLean DJ, et al. Novel vein closure procedure using a proprietary cyanoacrylate adhesive: 30-day swine model results. Phlebology 2012;27(8):398–403.

57. Almeida JI, Javier JJ, Mackay E, et al. First human use of cyanoacrylate adhesive for treatment of saphenous vein incompetence. J Vasc Surg Venous Lymphat Disord 2013;1(2):174–80.

58. Proebstle TM, Alm J, Dimitri S, et al. The European multicenter cohort study on cyanoacrylate embolization of refluxing great saphenous veins. J Vasc Surg Venous Lymphat Disord 2015;3(1):2–7.

59. Morrison N, Gibson K, McEnroe S, et al. Randomized trial comparing cyanoacrylate embolization and radiofrequency ablation for incompetent great saphenous veins (VeClose). J Vasc Surg 2015;61(4): 985–94.

60. Gibson K, Morrison N, Kolluri R, et al. Twenty-four month results from a randomized trial of cyanoacrylate closure versus radiofrequency ablation for the treatment of incompetent great saphenous veins. J Vasc Surg Venous Lymphat Disord 2018;6(5): 606–13.

61. Morrison N, Kolluri R, Vasquez M, et al. Comparison of cyanoacrylate closure and radiofrequency ablation for the treatment of incompetent great saphenous veins: 36-month outcomes of the VeClose randomized controlled trial. Phlebology 2019;34(6):380–90.

Printed and bound by CPI Group (UK) Ltd, Croydon, CR0 4YY

03/10/2024

01040306-0015